Techniques of Pleasure

TECHNIQUES OF PLEASURE

BDSM AND THE CIRCUITS OF SEXUALITY

Margot Weiss

DUKE UNIVERSITY PRESS DURHAM & LONDON 2011

Printed in the United States of America on acid-free paper ∞
Designed by Jennifer Hill
Typeset in Chaparral Pro by Keystone Typesetting, Inc.

Library of Congress Cataloging-in-Publication Data appear on the last printed page of this book.

CONTENTS

A NOTE ON TERMINOLOGY

In BDSM, terminology matters. The community recognizes itself—its practices, its desires—in and through a shared, yet contested, language. In this note, I do not attempt to pin down this complex and proliferating terminology with formalized definitions, but rather to give the reader a few conceptual signposts—some bearings—within the shifting discursive field that constitutes contemporary BDSM.

The terms *SM* and *BDSM* are used interchangeably to denote a diverse community that includes aficionados of bondage, domination/submission, pain or sensation play, power exchange, leathersex, role-playing, and fetishes. The community embraces a wide range of practices, relationship types, and roles, ranging from the more common (for instance, rope bondage or flogging) to the less so (playing with incest themes or playing at being a pony), yet all of these variations fit under the umbrella term *BDSM*.

BDSM is of relatively recent (and, many suggest, Internet) coinage. It is an amalgamation of three acronyms: *B&D* (bondage and discipline), *D/s* (domination/submission), and *SM* (sadomasochism). The use of *SM* (sometimes *S/M* or *S&M*) as the inclusive term predates BDSM, but BDSM is fast becoming the acronym of choice, especially in the *pansexual* community—the mixed BDSM community, made up of practitioners of various gender and sexual orientations. *Leather*, on the other hand, is used most often in gay and, in some cases, lesbian SM communities to describe an SM community that includes leather fetishism and motorcycle clubs (see also Kamel 1995; Rubin 1997). Some practitioners use the acronym ***WIITWD*** (for "what it is that we do") to encompass the entirety of BDSM practices; another inclusive linguistic term for the community and its practices and practitioners is *kinky* (with its opposite, *vanilla*). The community is also called *the scene*, which refers to a network of BDSM-oriented people, organizations, meeting places, dungeons, web pages, e-mail lists, conferences, and so forth. The scene is differentiated from *a scene*, which refers to a particular BDSM encounter. The SM scene stresses the modern mantra of BDSM: all BDSM practices should be ***SSC*** (for "safe, sane, and consensual"). BDSM practices are often called *play*, where play refers to any particular BDSM scene ("Jon and I played last night"), as well as to general categories of BDSM activities ("Sara is really into hot wax play"). BDSM gatherings that feature designated play areas are called *play parties*.

B&D, *D/s*, and ***SM*** each have their own linguistic histories. The *B* in ***B&D*** refers to *bondage*. Bondage has become an ever-more specialized technique—a highly technical, even transnational, practice. A recent craze for "Japanese rope bondage" (sometimes called *shibari*), an elaborate, aestheticized form of bondage, is one example of this emphasis on new techniques. Practitioners specialize in rope harnesses, suspension bondage, bondage on a budget, leather bondage, encasement bondage, and more. Classes, books, and workshops by San Francisco Bay Area experts have proliferated, and bondage remains a typical sight at play parties and events. The *D* refers to *discipline* or spanking, an outgrowth of the mostly heterosexual fetish-bondage-spanking communities that blossomed in the 1950s in the United States and Europe (Bienvenu II 1998). In many parts of the United States, the spanking community is separate from the BDSM community, and many spanking devotees do not identify with the SM community or its practices. Meanwhile, many SM practitioners view spanking as "SM lite," a sort of beginner activity. Spanking communities tend to be interested in formal discipline; practitioners are often heterosexual and married; and scenes involve minimal toys, clothes, or other SM paraphernalia, which is one reason it is considered "beginner" by some in the SM scene. At the same time, however, spanking, discipline, punishment, and caning—all classics of B&D—are also very common forms of BDSM play.

D/s, for *domination* and *submission*, refers to the explicit exchange of power. The phrase *power exchange* emphasizes that D/s relationships are explicitly about power (more than sensation, pain, or role play, for example), but also that they are an exchange: although dominant and submissive roles may be relatively stable, power is understood to be mobile, shared, or routed between practitioners during play (see also Langdridge and Butt 2005). D/s practices range from long-term, live-in *M/s* (*Master* or *Mistress* and *slave*) situations (where one has "ownership" of another in a variety of ways, sometimes including formal contracts of service) to short-term scenes between play partners (for example, a scene where a "naughty schoolgirl" has to write "I will not touch myself" on a chalk board, or a submissive must stand perfectly still while being tickled by his dominant). D/s practices might be a component of a scene or an overarching relationship structure; more specialized power exchanges include the collared slave who organizes her Master's business schedule, the submissive who gratefully cleans his Mistress's home, and the slave who is an always-available demonstration model for his *prodomme* wife's SM classes (prodomme is a contraction of "professional dominant," a term, like *dominatrix*, used to describe women who work as paid dominants. Men in this profession are called *prodoms*). These scenes and relationships are primarily about symbolic power; they may or may not involve physical contact or sensation.

D/s dynamics—the consensual exchange of power—are, as many argue, the foundation of BDSM play. As the sociologists Thomas Weinberg and G. W. Levi Kamel write, contrary to mainstream perception, "much S&M involves very little pain. Rather, many sadomasochists prefer acts such as verbal humiliation or abuse, cross-dressing, being tied up (bondage), mild spankings where no severe discomfort is involved, and the like. Often, it is the notion of being helpless and subject to the will of another that is sexually titillating . . . At the very core of sadomasochism is not pain but the idea of control—dominance and submission" (1995, 19). Practitioners and other SM researchers agree that sexual control, power exchange, or what Pat (now Patrick) Califia calls "the power dichotomy" or "imbalance" between partners is central to all BDSM (1994, 162; see also Alison et al. 2001; Langdridge and Barker 2007; Taylor and Ussher 2001).

In the community, *SM* has a double meaning: it can be used like *BDSM* to refer to the entire scene, and it can also be used comparatively, to refer to more explicitly physical or bodily practices, also called *sensation play* or *pain play*. Sensation play can range from very mild (being rubbed with a rabbit fur glove) to very intense (being struck with a single-tail whip). *Pain*, here, is a tricky word; basic to the dictionary definition of pain is its aversiveness, and thus no one who enjoys these activities would describe them as "painful" in this sense. In the scene, practitioners differentiate between "good pain" in SM and "bad pain," like stubbing your toe. They also use analogies to describe these sensations: the feeling that results from a flogging is like the relaxation of a deep tissue massage, the high of eating spicy food, or the cognitive release of meditation. Common examples of SM sensation play include flogging, caning, whipping, cutting, and temperature play. Most BDSM practitioners engage in some bondage, some sensation play, and some power play.

Although the term *sadomasochism* and the acronym *S&M* are more common in mainstream usage, within the scene, practitioners tend to use *SM* (and, less often, *S/M*). This points to the ways contemporary practitioners position themselves vis-à-vis the pathologization of sadomasochism in sexology, psychoanalysis, and psychiatry. Coined in 1890 by the sexologist Richard von Krafft-Ebing and popularized in successive editions of his *Psychopathia Sexualis*, the terms *sadism* ("the desire to cause pain and use force") and *masochism* ("the wish to suffer pain and be subjected to force") were classed as paraphilias, or sexual perversions ([1886] 1999, 119). Krafft-Ebing included "lust murder," the dismemberment of corpses, and what we would now call marital rape as examples of sadism; he linked masochism with flagellation, abuse, foot and shoe fetishism, and various "disgusting acts" (such as smelling "sweaty slippers" or eating excrement). This late-nineteenth-century definition remains remarkably current; the latest version of the *Diagnostic and Statistical Manual of Mental Disorders*, the standard diagnostic guide for mental health practitioners, defines "sexual sadism" and "sexual masochism" as psychopathological paraphilias, in which individuals "use sexual fantasies, urges, or behaviors involving infliction of pain, suffering or humiliation to enhance or achieve sexual excitement" (American Psychiatric Association 2000).[1] This history—and contemporary reality—of pathologization is why practitioners today tend to use *SM* and not *sadomasochism*: *sadomasochism* embeds the eroticization of pain within a psychiatric model of pathology, whereas contemporary practitioners understand their SM to be about mutual pleasure and power exchange.

Practitioners are also less inclined to use *S&M*. As the National Coalition for Sexual Freedom (NCSF; an advocacy group that serves BDSM and related communities) advises, if you are talking to the press about BDSM, "try to get the reporter to write SM, not S&M—that evokes the old stereotypes and we are trying to get around that. S&M stands for sadism & masochism while SM stands for sadomasochism; inherent in the word is the mutual necessity for both as well as the consent involved."[2] In this logic, *S&M* deemphasizes the relationality of SM power exchange; similarly, *S/M* still separates sadism and masochism (although it is preferred by some who see it standing for "slave/Master"). And, although theorists after Krafft-Ebing have debated whether sadomasochism ought to be considered a single desire or drive, or separated into two, many practitioners feel that *SM* brings the *S* and the *M* together, eliminating the slash.[3] This definitional complexity—where *SM* both refers to and resists an originary pathology, and where it is both an umbrella term for all dynamics of consensual power exchange and a narrower term referring to pain play—is part of the reason why *BDSM* is gaining adherents: for many practitioners, it seems more encompassing, and less problematic, than *SM*.

As this note begins to demonstrate, these linguistic terms shift over time; they refer to contested and contextual concepts used with different shades of meaning by different practitioners. This shifting discursive notation is representative of the ways such terms are used in practice. Because of this, I retain the notation my interviewees or sources use (*BDSM, S/M, S&M*, and so on); I also retain the terms they use to describe themselves. Some of these identity terms are more common: *top*, for example, refers to the person on the giving end of any form of BDSM; *bottom* is the corresponding word for the person on the receiving end. A *dominant* is the top in a more explicitly power-based relationship; *submissive* refers to the bottom. A *switch* is a person who enjoys both top and bottom, or dominant and submissive, roles. Other terms are less common, and practitioners use creative combinations to describe their interests and practices: a *pain slut* (a person who enjoys particularly heavy pain play), a *service top* (a top who gets off on pleasuring, or otherwise servicing, a bottom), or a *SAM* (a smart-assed masochist or a bratty bottom), for example. Thus, rather than providing a full glossary of terms here—an impossible task—I ask the reader to allow these terms and their referents and contexts to accumulate over the course of this book.[4]

ACKNOWLEDGMENTS

This ethnography, which began as my dissertation, would have been impossible to write without the support of the Department of Cultural Anthropology and the Women's Studies Program at Duke University. Antonio Viego's seminar on queer theories started me on this project, and Antonio remains one of the most compassionate, careful readers I have ever encountered. Anne Allison has been an amazing mentor, advisor, and friend, always managing to combine laser-point criticism with true support. Both Anne and Antonio have given me inspiring models of queer scholarship. Other faculty members at Duke—in particular Lee D. Baker, John L. Jackson, Ralph Litzinger, Charlie Piot, Naomi Quinn, and Robyn Wiegman—offered sage advice, a collegial atmosphere, and the critical support that made this project possible. I am lucky to have been able to work with such talented, generous, and kind scholars.

The Department of Cultural Anthropology provided funds for preliminary summer research, and support from my family made it possible for me to do this fieldwork. A yearlong Women's Studies Fellowship from Duke allowed me to stay in San Francisco and write, while visiting positions at Sweet Briar College, Duke University, and the College of William and Mary allowed me to revise the book manuscript. I owe thanks to all of these institutions, as well as to SOLGA, now AQA, the queer anthropology section of the American Anthropological Association, which provided a sense of institutional belonging at a critical time.

My students and colleagues at Wesleyan University provided the final intellectual context to make the completion of the book possible. My two departments at Wesleyan—anthropology and American studies—alongside the larger intellectual community provided more insights and inspiration than I can list. Thanks, most especially, to Henry Abelove, Tricia Hill, Claire Potter, Mary-Jane Rubenstein, and Anu Sharma, as well as the faculty members of the Feminist, Gender, and Sexuality Studies Program, who gave me the opportunity to present sections of this book in a very helpful workshop. Many people have read pieces of this book; others have offered insight and inspiration during the long writing and revising process. For conversations and encouragement along the way, I thank Liz Barnes, Robin Bauer, Evie Blackwood, Tom Boellstorff, Nan Boyd, Mindy Chateauvert, Lisa Duggan, Katherine Frank, Mary Gray, Bill Leap, Ellen Lewin, Martin Manalansan, Jeff Maskovsky, Bill Maurer, Alice McLean, Scott Morgensen, Gayle Rubin, David Savran, Susan Stryker, David Valentine, Brad Weiss, and Volker Woltersdorff. For reading part or all of this book in its final form, I am grateful to Gillian Goslinga, Naomi Greyser, J. Kehaulani Kauanui, Joel Pfister, Betsy Traube, Laura Weiss, and most especially Matt Garrett, to whom I owe more than gratitude. Thanks, too, to my two incredible readers at Duke University Press, whose helpful suggestions made this book far better than it would otherwise have been; to Ken Wissoker, who was both patient and motivating; and to everyone else at the press for shepherding this book along.

Most of all, I am forever in debt to the SM practitioners in the Bay Area who shared their insights and stories with me. I want to thank, in particular, the officers of the Society of Janus who facilitated my work in countless ways; Paul, whose intellect was an amazing field resource; Mollena, who was always both inspiring and fun; each of my interviewees who opened their lives to me and my tape recorder; and everyone else in the scene who made time for me, allowed me to come to events, introduced me around, and helped me in small and large ways.

This research would have been impossible without their generosity; it would have been a lot less enjoyable without the wit, passion, and spirited debates that make this community so remarkably rich.

Small portions of the introduction, chapter 3, and chapter 4 previously appeared in "Working at Play: BDSM Sexuality in the San Francisco Bay Area," *Anthropologica* 48, no. 2, 2006. Portions of the introduction and chapter 5 previously appeared in "Rumsfeld! Consensual BDSM and 'Sadomasochistic' Torture at Abu Ghraib," in *Out in Public: Reinventing Lesbian/Gay Anthropology in a Globalizing World*, edited by Ellen Lewin and William L. Leap (Chichester, England: Wiley-Blackwell, 2009). I thank Andrew Lyons, Harriet Lyons, Ellen Lewin, and Bill Leap, along with the publishers, for their enthusiasm and support for earlier versions of this project.

Techniques of Pleasure

INTRODUCTION

TOWARD A PERFORMATIVE MATERIALISM

I spent the summer of 2000 in San Francisco, trying to figure out how to do ethnographic fieldwork on BDSM. I started by looking up SM organizations online, slowly summoning the courage to e-mail my request for interviews to local groups. But I wanted to do participant observation, to attend some BDSM community event and get a sense of what was going on. I wasn't sure what to expect: black leather, for sure; motorcycles, tough women, chaps, and radical sex practices. I had gone to the fetish-themed night of a local club, Bondage-a-Go-Go, and, the next night, to the Power Exchange, a sex club with a dungeon area. But this, I thought, was "tourist" SM, so I was excited when I was invited to the "Byzantine Bazaar and Slave Auction." Held at the Castlebar dungeon in South San Francisco, the auction was a combination charity fundraiser and shopping and vending opportunity. As I browsed the website, I learned that the event would feature the chance to buy whips, floggers, canes, and other BDSM toys before a benefit auction, during which one could bid on tops, bottoms, and switches. A play party would follow the auction. We were encouraged to dress appropriately.

Since this was my first experience with the real SM scene, I scoured the Upper Haight neighborhood for a suitably "Byzantine" outfit, settling on a gauzy, shimmery nightgown. July in San Francisco is freezing, so, as I walked down the sidewalk to the dungeon that Saturday afternoon, I was cold as well as nervous. Inside, past the cashier (admission to the auction cost $5, the play party an additional $20), I threaded through a crush of people wearing leather vests and pants, corsets, slave outfits, saris, PVC and latex, or regular T-shirts and jeans. A side courtyard off the entry room served as a grill station for hot dogs and burgers, smoking lounge, and small vending area; people sat around picnic tables eating and chatting, while others browsed the toys. Past the entry room and down a small hallway were two smaller rooms. One was billed as a "harem room"; I gave the woman at the door a dollar and watched several belly dancers for a few minutes. A large table displaying all of the items to be auctioned off dominated the other small room: donated whips and floggers, paddles, canes, clothes, books, bondage paraphernalia, and the like.

Past the side rooms, I entered the dungeon proper. A huge room with high ceilings, the dungeon featured rows of furniture—crosses, stools, seats, cages, swings, and more crosses. Wedged between these stations were more vendors. I wandered around, looking at items. At one table, I examined a set of curved metal bars, neatly laid out in a zip-up, black leather case lined with red satin. I could not figure out what they were and finally asked. The vendor told me that they were sounds, for urethra play. I felt sympathetic pain and put the sound down, moving on to look at floggers, paddles, canes, cuffs. I bought a raffle ticket from a woman who offered me the chance to oil up a female wrestler; she pointed at the kiddie pool set up at the front of the dungeon room, where the oil wrestling was about to begin. There were at least 250 people there that afternoon, waiting for the auction to start. People chatted with vendors and acquaintances, trying out new toys on friends and partners.

My field notes report that I found everyone there surprisingly "NORMAL," which I rendered in all caps. By this I meant that the people at the Byzantine Bazaar that day seemed nice and friendly. My notes stress how "wholesome" the event felt to me: I was surprised that it was so easy to talk to people at this event, people I would only later get to know as members of the pansexual BDSM community. They all seemed excited about the upcoming play party, and they were welcoming, just having fun. But I also meant that they did not look like the radical leatherfolk I'd expected: they were middle-aged, overweight, professional-looking people and, although many were wearing black leather, the vibe was more afternoon barbecue and less biker bar.

When the slave auction began, I took a seat near the staging area, where I could overhear the event coordinators shepherding the people up for auction into neat lines, and making sure the index cards they held—which explained their sexual and SM orientations and limits—were in order. The auctionees approached the stage set up at the front of the dungeon and, one at a time, climbed onto a chair: the auction block. The emcee began the bidding: "Here is Darkstar! She is a het-flexible bottom, into canes, a total pain slut—hey, it's what she wrote! Limits: dead people, kids. Willing to be sold to either [man or woman]. Let's start the bidding at one hundred Byzantine dollars—that's ten bucks . . . do I hear fifteen? Fifteen to this lady in the corner, twenty?" As all the material for the auction and general community rules make clear, the winning bidder was not, of course, buying the person auctioned, or even the right to play with them. Rather, the winner bought the chance to negotiate with that person for a scene later, at the play party following the auction.

Forty-two bottoms, ten switches, and twenty-eight tops were auctioned off that day. Some people—especially the older male bottoms—were duds, receiving few bids. Others were superstars: one well-known heterosexual white top from the South Bay was being sold as a bottom for "one night only!" He prompted a frenzied bidding and strip show. As he stood on the block, the audience and the emcee coaxed him to take off his leather vest; his white shirt, revealing his white belly; and then his leather pants. He faced us, blushing, while we took pleasure in his discomfort, shouting for him to remove the final barrier: his tighty whities. When he did, the crowd roared; I had tears in my eyes from laughing along with everyone else in the room. He got some of the highest bids of the evening, eventually going for $750. Most people, the organizer told me later, sold for $50 (the auction raised $10,000 for the Earle Baum Center of the Blind, in Santa Rosa).

About an hour later, a young African American woman with a round face and closely cropped hair was led up to the stage by a tall, severe-looking white man who held the leash attached to her collar. She was the only person to appear on the stage with someone else, so the man explained that he needed to tell us, the audience, a few things about his slave. As she stood there, back straight, staring straight ahead, her master, addressing us in a tight, steely voice, said that she was fit. As he spoke, he yanked up her dress to display her shaved genitals, and he then turned her around. Still holding her dress above her waist, he smacked her ass so hard she pitched forward; the leash attached to the collar around her neck stopped her fall. Turning her back around, he said she was very submissive and guaranteed to make us happy. As he finished speaking, he stroked her head, petting and smoothing back her short blond hair. The audience was quiet throughout this display. When the bidding started, it was reserved; she did not sell for a lot of money. I was uncomfortable during this scene, and I felt sure that the rest of the crowd was, too. I strained to read the woman's expression, to see if she was all right at the front of the stage, but I couldn't tell.

Then a very butch Latina took the stage, a lesbian top to be auctioned off as a bottom. Though she was short, she stood tall on the chair, arms folded, legs spread, a defiant look on her face. The crowd taunted her, trying to get her to show her breasts. She smiled. She took off her vest. More shouting, and the bidding went up; obligingly, she took off an oxford shirt, revealing a long-sleeved T-shirt. Cheers and calls, and she delayed, until finally, with another smile, she took off the T-shirt. Underneath, another T-shirt. As the audience catcalled, she stood, removing layer after layer, pushing the bidding higher and higher. Finally, the last layer revealed a sports bra. We collectively held our breath as she started to lift the bottom edge of the bra—and underneath was another sports bra! The audience erupted into laughter; she had the last laugh.

Near the end, an Asian American man, young and tiny, cross-dressed in a red velvet dress, Mary Janes, and white lace gloves, stood docilely on the chair. The emcee announced that he wanted a mistress who would gender humiliate him: force him to cross-dress and then insult and mock him for this desire. The audience was not particularly receptive to him; no one shouted, and the bidding was slow. Maybe it was because we were tired, or looking forward to the play party, or maybe it was just that he seemed sad and small and quiet, way up there in front.

I tell this arrival story to begin to flesh out the ways that SM names a particular circuit between capitalism—the sexual marketplace and community entertainment of the Byzantine Bazaar—and performance—the racialized, gendered scenes at the Slave Auction. As I quickly found out during my fieldwork, the BDSM community is not the sleazy, underground scene portrayed on crime shows and made-for-TV movies; neither is it simply the transgressive zone of sexual emancipation that I expected to find. Rather, it is a formally organized community with very particular social and educational practices. This is not to say that there are no longer any leathermen in San Francisco, or radical queer genderfuck play parties, or other more-fringe SM events and scenes. But it is to say that the kinds of people at the Byzantine Bazaar represent a growing community—what is called the "new guard"—very different from both the men's "old guard" leather scene known as Folsom and the representation of SM in the public imaginary. The "fall of the Folsom," as Gayle Rubin puts it (1997, 107; 1998, 259), has given rise to a much larger community of practitioners of various gender and sexual orientations structured around SM educational organizations, classes, and workshops; semipublic dungeons like the Castlebar; and events like the Byzantine Bazaar.[1] During my fieldwork, practitioners, in an average week, could choose from at least five classes or workshops, six regular social meetings (called *munches*), several semipublic play parties, and two or three other events, such as SM book-release parties, fetish balls, or informal social gatherings. On average, the practitioners I interviewed spent fifteen hours a week doing SM-related activities. This is, as I will show, a technique-oriented community, made up of practitioners in their forties and fifties who are as likely to live in the South Bay as they are to live in the city of San Francisco. Most are involved in long-term relationships, either married or partnered; most of the men are heterosexual, while the women are bisexual and heterosexual. And the vast majority of practitioners are white with the means—or the aspiration—to buy the toys that, together with forms of self-improvement and technique, link community belonging with often-invisible race and class privilege.

At the Byzantine Bazaar, for me, the NORMALness of these practitioners stood in stark contrast to the performances that followed. Although the politics of racialized, gendered, and sexed performance was one of my original theoretical interests in this project, at the auction it became clear to me that, as scholars have argued for some time, politics could not be reduced to a dichotomy of transgressive sex radicals versus hegemonic straights. For how do we read the political effects of such scenes—of selling black bodies at a pretend slave auction in front of an almost exclusively white audience, or of mocking a straight, white, middle-aged man standing in his underwear in a "one night only!" inversion of male privilege? The positionalities of these practitioners were, I realized, linked in complex ways to the social and historical formations of race and gender, but also, in a more obscure way, to the subject positions produced within late capitalism. From the choice of scene, role, and scenario to the use of particular toys, such performances are both dependent on and productive of particular social, cultural, political, and economic formations. In other words, I began to understand SM performance as material. Rather than existing in a bracketed space of play, SM performances are deeply tied to capitalist cultural formations; rather than allowing for a kind of freedom from racial, gendered, and sexual hierarchies, such spectacular performances work within the social norms that compel subjectivity, community, and political imagination.

This is the community formation that I will trace in this ethnography. Departing from a Foucault-inspired analysis of the radical alterity of BDSM practice, I will show, instead, that BDSM sexuality—indeed, all sexuality—is a social relation, linking subjects (individuals, desires, and embodiments) to socioeconomics (social hierarchies, communities, and relations of inequality). In the technology-driven, purportedly liberated Bay Area, SM practitioners find a community where sex is seen as a skill, an accomplishment, and an array of sometimes-rigid techniques. It is somewhat ironic, then, that for many practitioners as well as social theorists, SM practice is imagined to transgress, or lie outside of, social relations and social norms. Much of the pro-SM literature produced by practitioners and theorists argues that BDSM is "transgressive" or "subversive." Working from Foucault's glorification of San Francisco's SM "laboratories of sexual experimentation" ([1982] 1996, 330), scholars like Karmen MacKendrick (1999) and Jeremy Carrette (2005) see in SM a "break" with both subjectivity and capitalist productivity. But to imagine SM sex as a break from social relations is to accept a logic that cordons sexuality off from the social real, variously imagined as capitalism, social norms, or the regulatory ideals that produce intelligible subjectivity. This creates the deep irony of a community organized around explicit codes of conduct and techniques, but whose very rules enable community members to imagine themselves, and their sex, as free from social regulations. By elaborating their own rules and regulations, BDSM communities simultaneously distance themselves from both a purportedly silent, "vanilla" (non-BDSM) sexuality and broader US social relations and regulatory norms.

The desire for sex to be free from social regulation characterizes not only BDSM, but also sexuality more generally: confined to the private, the deeply personal, or the psychological, sexuality often serves as a symbol of freedom, rebellion, or intimacy unbound to—and an escape from—structural social inequalities. This is phantasmatic but not inconsequential; imagining sex as resistance or opposition is one way that capitalist social relations are instantiated and validated. So, for example, these conceptions construct a private life that ought to ameliorate the alienation of wage labor, or a sense of individuality and true desire through which one might attain satisfaction (Hennessy 2000; Jakobsen 2005; Lowe 1995; Singer 1993). Thinking sexuality as a social relation, then, means understanding that sexuality is resolutely social, rather than private, or personal, or trivial. But it also means seeing the ways in which sexuality is a relation. It is not enough to contextualize it within a specific social, cultural, or historical moment; we must, instead, map the complex and often contradictory social dynamics that produce and are, in turn, reproduced within particular sexual cultures, practices, and desires.

I call such dynamics a *circuit* to draw attention not only to the dense connections between the bazaar and the slave auction—between capitalism and performance, public and private, socioeconomic and subjective—but also to the functionality, the effects, of these connections. Like an electrical circuit, which works when current flows between individual nodes, the circuits of BDSM work when connections are created between realms that are imagined as isolated and opposed. BDSM is a paradigmatic case for understanding sexuality as a conduit between domains that appear divided from each other: those conceptualized as subjective or private, and those understood as social or economic. The elaborate circuitry of BDSM energizes any particular BDSM scene, but it also provides the productive charge that constitutes the BDSM scene itself.

As I will argue, the relations between capitalism, social inequality, and sexuality are sometimes contested, sometimes contradictory, sometimes compensatory, and sometimes seamlessly enmeshed—but they are always productive. To understand this dynamic relationship, I deploy a broad reading of production, focusing on both relations of production (in the economic sense) and gender, race, and sexuality as productive performances. Bringing together the material/economic and the cultural/performative, I show how sexual formations like BDSM both compose and enact these social relations. The new BDSM community developed alongside post-Fordist transformations in capitalism, in concert with the neoliberal turn of the 1970s, when the first two BDSM organizations in the United States were founded (the Eulenspiegel Society, or TES, founded in 1971 in New York City, and the Society of Janus, founded in 1974 in San Francisco). BDSM is a form of social belonging facilitated—even produced—by contemporary US capitalism, especially consumerism and commodity exchange. At the same time, this economic shift relies on the production of other social hierarchies; differentiated subjects and niche communities are performatively produced in dynamic relation to capitalism. Following Miranda Joseph (2002), I bring together an understanding of the production of subjects through "performativity"—the "reiterative and citational practice by which discourse produces the effects that it names" (Butler 1993, 2)—with a materialist understanding of production as a dialectic of social belonging and inequality.[2] This method reveals the supplementary relationship between BDSM communities and capitalism: the ways in which community and capitalism depend on while also exceeding each other.[3] At the same time, it illuminates the supplementary relationship between BDSM practice and broader US racial, gendered, and sexual norms, norms that delimit the range of legible subject positions along with the rationalities that naturalize this social landscape.[4]

These relationships are not abstract or fixed; rather, the political, affective, or material effects of such circuits are dependent, particular, and variable. Indeed, because SM is a cultural, social, and historical mobilization of social power, it requires an ethnographically inflected *performative materialism* to track the on-the-ground dynamics that structure relationships between subjects and power. Performative materialism draws attention to relationships between the socioeconomic and the culturally performative, linking historical social transformations to local and subjective performances. The remainder of this introduction charts the key theoretical terrains of this ethnographic method, tracing the circuits between the subjective and the socioeconomic across different registers, and pointing to the ways that the method can enrich our understanding of contemporary sexual cultures like BDSM.

PRACTICE CIRCUIT TECHNIQUES OF SELF-MASTERY IN COMMUNITY

As I concluded my fieldwork in 2003, the Society of Janus, the largest BDSM educational organization in the Bay Area (often referred to as Janus or SOJ) instituted a cycle of introductory classes. Intended to introduce the novice player to the most common forms of SM, the seven classes, with suggested subtopics, were:

1 D/s (negotiation, collars and contracts, protocol, rituals, conflict resolution, slavery, punishment, models of power exchange).
2 Bondage (leather, rope, metal, plastic, jackets, harnesses, Japanese style, cages, predicament, suspensions, mummification/sensory deprivation, emotional aspects, pain, escapism, temperature and dis/comfort).
3 Impact (spanking, flogging, crops, canes, singletails, whips, Florentine [double] flogging, ranges from light to heavy, sting vs. thud, safety issues).
4 Electrical and medical (TENS units, Folsom units, violet wand, shock play, flyswatter, dog collars, cattle prods, light box, genitorture and genital play, monopole versus dipole, safety issues, piercing, catheterization, sounds, inflations, inspections, casting, shaving, playing doctor, body mod[ification]s, labial and scrotal inflations).
5 Sex play and sensation (fisting, anal, vaginal, CBT [cock and ball torture], oral, genitorture, tit-torture, enema, wax, chemical/spice, fire, ice, tickling, pinching, punching and kicking, biting, abrasion, cupping).
6 Psychological aspects (negotiations, relationships, polyamory, aftercare, violence, trust, land mines, personal fears).
7 Edge and fetish (fear and terror, breath, knife, cutting, branding, abduction, interrogation, rape simulation, body worship, uniforms, latex/rubber, foot fetish, corsetry and waist training, water sports).

This list begins to document the enormous range of BDSM practices and techniques—introductory or basic BDSM, no less—within the community.

The seven classes were distinguished from Janus's regular, more advanced classes, which, in the same few months, included "Total Enclosure Bondage," "Co-Topping: Sharing Is Good," "Erotic Knife Play," "Vaginal Fisting," "When Someone You Love Is Vanilla," and—my all-time favorite workshop title—"Tit Torture for an Uncertain World." The e-mail notice read that these classes were "not intended to make anyone an expert in a specific area, but to give the student an awareness of the spectrum of activities . . . and the basics of how to deal with it safely." Instructors, the notice continued, will "convey to the students the complexities of [each] area, the issues to be aware of, and where to go for further information." This expectation—that newcomers to BDSM will use such classes to begin their training or education—is made explicit in the following note: "The intention is that the twice-monthly Janus classes [the regular, nonintroductory classes] will continue to delve deeper into specific issues, techniques, styles and concerns while the Intro series will help the newcomer navigate the overall world of BDSM and help them integrate BDSM into their worldview." This somewhat odd phrasing begins to illuminate how becoming a BDSM practitioner requires not only BDSM interests or desires, but also a set of skills or techniques with which to navigate the BDSM world—a BDSM "worldview." In other words, becoming an SM practitioner, even if imagined to spring from a core or essential desire, requires self-mastery and self-knowledge that is bound to community rules, techniques, and perspectives.

One of my interviewees, Gretchen, a white, bisexual bottom/submissive in her early forties, described coming into her identity as "part of a journey toward self-mastering."[5] Similarly, Estrella, a white, lesbian femme top in her late thirties, told me: "[BDSM] is definitely an orientation in the same way my sexual orientation is not a sexual choice, it's just who I am, so that makes it an identity. And it's a practice in the sense that I do go to classes and I do take the practice of my craft seriously on the level of activities." At the same time, Estrella noted that SM is also a community for her, pointing to the ways that identity and practice merge with community: "It's similar to the way I grew into my lesbian identity: oh, this is who I am, other people do it, there's a name for it, and there are rules about it. And I can choose to learn those rules or not, be part of that community or not, follow those rules or not, but yeah, there's a name and now I know what I am." Estrella's comments reveal that BDSM is simultaneously an orientation or identity, a craft, a practice, and a community or social scene. This complex constellation of meanings is typical for BDSM practitioners, and it is this mix of information and subject production—BDSM as technique or skill and BDSM as worldview—that I understand as a Foucauldian "technique of the self."

In *The Use of Pleasure*, Foucault defines these techniques as the work "one performs on oneself, not only in order to bring one's conduct into compliance with a given rule, but to attempt to transform oneself into the ethical subject of one's behavior" ([1984] 1990, 27; see also Foucault [1984] 1988 and 1988; Mahmood 2004). Developed in the second and third volumes of *The History of Sexuality*, this work on the self, or *techne*, helps us think through the ways in which practitioners fashion themselves as SM subjects. This technique of the self is based on BDSM as a practice: a set of skills or a craft that must be learned and mastered. So, for example, many people see BDSM as something that they *do* (not something that they *are*), a sexuality organized around practices. As an obvious example, people who do BDSM are generally called "practitioners" or "players," not something like "BDSMuals." SM practitioners identify themselves in very specific and relational ways; my interviewees called themselves perverts, voyeurs, masters, masochists, bottoms, pain sluts, switches, dom(me)s, slaves, submissives, ponies, butch bottoms, poly perverse, pain fetishists, leathermen, mistresses, and daddies. For those who identified as tops, there were just plain tops, but also service tops, femme tops, switches with top leanings, and dominant tops. These SM orientations are typically modified with sexual orientation, relationship style or dynamics, and interests: "I'm a bi poly switch"; "I'm a het, sensual top"; "I'm a bondage bottom." In these combinations, the primacy of a fixed sexual identity as the ground of subjectivity is destabilized; instead, BDSM is an *identity in practice*, a deeply personal yet relational project of the self.[6]

This form of self-fashioning is organized around community codes of conduct. For SM is not simply a sexual activity; unlike most devotees of oral sex, for example, BDSM practitioners participate in a community that provides rules and techniques through which practitioners forge SM orientations. Many of my interviewees distinguished between "real" SM practitioners ("lifestyle," "heavy," or "experienced" players) and "weekend" dabblers ("bedroom," "unsafe," or "newbie" players). As Jeff, a white, heterosexual, dominant top in his late thirties explained to me, some people call BDSM "graduate school sex." It is this kind of educational mastery that differentiates—as Malc, a white, heterosexual mostly dominant in his late thirties put it—"people who are identified as BDSM practitioners and people who just do rough sex." Kinky people become real BDSM practitioners through participation in a social, sexual, and educational community that teaches techniques of the self alongside rope bondage and flogging skills. Indeed, it is this commitment to community, to SM as a form of social belonging, that differentiates the BDSM I researched as a community practice.

Although in recent years a growing number of scholars have written about SM, it remains the case, as Thomas Weinberg noted in 1987, that very little work focuses on SM as a community. Instead, most work on SM (or, often, sadomasochism) is interested in it as either an abstract problematic or an individualized orientation.[7] The former—work in philosophy, cultural theory, feminist theory, and literary criticism—theorizes SM dynamics or explores the political or ethical dilemmas posed by SM, but it does not locate SM practice in a particular socioeconomic or historical milieu.[8] The latter—work in social psychology, psychoanalysis, and sexology—dispels some of the more pernicious stereotypes of SM practitioners, but it does not link an individual's desires or practices to broader social formations.[9] In contrast, I build on Gayle Rubin's pathbreaking research on the history of gay male leathermen in San Francisco (1997 and 1998) as well as Thomas Weinberg's provocative suggestion that a large SM subculture will develop in a society that has an unequal power distribution, that has enough affluence for the development of leisure and recreational activities, and that values imagination and creativity (1995, 300; see also Gebhardt [1969] 1995). Fleshing out this tantalizing yet overly broad sketch with ethnographic analysis, I show how BDSM creates a circuit between self-mastery, technical expertise, and community belonging. SM, in other words, is a social technique, a practice that—in concert with SM toys, rules, and rationalities—simultaneously produces practitioners and community.

COMMUNITY CIRCUIT

FLEXIBLE SUBJECTS, COMMODITIES, COMMUNITIES

One evening in October 2002, I attended one of Mark's bondage parties. A white, heterosexual switch, Mark was one of the first people I interviewed during my fieldwork. Unlike many residents of the Bay Area,

Mark was born and raised in the region; like many of the pansexual practitioners I would meet, Mark worked for a large computer company down the Peninsula, in Silicon Valley. In his mid-forties, Mark was into what he termed "serious bondage": bondage play with expensive, often custom-made, leather and metal gear. Over the years, he had accumulated an extraordinary array of bondage furniture: heavy cages, a full leather table, a home-made bondage chair, a custom-sized leather body bag, numerous eye bolts for suspension play, and customized horizontal stocks. He began hosting regular parties for his friends in his Noe Valley Victorian home, to give everyone a chance to play with these toys.

When I arrived at the party, I stationed myself in the kitchen by the cheese and crackers and poured myself some wine. Leaning back against the stove, I surveyed the scene: Lenora, a bisexual college student in her early twenties in a Master/slave relationship, was laced into a very tight, full-length black corset and bound upright to a rocking chair in the living room, talking with other guests. Directly in front of me, between the kitchen island and the living room, Chris swayed from two eye bolts in the ceiling. He was strapped into a reinforced straitjacket and blindfolded, his crotch at our eye level. I heard what sounded like a vacuum cleaner in the front of the house, as the air was sucked out of a "vac sack" (a bondage device consisting of two layers of latex stretched on a frame eight feet by four feet, with a breathing tube for the person inside). Lady Thendara and Latex Mustang, her husband, stood close together off to the side, their eyes locked together as they cooed, post-scene. They had tried out the vac sack, Thendara explained to me later, completely sealing Mustang between the two layers of latex: a human version of vacuumed-sealed food. Speaking for her husband, Lady Thendara explained that he'd loved it: the restrictive feeling of the latex as it conformed to his entire body, and his feelings of helpless vulnerability when he was inside. Suddenly, Mark ran through the kitchen, holding a Hitachi Magic Wand vibrator aloft, its head covered with a latex glove, empty fingers fanning out. Ever the considerate host, Mark was satisfying what appeared to be an urgent need for a vibrator from the bondage scene participants in the back room.

Mark's house, a techie's shrine to the latest bondage toys and techniques, begins to suggest the deep imbrication of capitalism and community in BDSM. The house party is both a space of community and a site in which the very latest toys can be looked at, played with, and desired; a space made possible by commodities, and thus limited in its accessibility, but also a space where new bodies, desires, and relationships can be created and explored. Proliferating forms of desire, subjectivity, and embodiment like BDSM are themselves produced in and through the interrelationships between capitalism (especially consumerism) and community. In her analysis of "the gay community" in San Francisco, Joseph shows that community—often imagined as a more romantic form of belonging via identity—is instead "deployed to shore it up and facilitate the flow of capital" (2002, xxxii). Indeed, almost all of the practitioners I spoke with had invested between $1,500 and $3,000 in their toy collections, wardrobes, and, in some cases, play spaces. Commodities like bondage gear, sounds, and vibrators produce community; in this way, SM communities are not oppositional to, but rather complicit with, transformations in capitalism, particularly the consolidation of what is variously called late, flexible, informational, or advanced capitalism. Although different scholars emphasize different aspects of this shift, late capitalism is characterized by flexibility, new relations between production and consumption, a shift from Fordist to post-Fordist production, and the rise of new technologies and informatics (Castells 2000; Harvey 1997; Jameson 1992).[10]

These economic changes produce large-scale shifts in social organization: new social and cultural logics; new forms of community; and changed relationships between public and private, social and economic. In the field of sexuality, this has enabled new sexual identities, as new sexual practices, desires, and technologies have proliferated in the marketplace (Curtis 2004; Hennessy 2000; Lowe 1995; Pellegrini 2002; Singer 1993). From reproductive technologies and sex therapy to sex toys, phone sex, and pornography, the last few decades have seen a proliferation of ever-more-specialized niche markets, a shift that also heralds new possibilities for the generation and commoditization of social difference. With its endless paraphernalia, BDSM is a prime example of late-capitalist sexuality. The proliferation of commodities and the community-based knowledge to use them creates an infinitely expanding market for BDSM gear, which helps to produce both consumer-subjects who exhibit flexible desires and commodity-oriented communities that serve as flexible marketplaces.

Late-capitalist relations of production and consumption have also restructured bodies, subjects, and sociality. Linked to new forms of capitalism are more "adaptable" bodies, which absorb new techniques, technologies, commodities, and proliferating sexual pleasures as ideal consumers (E. Martin 1994). They also display a flexible tolerance of difference (racial, cultural, gendered, bodily) that make them ideal workers, especially in the technology and service economies (Hennessy 2000, 108–9; McRuer 2006, 2). This is not to say that such tolerant flexibility does not reproduce social inequality, but rather that such regimes regulate social normativity through shifting and flexible attitudes instead of rigid domination.[11] And a hallmark of such regimes is that they produce a sense of community and belonging through exclusions—which are often disguised or obscured through alibis of tolerance, class- or race-neutrality, and diversity.

To return to Mark's party, we can see SM as a community of consumption, where the latest bondage toys are produced for and produce flexible bodies, techniques of pleasure, and possibilities for the expansion of bodily sensations and play. Such possibilities are more available to those practitioners with access—material and social—to both the means to purchase these toys and the hegemonic forms of subjectivity that are normalized and reproduced by the SM community: the flexible —often white, heterosexual, middle-aged, and professional—high-tech workers of Silicon Valley. In this way, the BDSM community is produced in and through transformations in capitalism, but this community formation produces not only (commodity-oriented) belonging but also the ideal members of a community, an exclusivity based on both class and productive flexibility. The social hierarchies on which SM draws enable new meanings and social relationships, but these experiments are more possible and more accessible to those with class, race, and gender privilege: heterosexual men playing with sexism, white bodies at a charity slave auction, professional information technology (IT) workers with several rooms filled with custom-made bondage toys. BDSM, then, creates a circuit between social norms (especially whiteness, maleness, and heterosexuality) and socioeconomic relations (changes in class status, leisure time, technology, and spatial mobility), but it does so in ways that often disguise or conceal as much as they reveal.

In 2002 I attended a workshop on incest play at QSM, a classroom space and mail-order business in San Francisco. In the SM scene, although age play (adult babies, Daddy or Mommy/boi [boy] or grrl [girl]) is a relatively common form of play, age play with an incest theme is not. Estrella's workshop demo featured a "brother" and "sister" (adults performing as children of about eight years old); Estrella was "Daddy," arriving home from work. "He" sat on a chair at the center of the stage and began speaking to his children, asking them what they had done today and whether they would be nice to their Daddy this evening. Daddy coaxed the girl over with the promise of reading her a story. After the daughter sat on Estrella's lap, he began reading to her from a children's book. As the reading progressed, Estrella began adjusting the girl, positioning her more firmly against his crotch. Continuing the reading as the girl squirmed, Daddy began rubbing himself against the girl's ass, holding on to her hips. As the audience watched, Daddy pushed against the girl, cooing to his daughter ("Daddy likes it when you sit on his lap," "be a good girl for Daddy now," "stay still for Daddy"). As Daddy started touching his daughter between her legs (over her white cotton panties), he moaned, telling her she was a good girl and to "give Daddy a kiss now."

When I interviewed Estrella later, she told me that she had designed the class to respond to people who "look at age play as light, like SM-lite, because it's thought of as role play, it's thought of as pretend." When I asked her what about age play wasn't "pretend," she said, "Well, if you pick up a stick and hit somebody, there is no way that that's pretend." But, she continued, because the adults in the BDSM community have all been children, "those roles that we've all lived through can be very profound and very deep and very real." It is in part the fact that such scenes build on real-life experiences, attitudes, and cultural dynamics that lends them their intensity. But that is not all. Estrella is the mother of three teenagers, who live with her and her wife in their Alameda home. She explained:

> There are experiences that are from my being a mother that I probably use in age play, like that feeling of your kid going to sleep and you are stroking their head—that bond, that love, I think I tap into that in my

> acting that out with somebody. But I've certainly . . . I mean I wouldn't even think of, there is a line with your kids! It's really separate. I don't know how to say it, but it's separate. I've had plenty of bosses and never had sex with them, but I can do boss/secretary seduction, easy . . . I mean, things are separate because they're just separate.

By building on the familiar to construct something new, Estrella can create realistic play. But, at the same time, she emphasizes both that age play is "separate, really separate," from her real experiences as a mother and that it is a "very deep and very real" form of play.

This seeming contradiction makes use of what Gregory Bateson in a classic essay calls the "play frame" (1955). For Bateson, the play frame carries the shared understanding that what the players are doing is "just for play," not for real. Further, the frame, which says on the surface that what happens is just play, also enables what Bateson calls its opposite (but what may really be its mirror): what happens in the play frame is really much more than play. Like the anthropological concept of cultural performance, these frames construct a boundary around a particular performance so that it is, as Victor Turner puts it, "set-apart" from a more everyday social field (1986, 24).[12]

One primary way that BDSM practitioners create this framework of set-apartness is by imagining the SM scene as a "safe" and separate space: "safe, sane, and consensual," the motto of contemporary SM, becomes "safe" from social reality. In this fantasized split between the "real world" and the scene, SM's paradigmatic theatricality becomes important: sexual encounters are called "scenes"; one "plays" with one's SM partners; and roles, costumes, and props are a crucial part of SM play. But the way this disavowal via performance takes place is decidedly more complex than a simple theater analogy might have it.

Instead, understanding SM as a cultural performance shows us the ways in which such performances of social power can simultaneously draw on and disavow their social referents. The fantasy of the scene as separate, as set off or bracketed from the real world, acts as an alibi that enables practitioners to dramatize—while also disavowing—social hierarchies and institutionalized systems of domination, especially those of race, class, gender, sexuality, and imperialism. So, for example, BDSM is often about polarized roles: top/bottom, dominant/submissive, Master/slave. These roles are not fixed to a genital-sex-gender matrix; the practitioners I spoke with were adamant that there is no essential, generalizable, or immutable correspondence between one's body or genitalia, one's gender presentation, and one's BDSM practice. Some people in the scene enjoy roles "opposite" to their "real life" roles: the business man in bondage; feminized, cross-dressed heterosexual men (called "sissy maids"); female dominants with enormous strap-ons; adults in diapers; lesbian women as butch bois. Practitioners believe that gender in SM is "freely chosen," in accordance with liberal ideas of choice and agency; SM roles, in this analysis, have nothing to do with forms of social inequality. However, such scenes also require these very social norms to be legible; these performances are dependent on and productive of particular iterations of gender, race, and sexuality.

In SM this disavowal of a scene's dependence on social relations is installed through a refiguration of the public and the private. For practitioners, SM play happens in the private, a space of personal desire, individual relationships, and freely chosen roles. This construction of SM, then, is based both on a liberal subject—who knows its own desires, acts with autonomy, and freely consents—and on neoliberal rationalities that delimit this subject's sphere of belonging, of self, to the private. This private is not only opposed to the public, variously imagined as the law, vanilla social norms, or social space; it is figured as an escape from it.

This conception of neoliberalism is central to BDSM—neoliberalism not so much as a strictly economic theory, but as a form of governmentality, a contradictory and always local cultural formation that produces and validates subjects with marketized understandings of the relationship between public and private.[13] One crucial aspect of neoliberalism is that it creates and relies on racial, gendered, and sexual inequality, but justifies this social inequality as a logical outcome of purportedly neutral economic choice: *homo oeconomicus* as universal man (Brown 2005; Duggan 2003; Kingfisher and Maskovsky 2008; Manalansan 2005). A neoliberal valorization of free choice, individual agency, and personal responsibility works by obscuring the relationships between seemingly private identities (such as race, gender, and sexuality) and more public political and socioeconomic configurations; this can mask the ways that community performatively produces and reproduces social inequality.

Neoliberalism is a cultural formation crucial to contemporary sexual cultures. As a result, subject production is deeply tied not only to economic systems, but also to the shifting and culturally particular rationalities that justify the inequality produced by these systems. Imagining a split between a public, social world of "real" power and a private, individualized world of freely chosen fantasy can bolster the belief that SM scenes with race and gender have nothing at all to do with sexism or racism in the "real world." This refusal obscures the way that SM scenes like the incest scene are cultural performances that work by drawing on shared and meaningful social hierarchies of age, family, race, and gender. Moreover, just as late capitalism itself produces the transgressiveness of sex—its fantasized location as outside of or compensatory for alienated labor—the fantasy of the scene as a safe space of private desire justifies and reinforces certain social inequalities. Here, for example, practitioners' desire to escape the social ills of racism, denying that a charity slave auction like the one that opens this introduction has anything to do with historical slavery, reinforces the very whiteness of the SM community. This is what Howard Winant calls a "neoliberal racial project," a form of whiteness that disavows social and structural racism through a colorblind, individualist understanding of race (1997, 45; see also Gordon and Newfield 1994; Lipsitz 2006; Omi and Winant 1994; Wiegman 1999).[14] These disavowals use neoliberal rationalities of free choice, individual autonomy, and personal responsibility to obscure and sometimes reinforce forms of inequality. This can create opportunities to transgress, or feel free of, oppressive social norms while simultaneously restricting these possibilities to—and fortifying the position of—those with dominant class, race, and gender positions. When SM is seen as "just play," in other words, it can help obscure the dense circuitry between public and private, between oppressive social hierarchies and free, individualized desires.

Considering the politics of SM play and performance requires an examination of the ways in which BDSM acts within and on—appropriating, reiterating, reinforcing—these larger social systems of domination, not an analysis that assumes the a priori transgressiveness of alternative sexual practices. BDSM cultural performances can reproduce material relations of inequality through mimesis or repetition; they can also produce new racial, gendered, and sexual knowledges, positionalities, and possibilities through resignification.[15] *Techniques of Pleasure* reveals how SM scenes—and the SM scene—constitute and are constituted by social hierarchies, drawing attention to the multidirectional, awkward, and ambivalent circuits between social relations and sexual performances as they are lived, debated, and imagined. In this way, I explore BDSM as a series of sexual, social, and bodily practices that provide opportunities to remake and consolidate forms of subjectivity built both on capitalist practices of consumption and production and on the regulatory normalization of race, gender, and sexuality.

READING THE CIRCUIT

THE POLITICAL AND SOCIAL EFFECTS OF BDSM

This is the place to begin to read the politics of BDSM play. Cultural performances like the slave auction or the incest scene play with "real world"—and particularly American—social hierarchies. This is, in part, the reason why political, often feminist, critics of SM argue that SM slavishly replays either individual trauma (such as abuse) or social trauma (such as sexism), sometimes going so far as to argue that BDSM is simply the same as the violence it mimes. On the other side, SM supporters argue that SM is performed (thus not real), consented to (thus equalizing), or transgressive of normative vanilla sexuality and gender. Instead, BDSM performances produce the SM community just as they produce SM practitioners, but not in a "safe, sane, and consensual" vacuum—rather, in relation to economic, social, and cultural regimes and embedded systems of privilege and power. This moves us away from the bifurcation of power—performance as subversive versus performance as reenactment—and toward a dialectical reading of SM play as generated through and within social norms, and linked to multiple productions and disavowals of social power. In other words, SM play and performance not only display—often spectacularly—social relations, they also set these relations into motion, creating circuits between social norms and social power. These scenes are differentially productive and require an ethnographic eye to parse the multiple effects of SM scenes on differently situated practitioners, players, even readers.

Take, for my final example, a workshop I attended titled "Interrogation Scenes." The description of the class, circulated via e-mail, began with this teaser: "Do you enjoy having your bottom 'fight back' during play? Do interrogation scenes in war movies turn you on?" It continued: "Domina will explain what to do and what to avoid . . . See the ways you can make a scene like this believable." As is typical in BDSM classes and workshops in the Bay Area, the class began with a lecture. Domina, a white, bisexual, dominant/sadist prodomme in her late forties, stood in the front of the room wearing a California Department of Corrections shirt and jeans. She began by describing "consensual nonconsent" play —play with forcing themes—and suggested prisoner of war, rape, the Spanish Inquisition, and the Salem witch trials as potential themes for such play. Domina urged us to use a real-life context or historical event to create more exciting scenes; both setting and costuming choices are critical, she said: Nazi uniforms, for example, are "not PC, but they are powerful."

For interrogation, she told us, one can find a lot of very useful material on the Internet: Amnesty International's documents, an Israeli interrogation site, and—what she said was the treasure trove of technique —the declassified 1963 CIA manual known as KUBARK. Domina waved a printout of KUBARK at us while giving advice from its pages: the best way to stage an arrest, different kinds of sensory deprivation, how to create conditions of heightened suggestibility. It was 2002, and I had not yet heard of the manual; I was skeptical about this whole scene: that the document was real, that it was not just SM fantasy. Now, of course, in the aftermath of the Abu Ghraib controversy and several years of dispute about the legality of "no-touch" interrogation—torture—techniques, I know much more about KUBARK and its place in US imperial histories.[16]

As Domina talked, Richard and Denise jumped up from the audience —they had been sitting in the first row of folding chairs—and ran onto the stage where Domina stood; it was a surprise demonstration. Richard and Domina subdued Denise and tied her to the floor, cutting off her clothes. For the rest of the class, Richard, transformed into a slow, Southern "bubba," sat by Denise, leering with slack jaw, wet lips, and droopy eyes. Periodically he reached over to bound and naked Denise, grabbing at her nipples as she tried to kick him away. With this scene playing out behind her, Domina began to describe various torture techniques: water torture, breath play, electricity, making someone stand still without moving. "Threatening rape or body cavity searches is good," she said, as is anything that dehumanizes the bottom: give them a number, deny them bathroom privileges or toilet paper, deprive them of sleep, keep the room cold, don't feed them, or feed them tasteless or disgusting food, like boiled white bread or oatmeal mixed with peas.

Domina also gave us a few tips on how to maintain the fantasy of interrogation while "checking in" on the bottom. Staying in character as mean cop, for example, Domina might hold Denise's feet apart, a humiliating display for Denise, but one that would also allow Domina to check the temperature of Denise's feet to make sure that the rope around her ankles was not cutting off her circulation. Domina also told us we should have a prearranged signal with the bottom for something dangerous, which we should work out during negotiation. Before she put a real knife up to Denise's throat, for example, Domina grabbed her neck, their signal that the knife blade was sharp and that Denise should not move too much or struggle too hard.

These tactics allow for the management of real risk within the scene without breaking the fantasy. Using realism—real contexts, histories, emotions, and relationships—the scene becomes believable for both participants and audience. These spectacular scenes, like those that replay hierarchies based on gender, class, race, or age (often called "cultural trauma play"), use social or historical structures of exploitation as fodder for SM eroticization. In these scenes, the intensity of the play or performance is directly related to a shared national imaginary, a cultural backdrop of entrenched social power. Here, the interrogation scene works with forms of state power available as historical or cultural signage. These signs are flexible, mediated, and both public and personal: antique torture devices on display at a museum, war movies, familial military experiences, and photojournalist war coverage are all potential resources for creating an interrogation scene. BDSM scenes rely on this realistic quality—effective and believable, if not real.

How might we read a scene such as this, a mimetic performance of the kind of state terror that would come to light two years later in the Abu Ghraib scandal? Rather than stage an abstracted or formalized political reading, we might first linger on the question of effectiveness and effects. Drawing on Jon McKenzie's (2001) innovative theorization of performance, in which he argues that the contemporary regime of power/knowledge is organized around effective performance rather than Foucauldian discipline, I develop a method of reading that emphasizes the *performative efficacy* of SM scenes.[17] This method highlights performance as and of power: both the way power is performatively produced through flexible circuits and the way flexible circuits incite politicized performance. This conception draws attention to power as an injunction to perform creatively, quickly, and well, an injunction that is no more liberating than a rigid, modernist disciplinary power, but that is linked to the flexible subject formation and social organization of late capitalism. Performativity is productive, in other words, through flexibility—a flexibility tied to forms of capitalist production and consumption, as well as to social values and norms such as diversity and tolerance. Linking the material effects of a performance and the production of evaluative criteria through which effectiveness is measured, an analysis of performative efficacy thus focuses both on SM as a productive cultural performance (performatively producing SM subjects and communities) and on the political effects of such performances (the politics of performative productions). The key question is not "What are the politics of SM?" with its rote answer of "kinda hegemonic, kinda subversive" (Sedgwick 1993a, 15). It is, rather, "What is produced in this particular scene?"—a question that requires us to analyze how (and why) any particular scene works, for whom it works, and what the effects of a performance are for variously positioned participants.

I found the interrogation scene effective. Playing on and with my fears of *Deliverance*-style Southern men and drawling authority, it made me angry; I wanted to stand up and yell at Richard to get off Denise, to stop touching her, to leave her alone. I believed that Richard was this dangerous kind of man, even though I had met him before this scene, as he is Domina's husband. Yet the playing effectively produced real—although sometimes contradictory—bodily, emotional, and relational responses: fear, hatred, rage, arousal, trust, and betrayal. In this scene, the elaborate care taken to ensure consent and safety puts into place a circuit between a real or social referent and a scene realistic enough to be effective: arousing and involving for both participants and audiences. An effective scene creates a particular circuit that connects bodies and toys, subjects and histories, players and audiences through exchange: energy, commodity, affective, and power exchanges.

By dramatizing power in often spectacular ways, effective SM connects individuals with social and national imaginaries, and private fantasies with culturally legible social hierarchies. In so doing, it produces new sexualities, socialities, embodiments, and subjectivities, and it often reproduces not only the economic, cultural, and social regimes that are formed from and give form to SM performance, but also the unresolved contradictions and complexities within these regimes. Although such scenes are effective, they are not necessarily political, much less emancipatory. The interrogation scene, replaying imperialism in the name of eroticism, asks us to think through some of the political stakes of an analysis of SM, as it focuses attention on the nexus of sexuality and power that is both the source and product of BDSM. The impact of such involvement—whether an interrogation scene prompts a political critique of war, for example—must be explored at ground level, based on the social positionalities and epistemological frameworks of the participants. Particular SM scenes might, by making sex public, disrupt understandings of sex as private, of desire as asocial, offering practitioners and analysts a new vantage point on the contradictions of current social relations. They might also, by reprivatizing sex, create possibilities for a reentrenchment of subjects within such power structures, especially those that bolster the class, race, and gender inequality that is justified through neoliberal rationalities. SM scenes have differential effects; we cannot rest a political reading of SM on a formal dichotomy between transgression and reification of social hierarchies, but must rather ask about a particular scene's productive, performative effects on players, audiences, readers, and anthropologists like me.

At the Byzantine Bazaar and Slave Auction that first day of my real fieldwork, I was surprised by the kinds of people gathered at the event and the intensity of the staged slave auction. I struggled to make sense not only of the particular dynamics of desire and economics, and performance and positionality, that produced these practitioners and this event, but also of the relationships between the Bazaar as a sexual marketplace and the Slave Auction as racialized, gendered sexual performance. The performative materialism of *Techniques of Pleasure* is the result of this complicated arrival story, an approach that foregrounds BDSM sexuality as a social relation, a dynamic circuit between the subjective and the socioeconomic. Performative materialism enables me to link the proliferation and commodification of desire to the production and reproduction of social norms. Through this method, BDSM emerges as one of the ways that processes of subjectification are bound to normalized systems of inequality within contemporary capitalism. As I began to understand, SM is a practice of the self, a form of community and belonging, an impetus to consumption and lifestyle, and an eroticization of social inequality. *Techniques of Pleasure* both accounts for and disrupts what, at first, confounded me: the nondichotomous relations between normative and nonnormative embodied by computer programmers in leather, marketplaces of desire, and play scenes that dramatize and display—to uncertain political ends—US social hierarchies of race, gender, class, and sexuality. What I was seeing that first day, in other words, was the ways in which the performative or discursive is always deeply bound to the economic and the political, the ways in which subject formation is deployed within and alongside, but cannot be reduced to, forms of commodification. SM allows us to think anew the work these circuits do as they link sexuality with subjectification and desire, with leisure and consumption, with social difference and power, with economic relations and political rationalities—to rethink, in short, the socioeconomics of contemporary sex.

ETHNOGRAPHY AND PERFORMATIVE MATERIALISM

Techniques of Pleasure instantiates this performative materialism through ethnography. Combining socioeconomic and performative analytics, performative materialism insists on a method of reading that pays careful attention to the dynamic ways subjects are produced in and through social power. In order to read the effects—political, ethical, social, material, and affectual—of BDSM scenes, from the SM interrogation scene and the charity slave auction to the biotechnologies of flogging, we must analyze the rationalities, the cultural formations, that link a particular scene or individual practitioner with the larger social landscape. We need, in other words, an ethnographic reading that can illuminate the social relations condensed in everyday life, the thickness of social life on the ground, and the ambivalent effects of performance on multiply situated participants. My fieldwork method combined participant observation with open-ended interviews with diverse practitioners across the Bay Area. This combination of interviews and community-based fieldwork gave me a sense of the BDSM community as a whole—its internal debates, tensions, practices, pressures, and shared knowledges—as well as how differently situated individuals negotiate and make meaning within this community framework.

Between 2000 and 2003, I lived in San Francisco, attending, observing, and participating in a wide variety of community events. I served as the archivist for the Society of Janus, and so I attended organizational business meetings; I attended munches across the Bay Area, in San

Francisco, Palo Alto, Berkeley, Fresno, and Vacaville; and I spent as much time taking workshops on SM techniques and reading e-mails as I did going to dungeon play parties. I did, of course, attend play parties, ranging from large, semipublic gatherings hosted by organizations to small private parties, as well as other community-organized events such as film previews, book-release parties, charity events, flea markets, fetish store sales, slave auctions, fetish art openings, Christmas and Halloween parties, and the Folsom and Dore Alley Street Fairs. I occasionally went to fetish clubs and balls like the Exotic Erotic and Club SIN!, as well as local sex clubs (like the Power Exchange) and SM-themed club nights (like Bondage-a-Go-Go). As BDSM has grown, it has developed regional and national networks that are increasingly important in defining practitioners' sense of belonging. Therefore, I also attended contests and conferences both local and national (San Francisco Dyke Boi/Grrl contest, San Jose's Folsom Fringe, Washington, DC's Black Rose, and Boston's Leather Leadership Conference). As part of my fieldwork, I read e-mails from local, regional, and national mailing lists, and online and print SM magazines; and I watched movies, documentaries, TV programs, and ads that had some—sometimes tenuous—relation to SM. This array of events, attractive to different practitioners, gave me an overall picture of the new guard BDSM scene—its dynamics and its social networks.

To think through BDSM with the practitioners for whom this community is meaningful, I also conducted sixty-one interviews of two to four hours with diverse BDSM practitioners who have made this community a significant part of their lives (see the appendix).[18] My interviewees ranged from age twenty to fifty-eight, with an average age of forty-one; most were professional-class white people in long-term relationships (both monogamous and polyamorous). Because I focused on the organized SM scene, my interviewees were primarily pansexual practitioners who join Janus and women who join the Exiles (the women's or leatherdyke organization); this means that most of my male interviewees were heterosexual (although I did interview bisexual and gay men), while the women were more evenly divided between bisexual, lesbian, and heterosexual orientations (including two transwomen). Although racial dynamics within the SM community were a central interest for me, and I made an effort to interview nonwhite practitioners, the vast majority of my interviewees were white, and many worked in the

South Bay as computer programmers or IT consultants. My interviewees did range dramatically in how long they had been in the SM scene: I interviewed dungeon owners, well-known prodommes, and leading writers and community experts, some in the scene for over thirty years; I also interviewed newcomers, who had been involved for one or two years. The interviews were open-ended. I typically began by asking when the person had gotten involved with the organized BDSM scene and proceeded to discuss, among other things, the SM community and its tensions and dynamics, the politics of BDSM performance, and the local histories of BDSM. My interviews gave me an opportunity to try out my ideas and refocus my understanding; they also allowed my interviewees to direct and open lines of inquiry.

Combining participant observation with interviews gave me a deeper understanding of both the community (and its practices) and practitioners (and their narratives) than either one alone would have—enabling me to see how, for example, individual interpretations and community debates intersect, and how community pressures play out differently for practitioners depending on their race, class, and gender. It also allowed me to depart from the two most common frameworks for representation of minoritarian sexual practices like BDSM: the etiological and documentarian approaches. Neither approach pays enough attention to sexuality as a social relation, and thus neither can uncover the dynamic relationships between communities or subjects and the larger socioeconomic milieu.

The etiological approach, focusing on the causation of or motivation for BDSM desires, begins from the supposition that BDSM (and other marginalized sexualities) must be explained and diagnosed as individualized deviations. SM sexuality is commonly understood as pathological in both clinical and popular settings, but I am not the first to suggest that questions of etiology are, in the end, less interesting for what they tell us about so-called perversions than what they tell us about categories of normativity and the power those categories wield. Such vanilla-normativity does violence to sexual practices and desires like BDSM by cataloging, diagnosing, and, as Foucault puts it, "entomologizing" them ([1976] 1990, 43).

Like the etiological lens, a documentarian or voyeuristic approach also reentrenches a psychologizing, asocial approach to sexuality, in which personal proclivities and individual dynamics are severed from their social formation. Whereas in the former, BDSM is presented as individually pathological, in the latter, it is presented as a strange set of exotic practices. As Kath Weston notes, this approach partakes of the fantasy of the ethnographer as empiricist, as a "documentarian, a purveyor of distilled data" on what " 'the X' *really* do in the privacy of the shack, the hut, or the boudoir" (1998, 12, 25; see also Weston 1995b). Both etiological and documentarian approaches, then, not only belie the dense connections between BDSM and other social practices—sexual and otherwise—but they also construct a gap between SM practitioners and the researcher, author, and reader of this ethnography.

Both approaches simultaneously flatten out the tremendous range of meanings, motivations, interpretations, and desires within the BDSM scene (homogenizing the category of kinky)[19] and construct a chasm between the "normal" and the "nonnormal" or perverse (dichotomizing the categories BDSM and vanilla; see, for example, Rubin 1984). During one of the first classes I attended, Cleo, the instructor and a well-known prodomme, wrote a list of reasons why people play on a dry-erase board in the front of the classroom. Her list included: to fulfill a fantasy; to please a partner; to get "done," get high, have a big orgasm; to let go of control; to experience emotional catharsis or release; and to increase intimacy. Notably, reenacting a foundational trauma (of childhood sexual abuse, usually)—a common mainstream perception of BDSM's origin—is absent from this list. Instead, the list is not fundamentally different from the reasons people have vanilla sex. Indeed, the parallels between vanilla and BDSM sex, or the ways in which BDSM practice may resonate with other professional-class leisure pursuits like rock climbing, is further evidence of the fact that BDSM is not an individualized (and pathological) compulsion or a distinct set of exotic practices. Rather, in BDSM we see broader social, political, and economic formations: the links (and tensions) between leisure and labor; consumerism and desire; race, class, and neoliberalism; and politics and privilege. In this way, my ethnographic approach to BDSM neither psychologizes practitioners nor exoticizes these practices; instead, I pay attention to the multiple, variable, and complex meanings, interpretations, and effects of BDSM. Yet the durability of these two dynamics gestures to the way that representations of sexual difference effectively differentiate the us (good, vanilla subjects) from the them (the pathological or the perverse).

This problem of difference and distance besets most ethnographers, but perhaps especially those of us who work with alternative sexual communities. My field site—the familiar spaces of cafes and conference halls and the unfamiliar space of a dungeon—and my informants—white professionals who sometimes far exceeded my comfort zone—were both close to my home and far away. For example, my own discomfort during slave auctions and other cultural trauma play motivated my readings in the latter half of this book. But at other times, my positionality led to blind spots; because I am intimately familiar with some kinds of "technique" (I have bought more "how to" kits from Good Vibrations over the years than I care to admit in writing), I was initially simply bored by endless talk about the finer points of BDSM technique and toy craftsmanship. It took some degree of time and analysis before I was able to see just how important these conversations really were to the production of BDSM practitioners and community.

Similarly, my own relationship to BDSM practices draws attention to the insider/outsider border in fieldwork; as with most ethnographic projects, these dynamics were sometimes uncomfortable. One day, while giving me a ride to a women's play party at the Scenery, a semipublic dungeon, Lady Thendara—a white, bisexual top in her early forties—asked me, "So you aren't into SM yourself?" "No," I answered. "Hm. I would get so bored if all I had was vanilla sex." I doubt anyone thinks all they have is "vanilla sex"—sex that is bland, devoid of power exchange, technique, skill, and, usually, fun. Nonetheless, playing around the edges of BDSM does not make you "into SM"; instead, as I will argue, becoming an SM practitioner is about commitment, practice, and belonging to this social, sexual, and educational community in a serious way. Thus, when SM practitioners asked if I was "into SM" I always said no, as I hung around people who, unlike me, have made the SM community in the Bay Area home in a variety of ways. Some practitioners felt that I could never truly understand SM without doing it, but most appreciated my stance as a queer, SM-friendly nonpractitioner (often because they felt that it would give my research more scholarly legitimacy). And although I was sometimes the butt of semi-joking prodding or encouragement to try out some new toy or technique, or even plan a scene (usually with the person to whom I was talking), I found that the lose-lose situation of being, on the one hand, too close to or overinvested in SM or, on the other hand, too distant from or incapable of understanding it was more easily negotiated with SM practitioners than my academic colleagues. As Ellen Lewin and Bill Leap note, for anthropologists, "although doing research in New Guinea, for example, does not lead to the assumption that one must be a native of that region, studying lesbian/gay topics is imagined as only possible for a 'native'" (2002, 12; see also Weston 1998). In sexuality studies, even in queer studies, these assumptions about the researcher's identity are prevalent and problematic, continuously reproducing an imperative to either identify or disidentify with and as one's research.

My ethnographic approach resists the false dichotomies of distance as difference and closeness as sameness. Instead, I have placed the imaginations and experiences of my interviewees and their scenes at the center of this book in order to convey some of the appeal of SM practice and community for these practitioners—an appeal I locate in a particular social, economic, and cultural formation. And rather than highlighting individual practitioners' sexual narratives, I explore community debates, tensions, and points of convergence as openings to broader configurations of sex, money, and power, thinking critically about the dynamic relationships between subjects—their stories, narrations, and disagreements—and the socioeconomic relations that form and inform this community. My goal is to simultaneously convey the feel of the BDSM scene in San Francisco in the early 2000s (albeit in a nontotalizing, incomplete, and partial manner) and, perhaps more important, to use this depiction as a launching point to reflect on larger, US configurations of neoliberalism, community, commoditization, flexibility, and effectiveness. My ethnographic method, in other words, places the words and worlds of SM practitioners within our shared social landscape, highlighting the modes of subjectivity, the political and economic rationalities, and the cultural and community formations that make up everyday dimensions of social power in the contemporary United States.

CHAPTER OUTLINE

Techniques of Pleasure analyzes how SM community, practice, and performance produce a conduit between individual and social bodies, a circuit between the subjective (private desire, identity, individual autonomy, fantasy) and the socioeconomic (public community, social reality, collectivity, social power). In these circuits, BDSM names the specific ways in which practitioners situate themselves within and simultaneously reproduce larger social relations: iterations of public and private, community and commodity, self-mastery and technology, identity and social hierarchy. Each chapter traces these circuits as they operate in different cultural locations: cultural geographies of the Bay Area; contested terrains of BDSM community belonging: practices of self-improvement and technique; marketplaces of toys; exchanges of intimate bodily sensation; scenes of BDSM play and performance; and national discourses and ideologies of gender, race, and liberal subjectivity.

The first chapter, "Setting the Scene: SM Communities in the San Francisco Bay Area," shows how the current BDSM scene has developed in relation to large-scale regional, labor, and technological shifts in the Bay Area. Interweaving the cultural history of the new pansexual BDSM community and its practitioners with the economic history of the Bay Area, the chapter shows the supplemental relationship between the community and Bay Area (San Francisco and Silicon Valley) capitalism. In particular, I explore the tension between San Francisco's image as a tolerant, "queer" city and the reality of class and race inequality, including economic bifurcation, racial exclusions, and neoliberal redevelopment and gentrification. This tension resonates with neoliberal justifications of inequality within the BDSM scene; thus, this first chapter shows, at a regional level, the supplementary relationships between sexual community, economic policy, and ideological rationality.

Chapter 2, "Becoming a Practitioner: Self-Mastery, Social Control, and the Biopolitics of SM," focuses on the production of SM practitioners through techniques of the self. Analyzing the rise of SM organizations like the Society of Janus; classes and workshops on technique; and the proliferation of community rules focused on safe play, I show how these rules are ways that SM practitioners master themselves, becoming subjects of themselves. However, I expand this Foucauldian framework to show that concepts of risk and safety are also expressions of social privilege; they produce and justify the assumptive race and class locations (whiteness and professionalism) that the rules encode. In this way, I read the nostalgia that practitioners have for the old guard SM scene—when SM was more of an outlaw sexuality—less as a desire for transgression and more as a practice of the self, where the self is socially produced in accordance with both social relations and social privilege. Through an analysis of practitioners' ambivalence—their attraction to and concerns with the new guard scene—the chapter shows how the production of SM practitioners relies on the simultaneous production of social inequality.

As much as this nostalgia is a site of privilege, it is also an index of SM practitioners' desires for social connection, for the pleasure of play. Chapter 3, "The Toy Bag: Exchange Economies and the Body at Play," takes up this desire through an examination of the importance of—and community anxiety about—SM toys and other paraphernalia. The time and money required for such toys is yet another mark of the class privilege of SM; toys give practitioners access to new bodily pleasures and sensations, along with new possibilities for prosthetic social connections. Reading toys as a fetishistic displacement of social contradictions onto an object, I argue that the anxiety engendered by commodities shows us the primary place of the toy as a means of social connection, a contradictory relationship that requires broadening our understanding of exchange to include both commodity and power exchange. This account links the production of consumer subjects and communities to the creation of new, flexible pleasures, pleasures engendered by commodities.

Chapter 4, "Beyond Vanilla: Public Politics and Private Selves," investigates the neoliberal narratives of free choice and personal agency that SM practitioners use to justify play that parallels social inequality. Taking male dominant/female submissive gender play as the primary example, I analyze how the desire to transgress social norms enables practitioners to imagine a split between the public (oppressive social norms: white privilege, heteronormativity, and sexism) and the private (personal desire). This reading departs both from the anti-SM feminist argument that sees SM as a faithful copy of gendered inequality and the pro-SM argument that sees SM as fully consensual, fantasy, or queer play that transgresses normative gender. Instead, I explore the ambivalence generated by the mimetic relationships between gendered, racial, and sexualized social norms and SM roles, between the social real and the SM scene or play. This dichotomy relies on a narrative of self-empowerment, in which the freedom to sidestep or remake oppressive social norms depends precisely on the forms of social privilege instantiated through such norms. The ambivalence I track in this chapter is a method of reading the politics of SM play, attentive to the uncanny disavowals that structure the way practitioners know and do not know, name and fail to name, the social relations of power—grounded in material relations—that produce SM play.

The final chapter, "Sex Play and Social Power: Reading the Effective Circuit," sets my performative materialist method into motion with a series of close readings of the political effects of particular SM scenes. Focusing on cultural trauma play—specifically, play around race and ethnicity—I provide an ethnographic reading of slave auctions, Nazi play, an interracial mugging scene, and the "sadomasochistic" Abu Ghraib photographs. Although practitioners, like other Americans, are inclined to disavow the linkage between play with race and real racial inequality, I argue that these cultural performances are both based on and productive of material social relations. I foreground the performative efficacy of a scene, showing how and why a scene might work. This effectiveness, however, is politically multivalent; such scenes produce differential, variable, and uneven affective responses that link individuals with social and national imaginaries. These circuits between the social and the individual create opportunities for practitioners to both reaffirm and disrupt the fantasized break between the erotic and the political. Political effectiveness, then, is about whether practitioners connect their individuated, privatized erotic attachments to national histories of racialized belonging, and what happens when they do. *Techniques of Pleasure* ends not with a single, final analysis of the social politics of BDSM, but rather with an invitation, an opening—to explore, to linger on, the productive effects of sexual circuits.

ONE

SETTING THE SCENE

SM Communities in the San Francisco Bay Area

According to BDSM community legend, the very first munch took place in Palo Alto in April 1992. STella, a Stanford University student, posted an invitation to the Usenet newsgroup alt.sex.bondage: she would be at the outdoor patio area of Kirk's Steakburgers later that evening, and anyone who wanted to socialize offline should join her. This "burger munch" became the model for the munch: a social event usually involving food, held in a public place, open to newcomers, and with regular meeting times. During my fieldwork, there were over twenty regular munches, held not only in the cities of San Francisco, San Jose, and Oakland, but also in small towns, suburbs, exurbs, and newly created small cities across the Bay.

The largest munch, the Janus/San Francisco munch, attracted between fifty and a hundred people to a popular tapas restaurant on the second Saturday of each month. One of the smallest, the Mahogany Munch, a munch for "people of color and the people who like them," usually drew between eight and twelve people to a Mexican restaurant in Oakland on Saturday evenings. There are munches across the United States, in small towns and big cities, and in other countries like Canada, England, Scotland, and Israel. All munches are social events held on weekday evenings or weekend afternoons in public places, most often a restaurant. They are held weekly, biweekly, or monthly, and involve lunch, brunch, dinner, or drinks. They are publicized via e-mail lists and online calendars. And they are designed to be friendly, open, and welcoming to newcomers: SM play, fetish outfits, and nudity are prohibited.

The direct descendant of STella's original "burger munch" was held every Wednesday and Thursday night at 8:00 p.m., in a cafe in downtown Palo Alto. One night I arrived early and, seated with a few students working on their laptops, I watched as the cafe staff pushed large tables together and put out "Reserved for Munch" folded signs on each table. Around 8:00 people began to trickle in and sit at the tables; by 9:30 there were more than forty people, taking up most of the cafe. Sitting at one of the bigger tables, I looked around me. Most people who attend the Palo Alto munch live and work in the South Bay or Peninsula, so the people I saw there were middle-aged techies wearing khakis and T-shirts with dot-com logos. Everyone at the Palo Alto munches I went to was white; many were heterosexual and married.

The munch epitomizes the new guard pansexual BDSM community. This chapter explores the change from Folsom Street to Palo Alto, from the old guard to the new, providing a cultural history of this new scene and its practitioners in relation to the socioeconomic contours of the Bay Area. Developing Miranda Joseph's argument that communities are "complicit with capitalism" (2002, xxxiii), I show how the new BDSM community developed in relationship with—not just in the context of—economic changes in San Francisco and Silicon Valley. The rise of the Internet and Internet connectivity, the spread of informational capitalism and the development of Silicon Valley, new housing and settlement patterns across the wider Bay Area, and neoliberal city policies were crucial to the development of the new scene. At the same time, San Francisco remains the symbolic center of leather and SM: a queer homeland and a "wide-open town" (Boyd 2003). This symbolic meaning persisted even after the demise of the old guard scene, as San Francisco turned into a postcard city that few—and ever fewer of its queer, working-class, and nonwhite residents—could afford. This chapter shows how the production of this image is tied to material changes, such

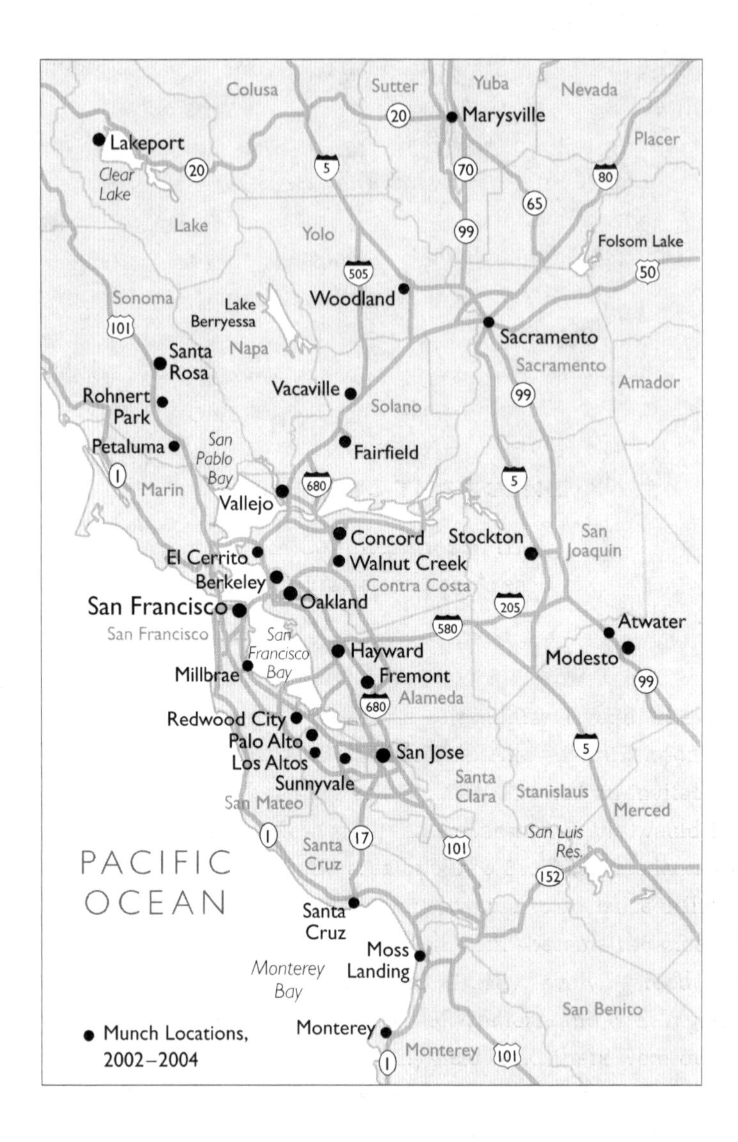

as escalating costs of living, redevelopment and gentrification projects, and racial housing segregation. As economic production moved from the city of San Francisco to the South Bay, the exurbs and suburbs outside the city grew, and tourism became San Francisco's primary economy. Tourism in the city (as elsewhere) relies on the spectacular display of difference, often racialized and sexualized difference. Thus, these material changes have produced an urban space that reproduces and solidifies class and racial exclusions through policies designed to make the city more "tourist friendly" (friendly to the flow of capital) and the display of—yet lack of support for—difference.

This is the material underpinning of the new pansexual community. The "fall of the Folsom" did not signal the end of BDSM in the Bay Area (Rubin 1997, 107; 1998, 259). Rather, these socioeconomic changes have transformed the SM scene. As I will describe, the new scene is networked and online, located in nebulous, diffuse, often suburban spaces: burger restaurants, cafes, online chat rooms, and e-mail lists. The new spaces of BDSM are less territorially defined than the Folsom leather and SM neighborhood. At the same time, BDSM organizations have transitioned from predominantly gay to predominantly heterosexual: new practitioners are more likely to be heterosexual or bisexual, middle-aged, white professionals than urban leather daddies and boys who populated the Folsom neighborhood. Of course, there are still leather daddies in San Francisco, and my interviewees included practitioners who are primarily identified with queer or more alternative scenes. However, the shifts of the 1980s and 1990s produced a flourishing new guard scene; and this scene, with its more normative practitioners, has become the organizational center of Bay Area SM.

In tracing this history, I show how, as Joseph puts it, "capitalism and, more generally, modernity depend on and generate the discourse of community to legitimate social hierarchies" (2002, viii). Reading the cultural history of the new pansexual scene reveals that the scene is compelling to its practitioners in part because it enables a particularly "neoliberal rationality" of privacy and privatization, personal responsibility, free choice, and individual agency and autonomy (Brown 2005). These discursive constructions, based as they are on material conditions, legitimate the social hierarchies of race, gender, sexuality, and class within capitalist social relations that form the subject of this ethnography. In brief, this chapter shows not only that the new SM scene is a community dependent on economic changes in a postindustrial Bay Area (just as this economy needs communities like BDSM), but also that this scene—as well as its practitioners—perpetuates race and class inequality as it fosters social belonging.

THE DEMISE AND REDEVELOPMENT OF FOLSOM STREET LEATHER

The history of SM in the Bay Area is epitomized by the story of the rise, fall, and redevelopment of the Folsom neighborhood. This neighborhood, known as Folsom, South of Market (Street), or South of the Slot, was the geographic home of the old guard leathermen. The old guard—the leather scene of the 1950s through the 1970s—describes a community of men who returned to the United States after the Second World War and settled in cities like San Francisco, Los Angeles, and New York. In the 1950s, these men created the first social space devoted to leather sexuality in San Francisco. Leathermen, as Gayle Rubin argues, had their own sexual and cultural style: a kind of butch masculinity, a fashion based on black leather and denim, and a sexuality that featured rough, often kinky sex (1997; see also Kamel 1995). Many belonged to motorcycle clubs, and the myriad bike runs and social events that the clubs organized formed the first backbone of the gay leather social world.[1]

Throughout the 1960s, bars and clubs devoted to leathersex opened in the South of Market neighborhood. The Tool Box, the first leather bar in the neighborhood, opened in 1962. The bar was "wildly popular" with leathermen and even attracted national media: the mural inside the Tool Box was the two-page opening photograph in *Life*'s 1964 "Homosexuality in America" cover story (Rubin 1998, 258). It was followed in 1966 by Febe's (a gay biker bar), a Taste of Leather (a leather and sex toy store), and the Stud (a leather-turned-gay hippie bar). In 1968, the Ritch Street Baths and the Ramrod, a bathhouse and a leather bar, respectively, opened. These bars and clubs were followed by others in the neighborhood: the Barracks, the Red Star, the Slot and the Ambush all opened between 1966 and the mid-1970s on Folsom Street; all were between Sixth and Eleventh Streets (Brent 1997; Rubin 1997 and 1998; see also Brodsky 1995 for details about similar clubs in New York). South of Market was a dense network of gay leather bars, stores, bathhouses, sex clubs, and cruising spots that lined Folsom Street—a leather "capital" (Rubin 1998, 258). By the mid- or late-1970s, the Folsom area (sometimes called "the Valley of the Kings") was one of San Francisco's largest and most prominent gay neighborhoods.

First targeted for redevelopment in the 1960s, the neighborhood came under sustained attack by the San Francisco Planning and Urban Research Association (SPUR) in the 1980s when it was labeled a "skid row neighborhood" and an "industrial wasteland" (quoted in Wolfe 1999, 708; see also Hartman 2002). In 1981, SPUR observed that Folsom Street had "a city-wide and national reputation of a particular segment of the gay population": the leathermen (quoted in Wolfe 1999, 718). As they wrote in 1985: "The oddest assortment of business activities share space, are neighbors, and do business with one another. It is not uncommon for artists, metal fabricators, restaurants, wholesale beauty supplies, bakeries and musical instrument repair shops to share the same building space. Neon artists, food processors, pawn shops, tourist hotels, auto repair shops and jazz and gay 'leather' clubs are oftentimes neighbors on the same block, particularly along the Folsom Street corridor" (quoted in Wolfe 1999, 722). This "blighted" neighborhood was the center of San Francisco's leather community, but it was also populated by Filipinos, senior citizens, Latinos, artists, and casual laborers who worked and lived in the mixed-use neighborhood. This is the historical context in which Mayor Dianne Feinstein, appointed after the 1978 murders of Mayor George Moscone and Supervisor Harvey Milk, advocated the redevelopment of the area in the late 1970s and 1980s.

Following on the heels of the redevelopment of Hunter's Point, the Western Addition, and the waterfront, this redevelopment was met with protest. Resident and neighborhood coalitions in South of Market fought against forced displacement, inadequate housing subsidies, and the lack of low-income housing available in the city (where public housing had a waiting list of thousands, many of whom had been displaced in previous redevelopment schemes). Yet in spite of this activism, several thousand residences were razed for the construction of the Moscone and Yerba Buena Convention Centers, displacing approximately four thousand households in the area. The Moscone Center opened in 1981 as a convention center. The plan for Yerba Buena was more elaborate; it included hotels, restaurants, high-end shops, plazas, museums, a sports arena, apartment buildings, parking lots, and office buildings. Located on top of the underground Moscone Center, Yerba Buena opened in 1993 with gardens, an arts center, children's play area, skating rink, food courts, and a Sony Metreon theater. For these two large projects, the city tore down residential hotels, eateries, bars, shops, light industries, warehouses, and artists' studios between Third, Fourth, Market, and Folsom Streets.

Several other factors combined with this urban redevelopment to destroy the Folsom leather scene by the mid-1980s. In 1981, a large neighborhood fire ravaged many leather spaces. Throughout the early 1980s, HIV/AIDS devastated this generation of leathermen (Rubin 1997) and public hysteria over HIV/AIDS forced the closure of all of San Francisco's bathhouses in 1984 (Bérubé 1996). Losing the sex clubs, including SM and fisting clubs like the Catacombs (in 1983), meant losing one of the most visible outposts of San Francisco's leathersex culture, along with the bars and clubs that supported the old guard leathermen's community. The combination of neoliberal urban development policies with misguided public health crusades (sex panics) made a potent and deadly combination—at least for public, street-level sexual culture. The golden age of Folsom came to an end by the early to mid-1980s (Baldwin 1998; Brent 1997; Rubin 1998).

As this short history makes clear, the demise of Folsom must be seen in relation to the economic transformation of San Francisco: the allocation of resources to tourism, downtown development, and office and residential high-rises, and away from art culture, local neighborhoods, and lofts and other spaces for low-income housing, work, and industry. This neighborhood, like New York City's Times Square before its redevelopment, was a diversified zone of sexualized contact across races and classes. As Samuel Delany observes, the redevelopment of Times Square for middle-class tourists demolished the porn theaters that had provided spatial support for rich social exchanges, amounting to a "violent suppression of urban social structures"—"economic, social and sexual" (1999, 153; see also Berlant and Warner 1998).[2] And, as Martin Manalansan argues, such projects are neoliberal; they "seek to delimit governmental intervention, increase privatization, and remove the safeguards of welfare services, creating a virtual free-for-all arena for economic market competition" (2005, 141). Privatizing public spaces has the greatest impact on the marginalized: poor, nonwhite, and queer residents and their less institutionalized communities, which become targets of anticrime and "quality of life" campaigns. Such projects, in other words, actively produce the city's citizenry as business owners and tourists, not renters or people who use the city's streets and dwindling public spaces.

In the 1990s, South of Market, now called SOMA, faced a new round of redevelopment in the form of the promotion of Multimedia Gulch, an area south of Folsom Street between Second and Seventh Streets, centered on the small city park called South Park. The buzz around Multimedia Gulch heralded new forms of labor in an increasingly information-based economy; the city promoted Internet services, publishing, and marketing along with interactive media such as graphic and computer arts, virtual communities, digital entertainment, and film postproduction. This sector accounted for 40 percent of San Francisco's new jobs in 1998. As George Raine notes in a *San Francisco Examiner* article, however, "the price of all this wealth, of course, is prohibitively expensive home prices for many, along with traffic congestion that saps energy and productivity and erodes the environmental quality that made the area desirable in the first place" (1999). Indeed, according to the San Francisco Redevelopment Agency, commercial rents increased from $6 to $60 a square foot during the 1990s (Borden 2000). Over one thousand "live/work lofts" with median sale prices of $270,000 were constructed in the neighborhood, driving out the few remaining low-income artists and blue-collar workers. New restaurants, the Museum of Modern Art (opened in 1995), and new luxury hotels also appeared, along with large numbers of media and IT businesses, including *Wired* magazine and Macromedia.

Although the end of the dot-com boom in the early 2000s gutted many of these Internet companies, SOMA bears the mark of this development. The area is known primarily for Yerba Buena Gardens, the Moscone Convention Center, and the Museum of Modern Art. Newly constructed high-rise "luxury lofts" and condos in SOMA and Mission Bay—such as Arterra, "San Francisco's first LEED-certified, green high-rise building," or the Infinity, two high-rise towers at Folsom and Main Streets—have been largely successful in wooing new residents "despite the sagging economy," as Judy Richter writes in the *San Francisco Chronicle* in 2009. In a NewGeography.com article, Adam Mayer notes that if South of Market seems "impervious" to the economic crisis of 2008, "part of this can be attributed to the continuing popularity of the city as a tourist destination for foreigners. Also keeping the local economy afloat is the investment in luxury real estate from those with disposable wealth purchasing second homes in this geographically desirable locale. Unfortunately, this does not spell good news for the city in terms of middle class aspiration and sustainable socio-economic diversity."[3] Current redevelopment plans for the area promise further privatization and rezoning, a continuation of neoliberal redistribution projects from the 1970s through the first decade of the 2000s.

Throughout these socioeconomic transformations, however, Folsom, now SOMA, has remained the symbolic center of SM and leathersex in San Francisco and beyond. This symbolism is partly anchored by a few remaining stores and bars: Mr. S, a large leather and SM store and manufacturer that first opened in 1979; Stormy Leather, a woman-oriented leather shop; and Leather Etc. But a Taste of Leather closed in 2008; and the Eagle bar, founded in 1981 and the oldest leather bar in San Francisco, is rumored to be closing in 2011. And these remaining outposts are nestled between big-box stores—an OfficeMax store abuts the Eagle—a situation Rubin describes as "ruptured territorial membranes" (1998, 266). There is still a strong gay leather scene in San Francisco. But, as Rubin argues, it is "thinner and more dispersed" than it was (1998, 268; see also Rubin 1997).

Folsom as the homeland of leathersex and SM is most visible during the two large street fairs held every year: the Dore Alley Street Fair (also known as the Up Your Alley Fair), which takes place in July, and the Folsom Street Fair, which takes place in September and is the largest leather event in the world.[4] Indeed, New York City's leather fair is called "Folsom Street East," and Folsom Street Events—the San Francisco–based nonprofit organization that runs the Folsom and Dore Alley Street Fairs—has licensed the name "Folsom" for street fairs in Germany ("Folsom Europe," in Berlin), Australia, and Canada. Begun as a neighborhood coalition devoted to anti-redevelopment activism, today the Folsom Fair is the culmination of Leather Week. The fair typically attracts 300,000 to 400,000 people to the area bordered by Seventh and Twelfth, and Howard and Harrison Streets; it is the third largest public gathering in California, after San Francisco's Gay Pride and the Rose Parades (Altine 1998, 6; Rubin 1997, 134). Tourists flying in for Folsom Fair can receive a discount on travel from American Airlines, as well as a special Folsom Street Fair rate at the Marriott in SOMA. Yet in spite of the neighborhood-specific history of Folsom, the leather pride flag flown above the city during the week is raised outside the Diesel store at Market and Castro Streets—in the Castro, not on Folsom Street or in SOMA. Turning now to a wider San Francisco context, I explain the origin of this situation—in which the devastation of a multi-use, demographically mixed neighborhood produced the Folsom Street Fair as a tourist event; and the image of San Francisco as urban, environmental, and progressive motivated the purchase of luxury condos by Silicon Valley workers and wealthy urbanites, even in an economic crisis.

SAN FRANCISCO A QUEER SODOM BY THE SEA

> We [San Francisco] were a sanctuary for the queer, the eccentric, the creative, the radical, the political and economic refugees, and so they came and enforced the city's difference.
>
> —REBECCA SOLNIT and SUSAN SCHWARTZENBERG, *Hollow City*

San Francisco has, throughout its history, cultivated a reputation as a "wide-open town," as Nan Boyd titles her history of the city, a "town where anything goes" (2003, 2). Since the days of the gold miners who flooded the Bay Area before California became a state in 1850 and the development of the Barbary Coast (the stretch of hotels, saloons, and brothels on San Francisco's waterfront that gave the city the nickname "Sodom by the Sea")[5] at the turn of the twentieth century, sexual license has been a key feature of San Francisco. Through waves of internal "countercultural" migration—the bohemians, Beats, hippies, and punks—San Francisco solidified its national reputation as a haven for alternative people, cultures, and communities.[6]

The *queerness* of San Francisco, suggested by the male miners, Barbary Coast, and the homosexuality of many of the Beats, was solidified by the end of the Second World War.[7] Servicemen and women who were stationed at military bases around the Bay or who worked in the shipbuilding, refinery, and other military industries in the Bay Area increased the city's population to 825,000 by 1945, over 48,000 more than its 2000 population.[8] After the war, many of these men and women remained in San Francisco, joining the city's nascent urban homosexual networks and frequenting designated cruising spots (D'Emilio 1983, 12, 22; see also Stryker and Van Buskirk 1996).[9] Spatially, these networks relied on the queer nightclubs and bars that had blossomed in San

Francisco after the 1933 repeal of prohibition in the old Barbary Coast area. Areas along the waterfront, in the Tenderloin, and in North Beach became primarily (although not exclusively) gay and lesbian spaces. The scene was mixed; for example, bar-based butch-femme lesbian culture included many sex workers (Boyd 2003, 40). Yet with lax alcohol regulation and tremendous graft, San Francisco's gay and lesbian—and sex worker and transgendered—bar scene along the waterfront was larger than any other US city at the time. San Francisco's prominence as a port city combined with these urban homosexual networks to make it especially attractive to gay men and lesbians after the war.

By 1959 *The San Francisco Progress* designated the city "the national headquarters of the organized homosexuals in the United States" (quoted in D'Emilio 1983, 121). The gay bars and clubs combined with political organizations like the Mattachine Society and Daughters of Bilitis to make gays and lesbians in the Bay Area visible as communities.[10] They were not, as Boyd points out, unified: bar culture and the homophile movements differed in style, goals, and political strategies. However, these overlapping components of gay and lesbian life—bars, organizations, magazines, and books—fostered a recognizable community even before the 1970s; Boyd argues that the gay community had become a self-aware political and social constituency by the mid-1960s. New activism (especially the formation of SIR, the Society for Individual Rights, in 1964) and highly publicized scandals involving payouts for liquor licenses in gay bars (called "gayola") brought homosexuality into newspapers and election campaigns. By 1965, facing unified political pressure, the police halted their bar raids. This nearly tripled the number of gay bars in the city between 1963 and 1968, bringing the total to fifty-seven—more than Chicago, Los Angeles, or New York (D'Emilio 1983, 121). The 1964 *Life* cover story "Homosexuality in America" solidified San Francisco's reputation as the "gay capital" of America. The story, which featured Chuck Arnett's mural from the Tool Box leather bar, encouraged thousands of readers to move to San Francisco, seeking a better, gayer life. Kath Weston describes the flight of gay men and lesbians across the United States to San Francisco in search of gay community in the 1970s and 1980s as the "Great Gay Migration" (1995a).

Today, San Francisco remains a homeland for queers. Gays and lesbians are estimated to make up between 10 and 20 percent of San

Francisco's population, a higher percentage than in any other US city. But more than this, for nonresidents, the city—as Cymene Howe argues—functions as a symbolic homeland: "Queers, who often experience exile from, and ostracism living in, their places of origin (nation-state, community, family, and so on), here [in San Francisco] find their 'return' in a pilgrimage to a homeland" during events like the Gay Pride Parade (2001, 44). Howe's work shows how the queerness of San Francisco draws on nationalistic ideas of identity and political community for queers near and far, while this queerness is mobilized during events to generate the tourism on which the city depends.

This is a complicated and contradictory queerness: San Francisco's image as progressive, free, and sexually liberated is produced by and for queer tourism. And even before tourism became San Francisco's primary industry in 1980, bars and clubs in the city capitalized on its reputation as America's Paris—a city of sexual freedom—with tourist-oriented entertainment designed to showcase sexual, gendered, and racial difference. At places like Finocchio's in North Beach, a former speakeasy operating from the 1930s to 1999, drag entertainment featured both queer and racialized performances. Exotic Chinese dancers, cross-race performances, and female impersonators were entertainment, while prostitution and companionship, purchased with drinks, were also available. These bars, clubs, and theaters showcased early drag king performers, but also geisha acts, hula, and Latin dance. Similarly Mona's, which opened in 1934 in North Beach, was the first lesbian bar in San Francisco. A bohemian bar, it featured male impersonators, singers, and, in the 1940s, Gladys Bentley, a black lesbian singer and piano player who became famous during the Harlem Renaissance (Boyd 2003, 68). Early tourism—so critical to San Francisco's economic development—was organized around the production and display of racial, gendered, and sexual difference for an audience consisting mostly of whites. This tourism fostered both the erosion and the reentrenchment of racial, gendered, and sexual social boundaries; it solidified a nascent queer community around these bars and clubs, and it also provided a spectacle of free and easy difference for the city's visitors and white patrons.

I describe these scenes of early touristic commodification because their echoes persist today. The city of San Francisco is itself a tourist attraction, besting Disneyland in the ranking of California attractions (R. Walker 1996). Tourism depends on San Francisco's reputation as the queer capital of the "Left Coast." It is part of the city's marketing: until recently, the city's official tourism website listed the Power Exchange (a sex club) under "mature fun," and "gay travel" is listed alongside "where to eat" and "maps." San Francisco is an important symbolic center of gay/lesbian culture in the United States, as was seen in the 2004 Valentine's Day issuance of thousands of same-sex marriage licenses, followed by marriage performances, in city hall. For this, Mayor Gavin Newsom, until then widely criticized (at least within San Francisco) for his probusiness, antihomeless policies, received national attention during the 2004 presidential election, portrayed as either the poster child of gay equality or the whipping boy of liberals gone too far, and standing in for the city as a whole.

San Francisco's sexual freedom is not simply symbolic; the city boasts the nation's first unionized peep show (the Lusty Lady, now a cooperative), a late-1990s development in the city that claims to have originated topless dancing with Carol Doda at the Condor Club, in North Beach in the 1960s. There are ongoing attempts to decriminalize prostitution, although the latest measure, Proposition K, was voted down in 2008. By 1980, Bay Area cities had the highest percentage of unmarried adults, single-person households, and divorced people, and the lowest percentage of family households, in the United States (Wollenberg 1985, 305). Many newcomers to the city were gay men and lesbians, but many were not; tolerance and (at least certain forms of) freedom made the city attractive to nontraditional people with a variety of lifestyles. It is for these reasons that Richard DeLeon argues that San Francisco is "progressive," citing domestic partnership laws, affirmative action, smoking bans, and safety standards as examples of San Francisco's progressive agenda (1992, 2–3). Indeed, the Bay Area is at the forefront of many progressive causes: curbside composting, surcharges for plastic bags at the grocery store, protection against gender discrimination for city employees, coverage of gender-reassignment surgery for San Francisco city employees, urban car sharing, and—in Berkeley—organic school lunches.

At the same time, however, these freedoms are part of the city's brand. San Francisco, as a 2008 NBCBayArea.com article put it, is a "live-and-let-live town, where medical marijuana clubs do business next to grocery stores and an annual fair celebrates sadomasochism." Here, again, San Francisco looks "tolerant"—the kind of place where "the sadomasochism fair draws thousands of tourists and a pornographic video company is housed in a former armory."[11] But the "progressiveness" of San Francisco is bifurcated: San Francisco is an important symbolic location for countercultural communities, while this symbolism conveys material benefits in terms of redevelopment and tourism. Meanwhile, in socioeconomic terms, the high cost of living in the city puts it out of reach for even middle-class residents, much less the young people who made the city queer. Indeed, a cover story in the *San Francisco Bay Guardian* questioned whether San Francisco is still a "gay mecca," since many queer people migrating to the city would not be able to afford the rents or find work (Rapoport 2005).

Further, as the brief history of San Francisco's tourist industry suggests, the city has long combined its sex-positivity with crippling racism. The extermination of Native Californians,[12] Chinese ghettoization, Japanese internment, and fierce labor and housing discrimination against African Americans sit uncomfortably with the city's long history of sexual tolerance.[13] Racism continues in the form of multiple ID requirements for patrons of color at gay bars in the Castro, most famously at S.F. Badlands (Buchanan 2005; see also Han 2007; Howe 2001; Ramirez 2003). Postcards of San Francisco feature the endlessly reproduced row of "painted ladies" on Alamo Square, in the Western Addition. This neighborhood, where I lived during my fieldwork, was one of the original targets of redevelopment in the 1950s and 1960s: the city's initial A-1 redevelopment project relocated 4,000 primarily Japanese and African American families, many out of the city proper, inspiring the name "Negro removal." Another 13,500 people were displaced in the A-2 project. San Francisco's black population has been in decline since, falling more than 14 percent during the 1990s. This gap between sexual tolerance and race and class exclusion—between symbolism and material inequality—relies on what Marina McDougall and Hope Mitnick call "theme park thinking," which transforms "the city into a series of picturesque facades" (1998, 153; see also Hannigan 1998; Judd and Fainstein 1999; Sorkin 1992). "Theme park thinking" often involves the staging of sexual license and racial or ethnic difference for an audience of tourists: Fisherman's Wharf with its chain stores and crabbers; North Beach with its Beat history and strip clubs; Chinatown, the largest in the United States; the Castro, with its enormous gay pride flag. These facades obscure, while depending upon, racial and class inequality.

San Francisco's famous quality of life—its openness, tolerance, and diversity—is, in other words, virtually unavailable to those who built the city, while its queerness has become a brand, used to attract affluent tourists and patrons while substantially undercutting social services and economic support for marginalized residents. In this neoliberal development, San Francisco has been remade into a city for large, multinational corporations; tourists; and suburban commuters—not the diverse people of San Francisco. Residents continue to be forced out of the city by a deadly combination of redevelopment and the rapidly changing Bay Area economy. It is this economy, located not in the postcard city of San Francisco but in the South Bay, that I turn to next.

SILICON VALLEY ECONOMIC POWER

San Francisco is the iconic center of the Bay Area, but Silicon Valley is the economic center. And it is these areas outside the city—less permissive, more family friendly, and even whiter than San Francisco—that have experienced major population and economic growth in the 1990s and 2000s and have driven larger socioeconomic changes throughout the Bay Area. The "capital of Silicon Valley," San Jose is the tenth largest city in the country; its population exceeds San Francisco's by at least 100,000.[14] From 1950 to 1980, while San Francisco's population declined by 12 percent, Santa Clara County gained a million inhabitants. This period of rapid suburbanization, produced, as elsewhere, through financial and federal public policies (urban renewal projects, federally funded highways, and home loan and business tax policies [see Brodkin 1998; Lipsitz 2006]), has transformed the spatial and economic landscape of the greater Bay Area.[15]

The movement of capital from San Francisco to Silicon Valley began in the mid-1940s and intensified throughout the next decades. Silicon Valley began with a combination of defense contractors, other industries related to the Second World War, and electronics companies—such as Hewlett-Packard, famously started in a Palo Alto garage in 1939 by two engineering graduates of Stanford. A naval station, Lockheed and Westinghouse plants, and housing, shopping, and factories followed, supplanting almost all of the orchards and farmland in the region. In the years following the war, Stanford University established industrial parks that lured IBM and GE, among other companies, to the area.

Combining research facilities, universities, venture capital, and land, the Peninsula started to boom in the 1950s.

In the 1970s, high-technology jobs and companies began to dominate employment in the Bay Area. The rapid pace of consumer electronic development and the invention of the microchip made San Jose one of the fastest growing cities in the United States. Silicon Valley in the 1970s had 20 percent of the nation's high-tech jobs and was the ninth largest manufacturing area in the United States (Wollenberg 1985, 309). By 1980, Santa Clara's population was 1,300,000—ten times its 1950 population. By the early 2000s, about a third of all the Internet businesses in the United States were based in Silicon Valley: more than 6,600 technology companies, including Cisco, Adobe, Apple, NASA Ames, and eBay, employing more than 254,000 people (Solnit and Schwartzenberg 2000, 14; see also English-Lueck 2002, 18). The IT industry—especially computer programming, software development, and network technology—grew at double the rate of other industries starting in the mid-1990s; in 2000, Internet and high-tech businesses accounted for 38.9 percent of new jobs—and 21.7 percent of all jobs—in the Bay Area. Even with the economic downturn, the US Bureau of Labor Statistics anticipates continued growth in these sectors: employment of computer scientists and database administrators, for example, is expected to increase 37 percent from 2006 to 2016 (US Department of Labor 2008).

These shifts resulted in the polarization of the US economy, especially in cities and metropolitan regions such as the Bay Area. As in other parts of the country, the service economy in the Bay Area has both high-paying and low-paying employment, but little in between. On the high end, computer and technology workers make well over $100,000 before their yearly bonuses; on the low end, workers scrape by in retail and service jobs (child care, personal care, and cleaning). The housing market reflects these economic changes. Highly paid technology jobs, combined with the influx of workers to these new jobs, led to the rapid escalation of housing costs in the Bay Area (Chapple et al. 2004); by the 1980s, the Bay Area had the highest housing prices in the United States. The dot-com boom of the late 1990s ratcheted up housing and other costs in San Francisco. In 1997, for example, the median monthly rent for a two-bedroom home was $1,600; two years later, it had swelled to $2,500 (Hartman 2002, 325). That increase, coupled with the rapid growth of Silicon Valley, has dramatically altered the Bay Area's economic and spatial landscape. In 2003, only 15 percent of San Francisco's residents could afford a median-priced home (median home prices in the city rose 40 percent between 1996 and 2000, to $328,000).

This growth, however, was uneven across the Bay Area. In the late-1990s, home prices increased more than 185 percent in San Francisco and across much of Silicon Valley, but in Solano and Contra Costa Counties prices rose less than 51 percent. San Francisco, Atherton, Menlo Park, Palo Alto, and Redwood City had among the highest home appreciation rates; Oakland, Concord, Richmond, San Rafael, and Vacaville had among the lowest. As elsewhere in the United States, changing housing patterns also produced and solidified racial and class segregation. Suburbanization across the Bay Area encouraged many middle-class whites to leave center cities and move to the suburbs, like Los Altos, Los Gatos, Walnut Creek, and Menlo Park. As a result, the Bay Area of the last decade of the 1990s exhibited clear racial and class segregation. In 2000, Richmond, for example, was 31 percent African American, 27 percent Latino, and 31 percent white, with a median household income of $44,210; Atherton was less than 1 percent African American, 3 percent Latino, and 85 percent white, with a staggering median household income of more than $200,000.[16] The white, professional class composition of new suburbs and exurbs around the Bay Area has been disrupted only by such factors as the immigration of highly trained computer professionals, often from India and China, on H1-B visas (Wolf-Powers 2001).

Silicon Valley's bifurcated economy drives housing, residence, and labor patterns across the Bay Area. As jobs and people relocate away from San Francisco, less expensive "edge cities" (Garreau 1992) and outlying counties have experienced tremendous growth. Between 2000 and 2002, for example, San Francisco lost 92,900 jobs; many of the 11,929 residents who left the city between 2001 and 2002 moved "to more affordable communities in neighboring San Mateo, Alameda and Contra Costa counties" (Hendrix 2003; see also Armas 2003). Between 2000 and 2004, critical dot-com bust years, San Francisco's population declined by more than 32,000, while Contra Costa County's population increased by more than 55,000 (Marcucci 2005). San Francisco bears the mark of gentrification, skyrocketing housing costs, and urban redevelopment; it is a city that few but Silicon Valley programmers can afford to live in. *Fortune*, naming San Francisco one of the five best cities for business, notes that "some people even refer to San Francisco as a suburb of the Valley" (Borden 2000). On the other hand, the edge city of Vacaville—a fifty-five-mile drive east of San Francisco past patchy growth, big-box landscapes, and browned weeds—experienced a 19 percent population growth between 1990 and 2000. The four outlying Bay Area counties—Contra Costa, Napa, Solano, and Sonoma—also grew; the population of Solano County, for example, grew 93 percent between 1980 and 2000.

These socioeconomic changes impact the social landscape of BDSM. It is perhaps not surprising, then, that the munch was founded in Palo Alto, or that there are munches in Vacaville, Hayward, Petaluma, Rohnert Park, El Cerrito, Walnut Creek, Fresno, and Yuba City, small cities and towns miles away from San Francisco. There are still munches in San Francisco, of course, but although the city remains the symbolic center of SM, it is no longer the spatial center. Many of my interviewees believe that San Francisco is more permissive and less conservative than the South or East Bay. Walking out the door in a collar or latex outfit might be less likely to result in social reprobation in San Francisco than in other areas, including San Jose. Similarly, the push to reinstate a semipublic dungeon in San Francisco proper after the Castlebar closed is also based on the sense that the city is the true home of SM and leather. But at the same time, a nearby, easy-to-park-at munch at Fuddruckers or Round Table Pizza makes much more sense for new suburban and exurban practitioners like Latex Mustang and Lady Thendara, whose lives—both work and play—are far from the city itself.

THE NEW GUARD BDSM ACROSS THE BAY AREA

Lady Thendara and Latex Mustang live in San Mateo County, on the Peninsula. They are married, in their early forties. Both are white professionals: Thendara is an insurance adjuster; Mustang is a manager in the computer industry. She is a bisexual top; he is heterosexual and identifies as a bottom/pony. Mustang has a child from a previous marriage who lives with the couple part of the time. They had been married one year when I interviewed them in 2002, having had a "kinky wedding ceremony" at an SM retreat where Mustang was in full pony regalia. They attend parties in San Francisco on the weekends, but they are regulars at the Palo Alto munch, just a few minutes from their home and offices. As Latex Mustang explains, they live in Menlo Park because:

LATEX MUSTANG: it's wonderfully central: from Menlo Park, you can go to activities in San Francisco, in San Jose, or the East Bay without thinking about it. It's a thirty- or forty-minute drive to just about anything you want to do. So that's true for cultural things, vanilla things, or kink things. You really have access to just about everything. And yet you've got a wonderful, safe bedroom community to go home to, where there's parking and . . .

LADY THENDARA: Good schools.

LATEX MUSTANG: . . . good schools. So it's really a wonderful compromise.

Thendara and Mustang are representative of the new guard SM practitioners in the Bay Area. Typically white, professional, and middle-aged, these practitioners often live in the suburbs or exurbs, and many work in tech jobs. Indeed, of the sixty-one people I interviewed, over a quarter worked in computer fields, most of them as computer programmers, software developers, or IT consultants; this was more than any other category of employment, including "other." The average age of my interviewees was forty-one, and many were in their fifties. Most were involved in long-term relationships (both monogamous and polyamorous): 25 percent were married, and 38 percent were partnered. The majority of the men were heterosexual, and the majority of the women were bisexual, although many bisexual women, like Thendara, were married to men. Eighty-seven percent of my interviewees were white, in spite of my effort to interview nonwhite practitioners. Finally, only about a third lived in San Francisco, while a quarter lived in Alameda County (in the East Bay), and another third lived on the Peninsula, in either Santa Clara or San Mateo County.[17] Although my interviewees were not, by any means, a controlled sample, their demographics reflect the people I commonly saw at parties, classes, and other pansexual events around the Bay Area. As Mollena—an African American, bi, submissive bottom in her mid-thirties—explained to me in a tone of regret, at a munch you find "Palo Alto people . . . middle-aged, middle-class white people" in "couples that are established."

But Thendara and Mustang are representative in more than demographic ways; they are the normative center of this community. These new practitioners and their scene are linked not only to the broader socioeconomic changes across the Bay Area, but most importantly to new technology: the rise of the Internet throughout the 1990s. The munch, for example, begun in Palo Alto, both epitomizes this scene and is a catalyst in the growth and increasing popularity of BDSM. Public, open to newcomers, and listed online, the munch makes it easy to find and join the SM community, in stark contrast to the closed, word-of-mouth old guard scene. The number of people joining SM organizations boomed in the mid-1990s, coinciding with the release of the first graphical (not text-based) web browser—Mosaic, released in 1993—and the increasing popularity of personal modems. Many practitioners were first exposed to an SM community on the Internet. They described first finding the community in AOL chat rooms, or by searching for "kinky sex" or "bondage" on the web. As Jay, a white, heterosexual switch with top leanings in his mid-fifties, explained, in 1994 when "the cyber era began . . . S&M [was] much more easy to find. It was the start of the munches, and . . . things really changed . . . when computer manufacturers started routinely putting modems in personal computers, more and more people started getting on the Internet." And once online, they found SM.

Like STella, founder of the munch, these practitioners were early Internet adopters, reflecting the wider public use of the Internet (or Usenet discussion forums) in the Bay Area. Although Internet use increased rapidly in the 1990s across the country, its growth was particularly intensive in the Bay Area. In part, this was because the Bay Area—primarily San Francisco and San Jose—already had dense Internet connectivity.[18] In 2000, for example, 72 percent of people in the Bay Area used the Internet, compared with 60 percent of Americans as a whole (English-Lueck 2002, 21). And today, in the Bay Area SM scene, there are hundreds of SM-related e-mail lists; my interviewees typically belonged to no fewer than ten. During my fieldwork, I joined twenty, including dungeon lists, a national activist list, lists for local organizations and workshop instructors, and party and other event lists. When I became a Janus officer, I joined that list; when I went through Dungeon Monitor training, I joined another. I do not think I was unusual; almost all community information, event locations, and news stories are communicated online, through online calendars, e-mail announcements, and web pages.

Facilitated by these social and economic changes, the growth and range of classes, workshops, organizations, munches, and play spaces available to BDSM practitioners is astounding. As Jay exclaimed, "There are leather stores, SM clubs in virtually every city . . . there are munches across the country, for God's sake! That this [BDSM] has become a social movement is something I never anticipated when I came into the community in 1975. I would have been happy if I had had one or two compatible sex partners and a small group that I could have gone to . . . Nobody anticipated that the community would get this big. I mean, for years there was one store and one club, you have your real minimal landscape, you had to know where to go to find people. Now look—it's huge and it's still getting bigger!" Part of this "hugeness" is the range of events a pansexual practitioner can attend throughout the Bay Area: munches, classes or workshops, play parties, BDSM book-release parties, fetish balls, charity slave auctions, kinky flea markets, organizational business meetings, and local contests. There are also events and venues positioned between this local community and what is understood as a more commercial, fashion-oriented scene: the weekly Wednesday fetish night at a San Francisco nightclub (Bondage-a-Go-Go) and a commercial sex club (the Power Exchange, with large basement dungeon area), open Thursday through Sunday. But the scene is also simply larger; as one index of this growth, the membership of the Society of Janus, the largest SM organization in the Bay Area, grew from 35 in 1975, to 250 in 1980, 450 in 1990, and 700 in 2000. And it is now just one of several similar educational, social, and political organizations in the Bay Area.

These new spaces of BDSM—the Internet, the suburban home dungeon, the national conference, the workshops on toys and techniques—are spaces accessible to, populated by, and produced for new white professional practitioners. In her ethnography of the culture of Silicon Valley, J. A. English-Lueck argues that the IT explosion has transformed everyday forms of life, from communication to subjectivity. Her ethnography highlights some of the key themes of this rapid change, especially new understandings of work as creative, technical, and personal: the center of one's life (2002, 22–23). Not only do people work at home, on weekends, and at night, but work itself structures their time and lives: as English-Lueck puts it, "life is a series of projects" (33), "work defines worth . . . based on producing technology, and embracing a fast pace and an open attitude" (25). This produces an intense commitment to work under the guise of flexible, casual, nonhierarchical structures (see also E. Martin 1994; McKenzie 2001).

These workers—casual, flexible, but always on call—make ideal SM practitioners. The casual dress code and flexible work schedule accommodate the many gamers, Dungeons & Dragons or Magic players, and Renaissance fair goers who work in the Peninsula's vast acres of cubicles, and head to munches and play parties after work and on weekends. For them, SM's combination of work and play, where working at SM practice is part of the pleasure of participating in this community, is attractive (as I discuss in the next chapter). And the influx of these practitioners, in the post-1990 Internet scene, has transformed the SM community into a different kind of community: one organized around and responsive to the desires of these professionals.

In the 1990s, the old guard cross-class Folsom scene, anchored by bars and clubs, was supplanted by a mediated, networked new guard pansexual scene. The story of SM in the Bay Area is part of a larger story about the relationship between San Francisco and San Jose, about San Francisco's sexual permissiveness—a haven for queer and alternative sex communities—combined with its declining role in the Bay Area economy. Bay Area SM communities have developed alongside the rise of IT industries in Silicon Valley, a high-tech culture that celebrates innovation, technique, and progress; a work (and play) culture organized around the productive demands of the information economy. And even after the dot-com downturn, the cultural changes wrought by late-capitalist economic shifts, especially in information technology and changing relations of consumption and production, have endured. As scholars like Donald Lowe (1995) and Linda Singer (1993) argue, the increased commodification of sexuality, the marketing of sexual identities, and the promotion of sexuality as a consumption-based practice have produced and nurtured various forms of sexuality, of which BDSM is but one example. Many BDSM community events are deeply tied to consumerism: workshops to learn new toy techniques, expensive parties that forge a sense of community. These changes are more durable than the ups and downs of any particular sector of the economy.

BDSM communities have also developed in the context of a "Left Coast" city and region—a center of progressive, tolerant diversity—that reflects an American belief in meritocracy and the California dream, even as it obscures material gender, racial, and class inequalities. This complex situation—in which the symbolic or discursive weight of San Francisco is dependent on material relations of production as well as on social inequality often masked through neoliberal rationalities—produces an SM community that, as I will demonstrate throughout this ethnography, perpetuates some forms of social inequality in the name of "community" belonging.

SOCIAL BELONGING, SOCIAL PRIVILEGE BDSM AS COMMUNITY

There is no doubt that SM functions as a space of belonging, a *community* with all of the vexed striving toward an ultimately failed inclusion that this term conveys.[19] Accompanying the profusion of SM clubs, e-mail lists, classes, and other social organizations is a substantial investment that most practitioners make in their SM community. In addition to spending much of their discretionary income on toys, practitioners also spend a tremendous amount of time being SM practitioners. For many participants, most or all of their friends and social circle are involved in the scene. Many people talk about "giving back to the community" through publications, websites, or classes; or by volunteering as officers of organizations or munch leaders. Even the nonstop complaining about the ways that the BDSM community has changed, always for the worse, indicates that SM practitioners view the scene as their community: a home or space of belonging. BDSM—along with online or virtual communities, hobby communities, and even exurban churches—is one of the new forms of community that have replaced the older forms Robert Putnam (2000) looks back at, nostalgically.[20] As Paul—a white, heterosexual, dominant top in his early forties—puts it, SM is a way "of being together," maybe to meet a partner, "but more so that I don't feel alone." He continues: "What's so funny is how frequently you will get a group of perverts and you will talk about almost everything except it [SM] . . . the joke is, of course, it's always computers: get six perverts together and watch five conversations start about the new operating system of such and such or handheld device, wireless whatever, interfaces, and all that. You know, we talk about politics, we talk about art, we talk about everything, movies, all kinds of crap." For Paul and other practitioners, the SM community is a place to get together and feel a sense of belonging, even when there is no sex involved.

At a munch, for example, SM play is prohibited. The Walnut Creek munch in Contra Costa County meets at Fuddruckers, a "casual dining chain." The e-mail note announcing the munch reads: "Fuddruckers is a family style restaurant. We will have reserved a private room for the munch but this is still a totally vanilla venue. Please respect the attendees and patrons by dressing appropriately for a vanilla venue and maintaining our confidentiality." Similarly, the TGIF—The Group in Fresno—munch instructs attendees to "leave your fetishwear and fetishgear at home. This is not a play party. It's a get-together for folks who share a common interest in BDSM. If you're shy or unsure of yourself, this is the perfect place to be . . . everyone is friendly and nonjudgmental." Robert, a heterosexual, white top in his early forties, described the first time he attended the Palo Alto munch: "Somehow or other, I met someone who told me about the munches. So I went to a meeting in a coffee shop somewhere in Palo Alto . . . a lot of these people are computer geeks so they were talking about what new chip is coming out and what research is happening, and language like this is really boring . . . It wasn't my optimal idea of a party. If it was a party, it was pretty damn dull." Yet Robert went on to start his own munch in Berkeley, rather than dropping out of the scene. Similarly, Phil—a white, heterosexual switch/bottom/slave in his mid-fifties—remains a fixture in the scene, although he is no longer interested in playing himself. He tells me: "It's a home; it's the only home I really have. I'm known, and I walk down the street in the community and people know who I am" (see also Newmahr 2008).

The ubiquity of silicon chip discussions in a sex-based community might seem odd, but it is one more example of the ways community does not exist outside of the relations of production, forms of leisure and labor, spatial geography, and other configurations of capitalism that it both depends on and reproduces. Indeed, it is precisely because this community is so bound to social and economic relations that it functions as a community. New media networks—Internet chat rooms, e-mail lists, and online calendars—and print media like organization newsletters, fliers, and cards posted on bulletin boards produce this new pansexual SM community and, with it, spaces of shared, imaginative belonging. It is not uncommon, for example, for people to request a ride to a doctor's appointment or help moving, advertise household goods, or announce upcoming weddings on local e-mail lists or at munches and other events.

At the same time, it should be clear that the word *community* does not refer to an idyllic, touchy-feely, or "romantic" homogeneous unit. Rather, forms of belonging institutionalized by community are themselves products of, and productive of, social relations. In SM, these cultural and material formations of community solidify and legitimate some forms of social privilege. Some SM practitioners—heterosexual, middle-aged, white professionals—are enabled to achieve a version of freedom that is constituted through participation in the SM community. However, as Manalansan puts it, "this kind of freedom is predicated on the abjection of other groups of people who are not free to consume" (2005, 143–44). Such versions of freedom are neoliberal; neoliberalism justifies inequality by discursively constructing the "we" of community as those who have the right to possess the city, defined in opposition to those "fenced out of these extremely private and privatized domains" (Manalansan 2005, 151). Neoliberalism—the solidification of understandings of privacy and privatization, personal responsibility, free choice, and individual agency and autonomy within market logics—simultaneously produces social belonging via community and legitimates social hierarchies of race, gender, sexuality, and class within communities organized in this way.

The SM community I describe in this book demonstrates just this dynamic. Consider the "public" play party. During my fieldwork, the Castlebar dungeon, in South San Francisco, closed, and the Scenery, in Hayward, opened (having moved from San Jose).[21] Many lamented the loss of a big dungeon in San Francisco, the symbolic home of SM and leather. At the same time, the Scenery's East Bay location was convenient and significantly cheaper. The public dungeon, alongside the munch, is a key site of SM community, one of the few places large enough to attract practitioners from across the Bay Area for play parties, grounding community in particular places as well as in play.

The public nature of such parties, however, deserves a second look. The new SM scene is, for practitioners, public in two ways. First, practitioners call SM play in community spaces public; it happens in front of other people who are playing, watching, and socializing. The Scenery, located in a commercial warehouse in a Hayward industrial park, had open play parties every Friday and Saturday night. To attend, you looked up the Scenery web page and e-mailed Larry, the owner, to request permission. Without much screening, Larry would respond with an e-mail containing an invitation, the address, and directions from across the Bay Area. You could also attend with a current member acting as your sponsor; that was how I went the first time. Entering the nondescript building, you first met Martha, Larry's submissive, sitting behind a desk. If you did not already have a Scenery membership card, you could sign up on the spot by paying a $10 membership fee, and then the party fee ($20 per person). As Larry—an American Indian, bi dominant/master in his late forties—explained: "because of e-mail, we are able to advertise to targeted groups—and when I say targeted, I'm talking about the leather community in particular—while we maintain a reasonably low profile within the general community as a whole." He continued: "We're able to keep it out of the—if you're not looking for it, we're not going to send it to you." The publicness of public play parties is thus immediately unraveled: the dungeon operates as a private membership club—you pay to join and attend parties. Furthermore, because of the assumption that everyone at the space is interested in, or at least supportive of, SM, the space is private in the sense of restricted, secluded, and safe from a (hostile) public world (see Leap 1999). Here, public SM has been "rezoned" as private through its function as social—public in the colloquial sense—belonging.

Second, practitioners see themselves as public when they have "come out" into the scene. This is not quite the same as the gay and lesbian coming out model; practitioners are generally closeted about their SM practices. Only a third of the people I talked with were out to people in their families, nonscene friends, or work colleagues; almost half were not out to anyone at all. Instead, outness, for many, was about being part of the organized SM community: attending classes, munches, parties, and community events, even with a scene name.[22] As Panther, an Asian American, heterosexual, dominant top in his mid-forties, explained, "I started getting a lot more active . . . that's when I really started coming out publicly. I started attending munches" as well as play parties, SM conferences, and classes. This kind of outness—"coming out" into the scene or being "out there" about SM (by teaching, organizing, even posting on e-mail lists)—does not happen after a ruptural move to the city, away from family, but rather by attending munches and parties near work and home, in strip malls or in dungeon spaces in industrial parks. In other words, in private—and nonurban—spaces.

For these reasons, I understand the SM community as *semipublic*, a term that draws attention to the ways a discourse of publicness can obscure the neoliberal privatization that produces and legitimates community belonging. As the next two chapters show, the new guard has transformed SM in the Bay Area, moving it from the city to the suburbs and exurbs; building a more professionalized, technique-oriented scene; developing formal classes and workshops; and working at SM as work on the self. These forms of belonging also reinforce social inequalities—obscuring the overwhelming whiteness of the SM scene and its attraction to play with racial inequality, and the social privileges that allow white, heterosexual men to play with gender norms—as my final two chapters reveal. SM is a community, but one that organizes social belonging through neoliberal governmentality. In the late-capitalist transformations of the Bay Area economy, it is not only the gentrification or redevelopment described in this chapter that has transformed the cultural geography of BDSM; it is also the cultural and political rationalities engendered by these changes. These rationalities are neoliberal: concepts of the public and private have been realigned, producing new subjects, new communities, and new inequalities. Neoliberalism enables social belonging through the production of certain visions of community, a belonging that rationalizes freedom as freedom to consume, and social inequalities like racism or sexism as either a thing of the past (especially in the purportedly tolerant Bay Area) or due entirely to individual actions or beliefs—not to social relations of power. Reading the cultural history of the Bay Area's SM scene, in other words, we can see the dense circuitry between capitalism and community, between spatialization and belonging: the ways in which the production of these new community practices and new queer freedoms rely on—and generate—material social inequalities.

TWO

BECOMING A PRACTITIONER

Self-Mastery, Social Control, and the Biopolitics of SM

This is a sample question from the website of the Dungeon Monitors Association (DMA):

> A top is doing a cutting on the bottom. They are using a tarp, containing the blood properly and the top appears to be exhibiting proper technique. The party rules say no blood play. You:
>
> a) interrupt the scene and politely tell the top that blood play is not allowed at the party and that they will have to stop.
>
> b) let it finish since they are doing it correctly, but when they are done inform them that they have violated party rules.
>
> c) bring the top some bandages to use when they are done.
>
> d) do nothing. They have already started so stopping it would be rude.

Founded in 1998 to "improve the quality of dungeon monitoring through education and the promulgation of standards," the DMA trains and certifies individuals to work at play parties as dungeon monitors, or DMs, across the Bay

Area. DMs become dungeon monitor trainees after successfully completing the full-day Beginning Dungeon Monitor Training Course: scoring at least 80 percent on a twenty-five-item multiple-choice test, with questions like the one above.[1] They become fully certified DMs after a six-month period as a trainee, during which they must log fifteen one-hour DM shifts at parties and take ten qualifying skills classes (documented and signed-off on in the log book given to trainees), obtain first aid and CPR certification, and maintain membership in the DMA. DMs patrol the play area at parties, watching to make sure that safe-sex and other party rules are being followed, and are on hand for any emergencies that may occur.

The DMA is an example of some of the social and structural changes that have taken place in the SM scene since the 1980s. Along with the socioeconomic and demographic changes I described in the previous chapter, the new pansexual scene is also much more formally organized than the network of old guard leathermen. Educational organizations and a vast repertoire of classes and workshops on SM technique; practices, like negotiation and the use of safewords, that stress safety and risk reduction; prohibitions on "edge play" and policing of the boundary between the safe and the dangerous; and the establishment of a "police" body of dungeon monitors are all recent developments in a community that, in contrast to the outlaw image of SM, appears almost obsessed with rules and order, safety and security.

Interestingly, as I interviewed practitioners and attended events, complaints about this obsession were ubiquitous: many in the scene feel that SM today is an overly rule-oriented, regulative community. This chapter analyzes the emphasis on rules and regulations, classrooms and guidebooks, safety procedures and dungeon monitors, as well as the community debates that such changes have engendered. Tracking the circuits between self-mastery or individuation and social control or community norms, I flesh out the ways in which people become SM practitioners by producing, policing, mastering, and debating the boundaries between safe (acceptable or correct) and dangerous (unacceptable or wrong) play.

These binaries rely on the social construction of risk. As Nikolas Rose argues, in the late twentieth century, "individuals, families, firms, organizations, communities" have been asked to "*take upon themselves* the responsibility for the security of their property and their persons, and that of their own families" ([1999] 2007, 247; italics in original). This shift both individualizes (via logics of choice, autonomy, and responsibility) and collectivizes (into newer "communities," each responsible for "'its own' risk management") risk and responsibility (248). The privatization of risk—coupled with what many have argued is a broader US ethos of anxiety, fear, or insecurity—has generated a range of practices organized around warding off or managing risk: body practices like going to the gym and dieting; hobbies like extreme sports and adventure tourism; spatial forms like the gated community and exurb; the growth of prediction and insurance markets; social shifts like self-help and life-coaching; and legal changes, like tort reform or bicycle helmet laws (see Ekberg 2007; Grewal 2006; Low 2003). Risk practices are also a potent generator of consumption: purchasing books, videos, services, and other commodities to make one (and one's family) safer and more secure both activates and alleviates a sense of vulnerability. This link to commodification is a reminder that safety is also a sign of social privilege; it is, of course, the people who live outside gated communities who are truly at risk. In this way, like the privatization of space I described in the last chapter, the displacement of health and safety onto private or privatized communities is one way that neoliberalism functions to justify material inequalities.

Risk management is biopolitical: a form of power "whose operation is not ensured by right but by technique, not by law but by normalization, not by punishment but by control, methods that are employed on all levels and in forms that go beyond the state and its apparatus" (Foucault [1976] 1990, 89). As Paul Rabinow and Nikolas Rose argue, biopower combines "a form of truth discourse about living beings and an array of authorities considered competent to speak that truth; strategies for intervention upon collective existence in the name of life and health; and modes of subjectification, in which individuals can be brought to work on themselves, under certain forms of authority, in relation to truth discourses, by means of practices of the self, in the name of individual or collective life or health" (2006, 203–4). Rabinow and Rose call for further analysis of biopower within particular cultural, historical, and social configurations. This chapter begins that work by exploring concepts of risk within the SM community. It highlights biopower as the "power relations that take humans as living beings as their object" and the "modes of subjectification through which subjects work on themselves qua living beings" (215): the self-mastery of becoming an SM practitioner.

Drawing on Foucault's work in *The Use of Pleasure* and *The Care of the Self*, I analyze this self-mastery as a form of subjectification, a "stylistics of existence" or "cultivation of the self." Self-scrutiny, self-control, and self-mastery are techniques that "one performs on oneself, not only in order to bring one's conduct into compliance with a given rule" but also to constitute "oneself as the ethical subject of one's sexual behavior" (Foucault [1984] 1990, 27; Foucault [1984] 1988, 240). Through techne, or "practices of the self," SM practitioners "monitor, test, improve and transform" themselves in relation to the SM community (Foucault [1984] 1990, 28). This technique of the self encourages practitioners to become subjects of themselves, to master themselves, even as it solidifies particular—white, professional—iterations of SM community.

As Foucault reminds us, practices of risk and safety are always tied to social power: techniques of the self were for men, and only slave-owning and married men ([1984] 1990, 22). These ethics, he argues, were not concerned with disciplining social inferiors (such as women) but were, rather, an "elaboration of masculine conduct carried out from the viewpoint of men in order to give form to *their* behavior" (22–23; italics in original). Although the time period that Foucault is considering—Greek and Roman antiquity, from the fourth century BCE to the second century AD—is obviously quite different from today, thinking about SM practice as a technique or care of the self is crucial to understanding how SM practitioners become practitioners by mastering rules of sexual conduct. As I will show, however, mastering the rules does not mean blind submission to community standards. Rather, as Foucault argues, "in this form of morality, the individual did not make himself into an ethical subject by universalizing the principles that informed his action; on the contrary, he did so by means of an attitude and a quest that individualized his action, modulated it, and perhaps even gave him a special brilliance by virtue of the rational and deliberate structure his action manifested" (62). An emphasis on mastery and distinction places community or social norms and individuation or self-mastery in tension. Social norms, as Judith Butler argues, provide a foundational horizon of recognition: "the subject forms itself in relation to a set of codes, prescriptions, or norms . . . that precede and exceed the subject . . . setting the limits to what will be considered an intelligible formation of the subject within a historical scheme of things" (2005, 17). Yet even though such norms "set the limits" of intelligibility, norms and subjectivity are supplementary; social norms and subjects constitutively depend on, but also exceed, each other. One of the key ways this works is through the individualization—not the internalization—of the rules.

The irony of this particular configuration in BDSM is twofold: ideologically, sexuality is imagined as a locus of freedom from the self, from social norms and conventions, from the state and other apparatuses of social control. Of course, as scholars have long argued, rather than a mode of freedom, sexuality is a primary form of social control, a way of locating individuals and relationships within grids of social meaning. Here, then, is a second irony: SM is perhaps the paradigmatic example of a sexual community organized around practices of safety and self-control, yet one that imagines itself (and is, in turn, figured) as radical, transgressive, out(side the)law. In this chapter, this irony takes the form of argument: read biopolitically, community rules and regulations—themselves dependent on neoliberal cultural formations—produce SM subjectivities by inciting certain forms of self-mastery. And in turn, practitioners resent the rules.

"KUMBAYA KINK AND BARNEY BDSM"

(BITCHING ABOUT) THE BDSM SCENE TODAY

In a speech Gayle Rubin gave at a graduation ceremony for the Journeyman II Academy on October 4, 1997, she argues against the popular BDSM dichotomy between old guard and new guard.[2] In this dichotomy, the old guard is formal, strict, apprentice style, and rigid, while the new guard is informal, casual, flexible, self-taught, and permissive. However, as Rubin puts it, "much of what is described when people talk about changes in the leather community comes down to more people, more money, and more commercialization." She continues:

> I began to notice some of these shifts in the mid-1980s, when the energy at public play parties seemed to change for the worse. Before then, many of the parties had been informal rituals of solidarity, pleasure, celebration and connection. People cared most about having a good time. Even in casual or recreational play, the focus seemed to be on

> the quality of the connection between the players themselves and on building and sharing an energy that whole rooms could get high on together. At some time in the mid-1980s, it seems that many people began to care more about what the audience saw than what their partners experienced. Leather had become trendy and popular rather than despised and stigmatized. Others seemed to merely go through the motions—SM too often became a mechanical exercise rather than an art form or a form of intimate communication. I'm not saying that there is no great public play today, but I often see a community that lacks some of its former style, grace, and values.

Rubin is describing changes she witnessed in the gay men's leather scene in San Francisco, but some of her observations can be generalized to the BDSM scene as a whole. For example, there is no denying the mainstreaming of SM fashion and style, or the large number of newcomers who came into the scene in the 1980s and 1990s. And although some might argue that SM is still plenty stigmatized, it may be less so as it becomes more mainstream (this is not, however, a simple dynamic; see Weiss 2006a). In lamenting these changes, Rubin also notes that play has become a "mechanical exercise," less intimate than it once was. Here she advances what is a common distinction among SM practitioners—between role-playing or public performance and authentic energy sharing or imitate connection—a distinction that I take up in more detail in the next chapter.

Many of the practitioners I spoke with agreed with these claims, even those who had never experienced the old guard scene. For example, Lady Hilary—a white, lesbian femme top in her mid-thirties—explained to me:

LADY HILARY: [The community] changed, and it needed to probably change . . . but I don't really support exactly what's happening now.

MARGOT: Do you have anything in particular that bothers you about . . .

HILARY: We're back to rules . . . the concept of safe, sane, and consensual was designed to throw the rest of the world off of our track, that's all. Have I ever brought harm to anyone? Never. Would I ever want to harm anyone? No. But part of that whole . . . mantra that everything has

> to be really sanitized is . . . it cuts the edge. It's not as hot, it's not as erotic, it's not as fun, edgy—and in turn, it's not as intense. The ritual of it is gone, and I saw that even when I first came into leather that there were people . . . [who] ran incredible teams to see, incredible power dynamics, and really good service and great hot beatings and great sex and then they'd get up and they'd be talking about the weather or the kids or the dog or whatever and there was no sacredness to what had just transpired. And I have a very hard time with that . . . with the lack of sacredness in sex . . . what's happening currently is sanitized, it's whitewashed, it's about how to do it right.

Hilary's complaints—that there are too many rules and too little intimacy, or that the scene today is "sanitized" or overprocessed in ways that detract from the connectivity of SM—are common. One memorable expression of this came from a leather conference I attended in Boston in 2003, where a presenter in a workshop on whether the influx of new practitioners was "diluting the SM community" called the current scene "kumbaya kink and Barney BDSM." Similarly, as one participant on a national SM e-mail list suggested: "Scene people are no longer sexual outlaws, nor a radical elite, nor the brave adventurers of the 60s and 70s. And, yes, instead of encouraging people to explore their SM sexuality on their own, today's community encourages them to explore it in the context of clubs; and clubs need rules; and rules restrict, even deaden, spontaneity. I see the Scene these days more like a kinky Kiwanis Club."[3] In my analysis, what "more people, more money, and more commercialization" have wrought is a different form of community: one less like a secret passion and more like a hobby with specialized magazines, websites and mailing lists, publishers, books, how-to films, classes, discussion groups, commercial and noncommercial locations, formal and informal organizations and networks, conferences, paraphernalia, tools and toys, clothing, technologies, tips, and rules and regulations.

Although practitioners today—even the newcomers—romanticize the old guard scene in ways that do not correspond to historical reality, these practitioners are correct that the scene today is very different from the scene in the 1970s.[4] J.—a white, heterosexual top in his early forties—told me: "I think the community's grown a lot . . . I have some concerns about that because the old guard had rules and they had a way of being and they had steps that one took, and you came up and you worked through a system, almost, to become a top and you had to know something to be a top." Before books, how-to classes, and the like, the old guard relied on networks to share skills and knowledge, and a system of training and apprenticing. As one old guard leatherman explains, "since there were no popular leather magazines, porn videos, or even books to inform the novice, everything was passed on by legend and word-of-mouth tradition" (Magister 1991, 96). The plethora of guides to negotiation, affect care (such as aftercare, or postscene emotional soothing), limits, and guidelines—combined with the formal rules and regulations of play at semipublic parties—have resulted in a scene that is more formalized in its knowledge production than it was in the 1970s and before.

This network of social rules and regulations is tied to the growth and popularity of SM, the changing demographics of SM and the Bay Area, shifts in the organization of leisure and the sexual economy, and HIV/AIDS and legal and state intervention into SM. For example, as SM organizations like the Society of Janus developed, the network of classes and workshops, experts and guides, has also grown. Teramis, an Arab American, lesbian slave in her mid-forties, explained to me that, when the scene was smaller, "closed-door word-of-mouth networking" controlled access to the community so that "the abusive idiot wouldn't be let in the door." Now, because the scene is so much larger and easier to find, "these self-control mechanisms have fallen by the wayside." "I see the community now struggling to find a substitute" form of regulation, "because the need to be self-policed is still there." In this vacuum, then, community-imposed rules and regulations perform the word-of-mouth policing functions on which the earlier scene relied.

The rules are also a community response to HIV/AIDS. The leather/SM scene in San Francisco was decimated by HIV in the early and mid-1980s. The second incarnation of the Catacombs, for example—the famous San Francisco SM and fisting club that many remember as the "community center for the S/M population" (Rubin 1991, 122)—closed during the bathhouse sweep of 1984, a public health/sex panic spurred by fear of AIDS (see also Rubin 1997).[5] BDSM parties and organizations responded to the AIDS crisis by requiring safer-sex practices and barrier protection at semipublic parties. These rules were subject to tremendous community debate; within Janus, this debate is known as the "great safe sex fight." In the late 1980s and early 1990s, Janus's safe-sex debates were also tied to how the organization would be perceived as responding (or not responding) to HIV/AIDS, and thus to the plight of gay leathermen in San Francisco. The tenor and form of this debate solidified Janus's reputation as a primarily heterosexual organization.[6] Implementing safer-sex rules at dungeon parties was the first codification of party rules and a more formal monitoring of sex play at parties. Paul, who entered the scene in 1987, explained to me: "my sense is that in the old days practically anything goes . . . AIDS obviously stopped almost all sex in dungeons."

A final critical issue is state and legal intervention. As play parties became larger and SM more visible, the chances of police busts and other legal interference increased. In 2001, for example, the National Coalition for Sexual Freedom (NCSF) reported that it responded to 461 complaints regarding child custody or divorce proceedings in which SM was an issue, and 392 cases of job discrimination based on SM practices.[7] A survey that the NCSF conducted in 1998 and 1999 indicated that, among the 1,017 respondents, 36 percent had experienced violence or harassment and 30 percent had experienced discrimination because of BDSM practices.[8] Add to this the high visibility of several police raids and arrests at semipublic play parties, and the desire for a more formally organized community becomes understandable. As Paul commented, "when things go public," the perception in the community is that "the state comes in and says, 'you damn well better organize this or we're going to do it for you.' And then some do-gooder with their heart in the right place will start saying, 'Well, we don't want that happening. Here, let me set up some rules.'" Intended, then, to protect community members from harsh legal intervention, some of the rules and regulations of the new scene are a response to the state.

Yet these new rules and regulations, this formalization and control, as Paul's words make clear, also reflect a neoliberal shift from state responsibility (for security, safety, and health) to individual and community responsibility for safety (Brown 2005; Duggan 2003; Lemke 2001; Rose [1999] 2007). As Thomas Lemke argues, summarizing Foucault's analysis of neoliberal governmentality, "neo-liberal forms of government . . . characteristically develop indirect techniques for leading and controlling individuals without at the same time being responsible for them. The strategy of rendering individual subjects 'responsible' (and also collectives, such as families, associations, etc.) entails shifting the responsibility for social risks such as illness, unemployment, poverty, etc., and for life in society into the domain for which the individual is responsible and transforming it into a problem of 'self-care'" (2001, 201). Security, here, is about producing and controlling subjects (making sure that the SM community is not accessible to "abusive idiots"), bodies (making sure that physical risks like HIV transmission are controlled), and citizenship (making sure that the community is organized in consistent, ideally legal, ways). These changes have important social effects; in regulating safety, for example, the scene also produces knowledge about acceptable practice and play. By offering classes on technique, the community has transformed the form of knowledge and learning from person-to-person to formalized education. By canonizing rules and regulations for safe play—negotiations, safewords, dungeon rules, play prohibitions—and by forming the DMA, the scene is also attracting and producing certain kinds of practitioners. In these ways, the production, regulation, and control of safety and risk produce SM practitioners and further reinforce the kinds of people—white, professional, suburban—who find a home in this SM community.

JANUS ENTERING THE SCENE

> Janus is considered an entry organization into the community because they teach people rules, they teach people how to act, how to do things.
> —MARCIE

The story of these technologies of SM—organized around training and knowing oneself, maximizing one's bodily pleasures and capabilities, and organizing one's relationships and intimacies in particular ways—must begin with the Society of Janus. Janus, founded in 1974 by Cynthia Slater and Larry Olsen, is the second oldest BDSM organization in the United States (after TES, founded in 1971 in New York City) and has transformed the social organization of SM in the Bay Area (for its history, see Truscott 1990; Weymouth and Society of Janus 1999). Before its founding, there were bars, motorcycle clubs, and informal networks of SM, fetish, and leather practitioners throughout the United States; there were also professional "session" (prodomme) houses and a few combination clubs like Backdrop, a club started by Robin Roberts in 1966 as a school of bondage photography, a social and educational club, and a professional domination house.[9] But from its beginning, Janus was an educational organization: Slater formed it to provide support and education on how to do safe SM.

Today, Janus sees itself as "an educational and support organization for adults interested in sexuality based on a safe, consensual, non-exploitative transfer of power between partners . . . We exist as an organization to learn more about sm, to share information among ourselves, to help build the sm community by providing a supportive atmosphere for ourselves, to get to know and enjoy one another, and to reach out to other interested, friendly groups and individuals."[10] In order to join Janus, one must attend an orientation session. The current structure of orientations was established in the 1980s, and remains much the same today. I attended the orientation session in June 2000, which was held at San Francisco's Fort Mason Center (a former military base now operated by the US Park Service). The orientees that day included one heterosexual couple in their sixties and four heterosexual dominant men in their fifties, along with eight Janus members as presenters (in 2004–5, monthly orientations attracted from seven to twenty-eight potential members). The presenters covered Janus's history and mission, and then each explained his or her interest and involvement with Janus and SM. Next we broke into small groups to discuss our experiences with SM and our interest in Janus. We were each given a membership form to fill out on the spot or to take home and mail in (between 65 and 80 percent of people who attend an orientation session end up joining Janus). After the meeting, the Janus members met to discuss whether anyone at the orientation should be denied membership. The orientation session is supposed to keep undesirable people out of the organization, although it is rare that anyone is denied membership.[11] As one member explains, "in the time since I have attended orientations, I have not seen anyone who was denied entry. We look for outright sociopaths and deviants of the wrong nature."[12]

Here Janus—fittingly—is balancing two goals: access (its desire to be supportive and welcoming to new members, and to build the community) and restriction. Of course, having to pass an orientation screening is not the only form this restriction takes; rather, as will become clear, a community organized around both formalized institutions (like Janus) and discourses of safety, risk, and security produces SM practitioners in particular ways and simultaneously reinforces ideal community membership. Taken together, this amounts to the formal organization of certain social norms.

Janus has almost always had a formalized organizational structure. In 1975, two years after its founding, the group began holding regular business meetings, electing officers, and producing a newsletter. It has formal bylaws that detail procedures for electing officers, running business meetings, and the types of program meetings Janus should have, among other organizational details. After I became the archivist for Janus in March 2003, I began attending the monthly business meetings, most often held in an upstairs room at a men's bathhouse in the Castro.[13] The first time I attended, I was surprised at the formal motions; Janus follows *Robert's Rules of Order*. Lady Thendara felt the same way: "I went to a Janus business meeting . . . I had never been to one before. They follow all these rules, I mean, there's all these kinky people and they're like 'No, you can't speak. He's got the table. He's made a motion.' It's very formal!" The members elect officers by secret ballot at the annual meeting; in addition to archivist, the officers include business meeting moderator, cashier, communication secretary, editor of *Growing Pains* (the newsletter), librarian, membership secretary, munch director, orientation director, outreach director, postmaster/mistress, program director, recording secretary, social activities director, treasurer, and webmaster.

Janus and the organizations modeled on it that followed in its wake —especially SMOdyssey, but also the gay and lesbian organizations that developed out of, in response to, or alongside Janus—have transformed the SM scene into one that is much more structured, formal, codified, and institutional than the old guard scene. As John Preston, author of the classic old guard leather novel *Mr. Benson* complains, the "sense of brotherhood among S/Mers" has been "replaced by a whole series of formal clubs, all directed by Robert's Rules of Order" (1991, 215), like Janus.[14] Even those who play key roles in Janus, like Jezzie and Anton, express some disappointment in this codification. Anton, a white, heterosexual master, and Jezzie, his white, bisexual wife and slave, both in their mid-twenties, explain:

ANTON: You have support groups and everything is very open and there's a lot of communication . . . People are trying to reduce the barriers to entry as much as possible, to be welcoming and friendly, and all in all, I must say it's a good thing. But there is something that you lose. There's this mystery and potency of something that is hidden and—and somewhat forbidden. Janus is, I think, the best educational organization that we have around . . . [It] is a wonderful networking resource and is very well organized and does a lot of great outreach, but it's not the slightest bit sexy. There's nothing sexy about Janus. I mean, you know, we meet in well-lit rooms in a circle of chairs and everyone introduces themselves and . . .

JEZZIE: Wear[s] name tags.

ANTON: Before it even starts, you come to an orientation where they tell you everything's going to be safe and you're okay. If you want to have a sexy group, a little clandestine advertisement in the back of the newspaper, meet in a dark room . . .

JEZZIE: Everybody act shady. Make it sound a little dangerous.

ANTON: I suspect that most of the people in the scene have at least some degree of [wanting] the forbidden or the dangerous. That's part of why it's interesting, and that's fading over time as things become more acceptable.

JEZZIE: It's a trade-off. You can't have it both ways. You can't be totally open and accepting and accessible and [also] be dangerous and edgy and forbidden.

This disappointment—that SM isn't as dangerous or dark or sexy in an era of formal rules and organization—is nostalgia for a time when SM was more outlaw. I explore this desire further below; here I want only to note that Janus, and organizations like it, have produced a new scene organized around, as Marcie—a white lesbian switch in her forties—puts it, teaching people "rules," "how to act," and "how to do things." And in this kind of training, Janus led the way with classes.

From its beginning, Janus focused on classes: "dungeon tours, enemas, uniforms, role-play scenes, negotiation, dungeon safety, whipping/flogging technique, and basic rope bondage" were some of the workshops and classes taught in its first few years (Weymouth and Society of Janus 1999, 7). Since the 1990s, alongside the growth of the community and the increased availability of SM toys, there has been a proliferation of classes and workshops. There are how-to classes on techniques and skills, but there are also classes on aftercare, setting the scene, and negotiation. Although the proliferation of classes in the Bay Area is related to the appearance of new organizations, it is also tied to the late-capitalist expansion of self-help, training, and guidance industries focused on sex and romance.

During my fieldwork, I attended a variety of classes, including "The Art of Negotiation," "Hot Wax Play," "Spanking," "Fire and Ice Play," "Aftercare," "Processing Pain," "Spirituality in the Scene," "Terror Play," "Resistance Play," "When Someone You Love Is Vanilla," "Beginning Rope Bondage," "Caning," and "How to Co-Top." Most classes follow a basic structure: introductory and safety material, more-detailed information, a demonstration, and Q&A. They are held after work during the week, or on weekends, at local dungeons, stores, spaces rented by organizations, and at QSM. The classes cost up to $25 dollars a person, and typically run about two hours. At most of the classes I attended, there were between eight and twenty-five people present, most in work or casual clothes—unless it was a weekend class before a party. This proliferation of formal classes marks a shift away from person-to-person, apprentice-style learning (where, for example, a potential top would first be trained as a bottom by an experienced top, and later learn various skills from masters recognized in the community) toward the institutionalization of BDSM education. Guy Baldwin, one of the original Janus members, writes of the old guard scene: "None of these rules [for example, on what to wear or how to do SM] is taught or explained to anyone except by innuendo, inference, or example. Erotic technical information is only shared among peers" (1999, 77).

In contrast, in the new scene, as Latex Mustang explains:

> There's this huge tension about something that's supposed to be so driven by energy and so spontaneous, and so coming from the inside of you, and in some ways happens so organically—and then having to bring it under the structure of a classroom. But I think that's what separates us out from the unsafe, bedroom players who try to experiment with this on their own and then sometimes kill themselves. Sometimes they don't really have the opportunity to experience this to its fullest because to get to that next level takes a level of education for sufficiency, equipment, that you can't get without learning from the masters. And it used to be that that stuff was taught in the gay communities back in family houses, where there was a whole structure to the family. And I think the heterosexuals have evolved a much more open system of, basically, you want to do it, you pay your money, you get in, you can go to the conference.

The institutionalization of SM technique, a more open system according to Mustang (as long as you can pay your money—the subject of the next chapter), is both regulated and standardized.

As Paul puts it, all of the BDSM books, manuals, how-to videos, and classes exert a "normalizing influence" by "teaching everybody how to do X" in the same way. This turns SM practice into a technique, a skill for which there is "OTW"—one true way that things are supposed to be done ("Keeper of the OTW" is a mocking community shorthand for a person who is excessively invested in this viewpoint). Preston argues that these workshops and classes, along with what he describes as "'objective' means to establish someone's accomplishment or level of achievement," have destroyed what was an "anarchistic," "anti-establishment," and experimental leather scene (1991, 215–16). He writes: "Leathersex has . . . lost its edge. It's been codified, measured, and packaged. The magic of trusting one person, a mentor, and letting those one-on-one bondings spread out until a brotherhood was formed has been replaced with impersonal how-to manuals" (214).

Many argue that, because the classes emphasize toys and techniques, the new SM scene allows people to engage in SM without feeling, just by following the rules (and buying the toys). An overemphasis on technique instead of the old guard understanding of intimacy, energy, or magic between players has produced, as Baldwin remarks, "the era of the tyranny of technique," what Gayle Rubin calls "paint by number"

BDSM.[15] Mocking the "swelling curricula" as formula without heart, Baldwin argues that the energy of SM organizations is directed toward teaching how to do SM "'properly' which meant technically correct." The nostalgic view that condemns the new scene sees "the rules"—classes, workshops, organizations, play regulations—as an impediment to freedom and authentic social connection or intimacy. Instead, I read "the rules" as inciting certain forms of self-mastery: the mode of subjectivity that is being practiced alongside one's rope-tying skills.

As BDSM has become more mainstream, more organizationally focused, and more professionalized, practitioners work on their SM in self-conscious ways, mobilizing American discourses of self-improvement and education that dovetail with the emphasis on self-cultivation of Foucault's practice of the self. Today SM practitioners learn how to be practitioners by attending a discussion group for newcomers, going through an orientation like Janus's to become a card-carrying member of a BDSM organization, and taking classes on basic topics such as flogging, spanking, and aftercare. They graduate to more advanced topics (for example, edge play, suspension bondage, and Master/slave relationships), attending play parties and munches as they become more involved and integrated into the scene. Eventually they may become teachers, munch leaders, recognized experts, or officers in SM organizations. As Hailstorm, a white, heterosexual top in his mid-fifties, explains:

> As a top, you have to know what you're doing. It's like going to driving school. You have to learn how to do it because number one is: you could hurt somebody. But the other thing is: it shows you're serious. Like, if you go to college, get a degree—well, you may be a smart person, but you went the nine yards to be certified and got the sheepskin to prove that you're a player, you're serious. That's what it's like in the dom world. If you're serious, your confidence will show it in front of everybody. You do the workshop and then, of course, you get to the level where you can become a teacher and teach a workshop, which I've done, and then, of course, you're way up there: "Oh, this guy's a teacher, he's a master, he's a guru. He's the person you go to on the top of the mountain to learn how to do all this stuff." You're on top.

Indeed, teaching classes is one way to gain status as an expert or authority. Many people I interviewed told me about the classes they taught as a way of establishing themselves as local bearers of knowledge. One person bragged about how he attends the same munch as the "guy who wrote the book" on electrical play and a "guy who teaches classes nationally on role-play." Lady Thendara explained that after teaching classes, she and Mustang are "known" in the community. And almost everyone told me about the classes they planned to teach.

This kind of community expertise positions some practitioners, as Rabinow and Rose put it, as "authorities considered competent to speak" the truth "in the name of life and health" (2006, 203). So, for example, Jay Wiseman—a local safety guru, author, and expert—actively campaigns against breath play (play with breathing restrictions) in the scene. He has posted numerous essays on the subject on local and national e-mail lists, in addition to the essays in his books and on his website. Wiseman, a former EMT, believes that breath play is never safe: "As a person with years of medical education and experience, I know of no way whatsoever that either suffocation or strangulation can be done in a way that does not intrinsically put the recipient at risk of cardiac arrest" (see also Downing 2007).[16] Wiseman argues that there is no precaution one can take to make breath play safe (unlike bondage, which is safe as long as the bond is not tight, or electricity play, which is safe as long as it's not above the waist). During my fieldwork, Sara told me that Wiseman picketed a class offered by a South Bay woman on breath play. In her description of what had happened, Sara, a friend of the teacher, mocked Wiseman's concern with health and what she called his "middle-class mores."

Here again, not everyone agrees with the experts or masters. Some argue that the proliferation of classes and how-to books and films means that almost anyone can become an "instant expert." Some worry that one cannot learn proper technique from reading a book or watching a demo in a class. For example, Meg'gan—a white, lesbian butch bottom/sometimes switch in her late twenties—told me that she was less comfortable as a bottom now that there isn't "that same kind of hierarchy that there was," and a woman can "just get a flogger and start flogging": "You don't know anything about flogging. Are you going to throw your wrist out? How badly are you going to bruise someone? Are [they] going to throw their back out? I mean, there's a lot of things that can happen." Others, like Stephanie and Anthony, both white, bisexual dominants in their mid-fifties, simply mock this aspirational SM:

STEPHANIE: You want people to recognize you as some sort of expert or fount of knowledge . . . it brings prestige and status to you . . .

ANTHONY: . . . Bob is the guy that I think about . . . because he's walking around in the scene kind of quiet and shy . . . and then he goes to Black Rose [a large conference/convention in Washington, D.C.] . . . and comes back with a T-shirt, and the next thing you know, he's teaching a singletail class and he's, you know, Mr. Singletail . . . It looked like there was a career path for him, and he seemed very ambitious about doing all this stuff. For some people, it's not just a hobby and something to do on the weekend. For some people, it really is like they are really serious about this.

MARGOT: How would you describe that?

STEPHANIE: A career pervert.

Although it is easy, as Stephanie does, to snicker at this "career path"—a career, I should note, where income is limited to cultural capital—the transformations in the scene extend beyond those practitioners interested in becoming community leaders or experts. Rather, SM practice provides an opportunity to fashion oneself in relation to these social norms, where "relation to" does not entail blind adherence, but rather a form of work on the self, a testing, monitoring, and transformation that can, as we will see, include rejecting the rules.

BECOMING AN (SSC) PRACTITIONER

COMMUNITY RULES AND SELF-MASTERY

Mollena described her initial foray into BDSM to me: "I became really geeky about it; I was on the 'net, I researched everything, I found the books and went out and bought them . . . I really spent a lot of time and did a lot of personal research and introspection and a lot of writing about it." After finding the Society of Janus and the Exiles, Mollena attended an orientation session and started going to classes and munches. She continues: "At the Berkeley munch I met a bunch of other people, and I was invited to my first play party, and it sort of blossomed from there. The involvement purely is not enough; to get you really, fully involved, you have to really work at it. It's like a project, you know?" Similarly, Chris, a white, heterosexual dom in his mid-thirties, explains that he and his wife use their relationship "as an opportunity for general work" on their marriage and their individual "growth and development" as SM practitioners. To achieve this, they set up explicit goals, monitor their progress, and make daily plans, such as "daily affirmation, daily motivation, exercises that we do," each designed to work on actualizing specific goals (such as behavioral training) in the context of their BDSM relationship.

For these and other practitioners, BDSM is a project, a practice of developing oneself as a skilled practitioner, of learning how to be a practitioner (see Weiss 2006b). Becoming a practitioner takes work on the self: finding the community, attending events, learning techniques and skills, and educating oneself. These practices are forged in relation to the community norms and rules, but—as Foucault emphasizes—it is not a question of complying with the rules, but of transforming oneself through one's own interpretation of the rules. As he argues, the proper use of pleasure, one's self-mastery in relation to pleasure, produces a "solid and stable state of rule of the self over the self" ([1984] 1990, 69; see also 91–92). This rule is less a strict rule of conduct and more about individualizing, moderating, and elaborating conduct, subjecting the self to his own moral mastery. Foucault's understanding of self-mastery in relation to the rules of pleasure is useful here, as SM practitioners also learn to elaborate codes of conduct, to subject themselves to a kind of self-mastery that is supplementary to, rather than in strict compliance with, social and community norms. As Foucault argues, in time, these practices of the self "evolved into procedures, practiced and taught. It thus came to constitute a social practice, giving rise to relationships between individuals, to exchanges and communications, and at times even to institutions" ([1984] 1988, 45).[17] The rules, worked on as part of the labor of becoming an SM practitioner, also produce this particular SM community and the circuits and exchanges it endorses.

Working at BDSM play is also work on the self: it produces and consolidates subjectivities and communities. It is deeply class-inflected, relying not only on the income and time to attend courses and conferences, but also on shared forms of community recognition—education, expertise, and mastery—that are most available to professional-class practitioners. This exclusivity, however, is displaced and obscured in community discourse; these forms of recognition are hegemonic precisely because they construct an ideal, class-restricted community member (the professional practitioner with sufficient means and proper education) toward which other, nonaffluent practitioners aspire. Universalizing ideologies, therefore, normalize such careful work on oneself and one's pleasures. Bailey, a white, heterosexual bottom in her mid-forties, explains that she got into the scene after joining a local SM e-mail list: "I found out about munches. I started showing up, and from there I just networked the hell out of it. So I've been active in the public community in the Bay Area going on six years now. Two years ago I did six national events. Last year I probably did four . . . [although this seems like a lot], more-educated people, more-knowledgeable people, more-affluent people tend to be at the national conventions. And I'm like, 'Well, I want to learn more. That's why I'm going.'" Thinking of the rules in this way focuses attention on self-mastery and knowledge as an active practice of modulation, testing, analysis, and self-cultivation.

This form of self-mastery, of techne as crafting or practicing oneself, is articulated especially strongly around the rules, especially rules—like Safe, Sane, and Consensual—that require practitioners to forge their own practices of safety. Safe, Sane, and Consensual (SSC) is the mantra of SM in the United States today. Coined in 1983 by david stein, as part of the statement of purpose of GMSMA (Gay Male S/M Activists), the slogan was popularized across the country and is now widely endorsed by BDSM organizations.[18] Stein notes that the slogan was originally understood to distinguish "defensible" SM, practiced on "willing partners for mutual satisfaction," from "harmful, antisocial, predatory behavior," "the coercive abuse of unwilling victims." Beyond being a motto, however, Safe, Sane, and Consensual has become critical to the social organization of SM; it is the primary way practitioners distinguish between good, safe, acceptable SM and bad, unsafe, unacceptable practice. To ensure that the community of practitioners corresponds to SSC rules, several practices have become standardized; the two largest, most institutionalized are negotiation and using safewords.

Although it is likely that old guard scenes involved some sort of negotiation, today, all BDSM scenes are supposed to involve fairly formal negotiation.[19] Like the infamous Antioch College rules that required explicit and specific verbal consent for every sexual act, negotiation ensures that there will be informed consent throughout the play, and that each player's desires and fantasies will be responded to in the course of the scene.[20] Unlike the Antioch rules, negotiation is supposed to be done before the play, thus requiring anticipatory foresight. During negotiation, one should divulge any emotional, physical, or sexual information that may be important (for example, one should tell one's partner about the child abuse that may crop up and force the scene to end abruptly, or how one's carpal tunnel syndrome might impact bondage, or that the word *slut* is acceptable, but *whore* is not). One should also explain the kinds of SM play one particularly likes. Finally, one should describe one's limits; the most common limit is "dead people, kids, and shit," although there are many other limits.

SM guidebooks explain how to negotiate with a partner in excruciating detail; Wiseman's *SM 101*, one of the most popular, has a ten-page "long form" for negotiation that lists sixteen categories with spaces so that practitioners can fill in the blanks with their own desires, limits, and protocols. The categories include people involved; place; how long the scene will last; emotional and physical limits; presence and kind of sex and safe-sex procedures; presence and kind of bondage and pain; what, if any, marks can be left; and safewords (Wiseman 1998, 58–62). Many people rely on verbal negotiation, but many others use these highly formalized checklist negotiation forms to plan a scene.

Similarly, the use of safewords—words like *red* or *safeword* or *pineapple* that are unlikely to come up during a scene—was introduced in the 1970s and has now become a crucial part of contemporary SM. Wiseman recommends having two safewords, "one for 'lighten up' and one for 'stop completely.'" He adds, "I also strongly recommend using the 'two squeezes' technique. If the players will use a gag or a hood, they *must* agree upon non-verbal 'safe signals'" (1998, 62; italics in original).[21] Semipublic play parties almost always have a house safeword, usually *safeword* or *red*. Viewed as a last resort, safewords function as an out for when the scene has gone too far—when it has exceeded the boundaries of either player. Thus, like negotiation, safewords have become an institutionalized procedure of safety.

Many practitioners find this level of planning and negotiation ridiculous. Lady Hilary, for example, explained that "rules now are for safety." "Not that safety's not important, but . . . none of the rules enhance the dynamic. 'Oh, let's over-process how we're going to play. So you want to be spanked five times—okay, fine, but six I can't do.' And then I have to do this, so that's how some people negotiate a scene. It's now lost the tension." Pam, a white, bisexual slave in her fifties, described coming out into the scene in her twenties, when "it wasn't a bunch of negotiation." "I found who he [gesturing to Vince] was as a person and his character and everything else and that was enough to serve him." With the new players, she explained, you sit down and negotiate "an hour and a half for a twenty-minute scene." "And I'm just like . . . 'you're boring the shit out of me.' " Pam is in service to her master Vince, a white, gay man in his mid-forties; they play without safewords or negotiation because, as she explains, "he knows just where I am at every moment, and plus if something does happen that he's not aware of, I can just say it. I don't have to go 'beige' or 'yellow' or 'green' or whatever the hell they're all doing." Vince agrees: "I think that we can think about sex or we can have sex. And so my question and my process has always been 'Is this someone that I can connect with? Can I sense you? Can I feel you?' . . . If that's possible, then I don't really need to negotiate because all I really need to do is pay attention."

Here, practitioners' concern that the more mechanical exercise of negotiation destroys the heart of modern BDSM parallels the mainstream press's response to the Antioch rules. Like the excessive zeal of mandatory bicycle helmet laws, the rules were seen as political correctness gone awry. These critics of both safewords and negotiation argue that by codifying very specific ways of doing SM, the intense connection that SM can create between partners is destroyed, that excessive negotiation will diminish interpersonal intimacy. Taking sex, a practice that is supposed to be spontaneous and magical, and delineating and codifying it seems counterproductive to many. Indeed, this is one of the most common vanilla responses to SM that I hear: how can a scene that is negotiated ahead of time be hot, believable, or fun?

There are two related ways to approach this question. The first is to note the pleasure that inheres in the rules. So, for example, in a front-page news story in the *New York Times* on the Antioch rules, Jane Gross reported that students liked the policy. They thought that talking about sex was erotic, that it was more about setting up "ground rules" than a rigid checklist, and that the policy effectively addressed rape (1993). In this case, negotiation is a practice that carries with it some unintended pleasures: the pleasures of describing one's desires in detail, for example, a pleasure (bound to safety) that many people—especially women who have sex with men—emphasized when contrasting SM sex with vanilla sex.[22] The second approach, which I follow here, is to note that community pressure to be safe, sane, and consensual does not ask practitioners to blindly follow the rules, but rather to negotiate their own relationship to these rules, to define safety and risk for themselves. This work creates a relationship between individual subjects and social norms, a relationship in which one's enactment, disavowal, or disregard of the rules is a form of self-subjugation and self-mastery in accordance with professional-class standards. This provides one way to read SSC SM and the rules as technique, allowing us to see the community debates about the rules and their pleasures as themselves part of the construction of SM practitioners.

For example, many of the BDSM practitioners with whom I spoke agreed that Safe, Sane, and Consensual was a simplistic slogan, but they had varying opinions about its value. Most thought that SSC was a good policy, but that it couldn't really be followed to the letter. Many also felt that it was, as Teramis puts it, "an easy sound bite for newbies to digest . . . a good tone to strike for the masses," or "created as outreach or propaganda, and I think it's best in that role," in Anton's words. Others liked it for its usefulness in conveying to medical professionals, psychologists, or the police the difference between BDSM and abuse, rape, torture, or violence—as well as between BDSM practitioners and psychopaths.

A few unconditionally liked the phrase. For example, Monique Alexandra—a Latina, bisexual bottom/submissive/masochist in her mid-thirties—thought that the use of negotiation and safewords in the community made her feel comfortable and, more important, safe: "I want things that are exciting, but I want to know I decided to have that done, and that at any point I can say whatever the codeword is and it will stop . . . Safety is very important to me; I would not play with anyone who has the attitude 'I won't negotiate because it's boring.'" For some, the emphasis on safety reduced the fear that people coming in to the scene may experience, but it didn't make BDSM any less erotic. As Mustang explains: "Safe doesn't mean you're driving around in your Suburban . . . Some of these people are pretty far out on the edge . . . It's people doing things safely and yet still getting what they need." For him, community resources, experts on things like "rope or whipping or electricity," and medical doctors and lawyers who are "kink aware," are all aspects of community development "not available ten years ago."[23] This development means that there is "community support to say, 'here's what edge play is, here's what it means, here's the things you need to do, here's what you can't do, and here are the risks you're taking when you do it,' so there's informed consent." "I think that's a wonderful thing . . . It's what saved me."

Yet many people pointed out that there was no way to be truly safe, sane, or even consensual. For example, Chris told me that "we need some way of distinguishing this [SM] from abuse." "[But] my opinion is also that we've picked the wrong three words. I can't think of any activity . . . that I would wholeheartedly call safe . . . [and] the definition of sanity is actually a legal issue." He continued, half joking: "Now if it were something like informed, consensual, and involving a level of risk that was comparable to, say, everything that everybody on the planet does, I'd be all for that." For this reason, many prefer RACK (risk-aware consensual kink), a term coined by Gary Switch of TES in the late 1990s.[24] Teramis argues: "You can't define for somebody what's safe for them. You can't define if what somebody's doing is sane for them. [What matters is] that I'm aware of the risks, I'm informed, I've given consent, and it's making me happy."

Practice—being "informed," learning the risks, being educated—leads here to less safe, sane, and consensual SM, but this is not surprising. Rather, it is through these community practices of education, classes, orientations, and the like that practitioners take responsibility for their own practices of safety, that they map out their own relationship to the rules. So, for example, Domina and Hayden told me that they play without limits or safewords, as do Jezzie and Anton. Jezzie explained that she initially needed SSC to feel comfortable in the scene, but then she "kind of outgrew it." "Safe, well, what if I knowledgeably want to do something risky? Sane, what the hell does that mean? I mean, I'm in the mental health profession!" For her, SSC is "like training wheels." Once one is a part of this community, having learned social norms through educational structures, one should "outgrow" or cultivate one's own rules.

This is why many, like Annalee—a white, bisexual genderqueer/pervert/voyeur in her early thirties—insisted on their own definition of the terms. Annalee explains: "I'm a fan of consensual sex, however you each consent with your partner. You can each consent like, 'okay, I consent to having you push my boundaries until I say *red*,' which might not be somebody else's definition of safe, sane, and consensual, which would be like, 'we will agree on ten acts to be performed in this order.' I'm not a fan of the 'ten acts in this order.' I just think it's too much to remember . . . If I'm playing with friends, or partners, we know each other well enough that we can push these limits and [do] whatever the hell we feel like doing. There's a lot of safety built into it, and that's how I define safe, sane, and consensual." All of these debates point to the ways practitioners work with and customize the rules and definitions of safe, sane, consensual, and negotiated. The rules provide a social structure, a scaffolding, within which people cultivate their own ways of being practitioners with—and against—the rules.

RISK AND SOCIAL PRIVILEGE

In a speech critiquing the SSC mantra of contemporary BDSM, Alison Moore argues that "when we invent these sorts of simplistic slogans to differentiate our behavior from nonconsensual violence, what we end up with is often a set of definitions that do not reflect anyone's way of doing SM." She continues: "For me the whole beauty of SM play is that it doesn't always make sense, that it does take us outside our 'safety-zone,' that it is frightening; it taps into the purest essence of sex which is ultimately chaotic, chthonic, exhilarating, exuberant, a dizzying abyss, an electrifying scream . . . There is no political slogan to describe this."[25] Moore neatly summarizes the desire that many people have: to have sex that is unsafe. SM sex is already edgy sex, in that it is—to the general public, at least—forbidden, dark, and prohibited. It is also risky, although generally no more physically risky than football, rock climbing, or other sports. Maintaining this allure of the clandestine, outlaw, or dangerous is important to practitioners, and this is one reason they remain ambivalent about the rules, as well as the cultural mainstreaming of SM fashion and, to some degree, practice.

At the same time, practitioners are quick to rely on precisely the binaries established by SSC to assert that SM is not what stein referred to as "harmful, antisocial, predatory behavior," and what many would call simple, sociopathic sadism. The rules, then, solicit a complex technology: they create a social context within which SM practice is understandable—as sexual and as desirable—and they also demand that individual practitioners chart their own relationship to that edge between safety and risk, control and the "abyss."

Here, risk must be understood as productive and desirable, not merely aversive. This is, in part, a critique of the "risk society" thesis of Anthony Giddens and Ulrich Beck, which—in the words of Merryn Ekberg—suggests that societies like the United States are characterized by a "collective consciousness of anxiety, insecurity, uncertainty and ambivalence" that produces "an ethos of risk avoidance" (2007, 346, 344). As Ekberg puts it in a review essay, these understandings posit the risk society "in contrast to primary, industrial modernity, which was characterized by the safety, security, predictability and permanence of inherited traditions, such as class location, gender roles, marriage, family, lifetime employment and secure retirement." The risk society, however, "is characterized by a dislocation, disintegration and disorientation associated with the vicissitudes of detraditionalization" (346).

Although many scholars agree that risk, anxiety, and security are key discourses in the contemporary United States, this universalizing metatheory has come under attack in recent years (Zaloom 2004; see also T. Baker and Simon 2002; Mythen 2007). First, as Ekberg notes, "communities have not disappeared [due to social dislocation], rather they have reformed around risk and safety . . . risk is now the collective bond holding communities together as imaginary risk communities" (2007, 346). Second, imagining a "collective consciousness" of risk aversion "negates the possibility of a risk-seeking culture" (362). The desirability of risk—its pleasure and benefits—is part of this ethos and combines with the community- and subject-producing aspects of risk. As Caitlin Zaloom argues in a essay about risk in the Chicago Board of Trade trading pit, risk produces Chicago traders as subjects: "In the pit, a particular kind of self is manufactured in relation to financial action. Risk is the key object for traders in their individual projects of self-creation and re-creation . . . these practices encourage the production of subjects who can sustain themselves under high-stakes conditions" (2004, 366). Practices of risk "describe a capitalist ethic that centers on the mastery of the self under conditions of hazard and possibility" (366; see also Celsi, Rose, and Leigh 1993). Risk enables the production of self-mastery, but these forms of self-creation also rely on an evaluative community. As Zaloom notes: "Trading provides the opportunity to develop and perform self-control and determination for all who are watching" (2004, 379).

In SM, risk is similarly productive; building and mastering BDSM skills produce new subjects in relation to an evaluative community. The community evaluates one's education, trustworthiness, experience, and skill. So, for example, Bailey explained to me that a DM at a party once stopped her friend: "One of the things he's very good at and he teaches is Japanese rope bondage, in particular suspension bondage. And . . . the last two years in a row they stopped the scene before he [had finished the] suspension because they didn't think he was safe. And if there's anyone I would trust to do that, it would be him. He knows his stuff." Here trust is based on knowledge and skill, in terms of one's public persona. Waldemar, a white, bisexual mostly top in his early thirties, explains that he has no problem making play dates: "I'm well known, and people trust me and they like what I do." Francesca, a white, bisexual, pain slut bottom in her late forties, explains that if she were playing with a friend, she "could probably take a lot more stressful [forms of play]." "It's a matter of trust, how much do I trust this person? And trust is based on knowledge for me."

Concepts of risk also entail "edgework," or "the personal exploration of the limits of both the context and the individual's ability to control it" (Celsi, Rose, and Leigh 1993, 16). Here, as Richard Celsi, Randall Rose, and Thomas Leigh note, in an essay exploring the motivations of skydivers, "many high-risk performers learn to like working at the edge of their abilities, 'to push the envelope'" (16). Skydivers want "thrills," but also "high-risk performers seek controllable risk contexts where their abilities can be challenged" so that they can "attain mastery, self-efficacy, and flow" (16). Of course, the edge is not a fixed limit; it changes based on ability, knowledge, experience, and confidence level. Hence risk is not to be avoided but managed; not a static relationship, but a boundary of self-improvement and skill.

In SM, edgework might be productively discussed in terms of edge play, a category of play that is physically or psychologically risky or dangerous (see also Henkin and Holiday 1996, 66). Examples of edge play include suspension bondage, electricity, cutting, piercing, branding, enemas, water sports, scat, breath play, knife play, blood play, gun play, terror play, intense humiliation, race and cultural trauma play, singletails, and fire play—all kinds of play in which the risk of physical or emotional damage are fairly high. Patrick Califia adds to this list mind games, consensual nonconsent, abduction and kidnapping, catheters and sounds, and scarification (2002, 193–215). The management of risk is central to the classification of edge play. Some of these play forms are edge play because they risk unintentional physical harm, such as falling during suspension bondage. Some risk long-term bodily damage, death (for example, heart stoppage with electricity play and suffocation during breath play), disease, or psychological trauma. Yet these definitions are not stable; familiarity changes what counts as risky SM. For example, many participants think play piercing is no longer edge play because so many people do it, and the techniques have become standardized. Single-tail whips, too, became trendy during my fieldwork, and there were many classes on how to throw or crack them correctly; this made the use of singletails at semipublic parties much less edgy. Breath play, on the other hand, is widely prohibited, at least for now.

The desirability of managed risk, in edge play, is an opportunity to fashion oneself as a person with skills and knowledge in relation to SM as a risk community. This is why many people told me that they do breath play, but not *that kind* of breath play. Domina, for example, told me: "I don't do much in the way of breath play. I might put a gas mask on somebody and put my hand over the intake, but I don't believe in breath play because you can kill people doing it."[26] Anthony described a scene in which a woman was encased in Saran Wrap: the top wrapped it around her body, over the top of her head, and finally across her face. The top then "ripped it off [from the roll] and walked away and left her there flopping and struggling for breath, and then finally when the thing [Saran Wrap] started sucking way in [to her mouth], he pops his finger in it." Anthony has adapted this scene for himself, using a latex mask that he rips off just in time. But then, he tells me, "in reality I'm only holding her nose for maybe twenty or thirty seconds; it's not really that long at all. It's not really breath play." For Anthony, the scene had what he termed "symbolic value," but it wasn't "really all that edgy." "I do some knife play, but I don't really slice anybody up. I'll cut a couple layers of epidermis and then blood will pool up on the cut." These practitioners, by claiming that their play isn't *really* dangerous, are actively redefining their practices as manageable—SSC—risk.

Other practitioners enjoy imaginatively violating community standards. There are community jokes and T-shirts that say "unsafe, insane, nonconsensual," an homage to the outlaw quality of SM play. In our interview, Vince explained that he and Pam "play with the edges, we play with that monster." Pam clarified the point: "It's kind of like running a marathon or climbing a mountain, it's like 'Can I do it? Where are my edges? Where do I stop? Where do I start?' . . . If you always stay in your safety zone, how do you know what you can do?" SM play, for these practitioners, *should* be unsafe, a place where boundaries and limits can be pushed outside of a personal safety zone.

Yet these practitioners also forge an ethical relationship with the self based on techniques, self-mastery, and community norms or rules. Sybil—a white, bisexual dominant/mistress in her mid-fifties—told me: "This whole thing about 'edge play' is a joke. Edge play is not heavy, it's what's heavy to you. So edge play is . . . blood and heavy whipping . . . to some people, [but] that's not all there is to edge play. If you have a phobia of needles, that's edge play. If you're freaked out because you're a woman and I don't want you to wear pink lingerie, that's edge play. Whatever makes you nervous and you don't want to go there, I want to go there 'cause that's where the exchange of power comes from." Sybil's comments show how community rules incite individual or personal responses: the self-cultivation of practice. The point here is not that breath play or edge play is strictly prohibited, thus inciting the desire to do it. Rather, self-mastery as a practitioner requires the production and subsequent personal refinement of community rules.

As Liz Day notes, all the authors in the SM essay collection *Leatherfolk* (Thompson 1991) claim that SM is transgressive (of nature, culture, materiality, and discourse) because it is "outlaw" (Day 1994, 243). These essayists, like the practitioners who argue that SM is (or should be, or used to be) outlaw, read the limitations imposed by community rules as a coercive form of disciplinary power, forcing practitioners to choose between replication (obeying SM community rules) or transgression (operating outside of, or in violation of, these rules). Rather, these community debates about edge play, risk, and safety produce knowledges that, in turn, encourage practitioners to position themselves in relation to these rules and thus this ethical community. In edge play, then, pleasure comes from defining and marking the boundaries and limits of what can be done; in policing and enforcing these boundaries in the community and in one's own play; and in mastering the rules—the knowledge, skills, and techniques of self-improvement—that make being a practitioner possible.

Here, risk is not aversive, nor does it stand outside of or serve as an escape from the demands or "constraints of modern social routines" imagined as boring, banal, or routinized (Zaloom 2004, 365). Although these practitioners—like high-risk hobbyists such as rock climbers and skydivers—imagine their practice as a break from the "real world" that is simultaneously closer to their authentic selves, the management of risk is actually a way of aligning their play selves with "real life." Indeed, imagining a risk community as a break from the real world is, as I will discuss in the last two chapters, a way of bracketing off SM play as a priori "safe" and "fantasy." This bracketing works as an alibi to screen off SM as safe precisely when it is most productive—of selves, communities, and social inequalities.

In this way, rather than a general ethos or collective consciousness, risk functions to produce differentiated subjects. As Bruce Braun writes, white, middle-class people "constitute themselves as middle-class and white precisely through the externalization of as many risks as possible . . . and through barricading themselves from many others . . . hence, if you are white and middle-class, 'risk' is something you take on voluntarily, not something you are subject to" (2003, 199). Therefore, he argues, adventure-sport advertisements both construct the "proper" risk-taking subject and naturalize racialized and classed hierarchies (199; see also Simon 2002). Representations of risk and ability do not passively reflect but rather justify social inequality. In SM, the ability—or desire—to take on a socially constructed risk is one way in which the community is produced as white and middle class, and, cyclically, continues to appeal to—and produce—these same practitioners. Thus, for example, Wiseman's "middle-class mores" position him as an expert or authority, able to prohibit or permit certain behaviors. But other practitioners' ability to disregard his (and others') expertise is based on their own attainment of knowledge, their self-cultivation as professionalized community members.

(DUNGEON) MONITORING MAKING PRACTITIONERS RESPONSIBLE

The plethora of rules and regulations in the community is related, in part, to the legal challenges that BDSM play presents. Part of the social context for this is the transfer of responsibility from the state to communities and individuals. This transfer owes its legibility to a neoliberal cultural formation that is part and parcel of the new SM community—the privatization of risk, responsibility, and safety. As Wendy Brown argues, neoliberalism produces subjects "controlled *through* their freedom" (2005, 44; italics in original). This freedom is the freedom to take risks, but it is also, critically, the freedom to be held responsible for one's choices and one's own health, well-being, and safety. Managing risk therefore emerges as precisely the responsibility of the SM community and its practitioners. House rules—rules for semipublic play parties—are a good example of these shifts.

The first private party I attended was held in Vallejo, a small city forty-five minutes east of San Francisco on I-80. The party was held in a brown ranch home in a cul-de-sac, in the middle of a new housing development. The house had a large back deck with a pool, and a beautiful view of brown California hills. The party was a regular, once-a-month event called "the Valley." From noon to 7:00 p.m., guests—who had each paid $20 for the afternoon—ate hot dogs and burgers on the deck, socialized, and played in one of the several rooms open in the house. I secured an invitation by e-mailing the organizer, and she sent me the house rules as well as an indemnity form to sign and bring along to the party.

The Valley's house rules are quite similar to those presented at the door of the Castlebar, the Scenery, and every other semipublic play party I attended. Critical to the rules are concerns with safety, both physical and emotional; consensuality, safewords, and informed consent; propriety, privacy, and secrecy; and separation of play and social areas. The Valley's rules also prohibit certain forms of play and behavior (drugs and alcohol, sex without barriers), and require participants to notify the Dungeon Monitor before starting others (blood play, watersports, and wax play). This is similar to the Castlebar, where the rules require that DMs be informed before any "loud, disruptive, or messy scenes," full suspension, blood play, or fire play; prohibit uncontained blood, scat, and piss play, unsafe behavior, professional (paid) scenes, drugs or alcohol, audio or video taping, and firearms; and require barrier protection (condoms, gloves, plastic wrap) for all insertions. Janus and Scenery parties have similar rules and requirements.

In our interview, Larry explained the Scenery's prohibitions on breath play: "Breath play to me is asking to kill someone . . . I've lost several friends to breath play. I don't want that to happen in my space, [and] neither would my insurance company." Larry's concerns centered on the legal risks of these forms of play. Interestingly, given that many community debates have focused on requiring safer-sex practices, Larry did not require the use of barrier protection. When I asked him why, he explained that the California state legislature had changed a law so that now "consenting adults have the right to consent to expose themselves to other folks without leaving liability on a third party." Although the Scenery makes condoms, dental dams, and gloves readily available, he said, "if they choose to play together unprotected, that is their own personal decision . . . I don't think that's my choice. I don't think that's my business." Larry's concerns about insurance and third-party liability are informed by his understanding of consent: a shift from a broader social configuration of risk and responsibility to a "personal decision" based on negotiated consent to risk.

In response to widely publicized raids on semipublic parties, community organizers are increasingly concerned with establishing their indemnity, as legally as possible, in order to protect the party space, the owner, and the players from police and legal action. Most semipublic play parties include an indemnity statement in the house rules and consent form you sign when entering the party. When you sign the membership application form at the Scenery, for example, you are agreeing to a series of statements, beginning with declarations that you are of legal age and that you understand that the party focuses on BDSM and is sexually explicit. The next four statements are: "I am not offended by this conduct"; "I am freely and voluntarily choosing to attend and participate in this event"; if I am "touched, hit, penetrated, spanked" and so forth, it is because "I have specifically and freely and voluntarily consented to these acts"; and finally, "my feelings are not and will not be hurt" by any of these acts. These statements move from the establishment of personal interest to statements about consensuality and freedom from force or coercion, and finally to the management of "feelings." The last part of the document affirms that SM is a form of acting or fantasy; done for entertainment, sport, or hobby; a "time-honored form of performance art"; activities with psychological and therapeutic value; and an "important political statement" about sexual freedom. This document does not only lay out the party rules; it is intended to protect the Scenery from legal action. For example, the statement that SM is performance art with "serious artistic and literary value" seems to be a direct response to legal definitions of obscenity as materials lacking "serious literary, artistic, political, or scientific value."[27] Other statements are concerned with spelling out, in detail, that all activities are freely and voluntarily chosen and specifically requested, and that no one is being forced to participate. These statements seem designed to ward off prosecution in the event of a raid.

The Valley is unusual in that the organizers ask partygoers to sign a separate indemnity form. This form, titled "Agreement and Release of Liability," contains five sections. The first is a paragraph on voluntary participation ("I am freely and voluntarily choosing to attend") that is similar to other party forms. The next four sections establish, with increasing specificity, the house owners' indemnity. The second section requires you to initial after a statement that reads, "I assume full responsibility for any and all risks of property damage, personal injury or death"; the third is a statement that you "release, waive and forever discharge" the party hosts and anyone connected to the Valley from any legal claims, actions, or suits. The fourth section asserts that you agree to "indemnify and hold harmless" everyone connected to the party, while the fifth and final section states: "I am aware that this is a release of liability and a contract between me and the Valley and/or its entities and that I am giving up many legal rights and remedies by signing it."

Whether such forms would actually stand up in court is a matter of debate, since the basic legality of consensual BDSM is uncertain. In part because of developments in laws concerning domestic violence and rape, it is unclear in most states whether "victims" can legally consent to "abuse."[28] Just before I started my fieldwork, police raided semipublic play parties in San Diego and Attleboro, Massachusetts. The cases—the San Diego Six in 1999 and "Paddleboro" in 2000—energized practitioners and activists across the United States.[29] And although most of the charges were eventually dropped, the cases demonstrated the tenuous legal ground of semipublic BDSM parties and dungeons. Club X—the San Diego club that was raided—rewrote its "Agreement and Release of

Liability" form to more explicitly assert voluntary participation, as well as personal responsibility for risk, liability release, and indemnity.

Consensual here, as a key term of contemporary SM, means more than free from coercion; consent becomes, in these rules, a way to insist on the voluntary participation in, and thus participant's own responsibility for, SM play. This logic has produced the current situation, in which practitioners are asked to be responsible for their own behavior and any risks they take on, and thus resent "the rules." So, for example, Stephanie complains: "We used to be able to do a lot more than we can do now. Now, you draw blood, there are fourteen DMs all over you. Or you've broken the house rules or . . . you've got your hand in somebody's cunt, [a] DM is right there: 'Get a glove on.' I'm like, 'Just back off!' I understand the need for DMs, but I think there's a little policing thing that's happening more and more, and I think that that's changing and that's one of the reasons we don't play at some places. I mean, I just don't want to have the police on me all the time . . . it ruins the scene if somebody is there with a magnifying glass of rules and regs over my shoulder all the time." Stephanie is resentful because she is already educated. She has, in a way, outgrown the rules: "We do play on the edge, we do do breath play, and we do use knives and needles and all that stuff. We're very competent with it, and we know exactly what we're doing." "There are a million rules for what you can do in public spaces," she continues, but "I also don't feel like I have any responsibility to have to protect anybody from themselves." This is because Stephanie, like many other participants, does not want the people who make or enforce the rules to try to protect her or her partners. But even those who complain about the community rules are taking it upon themselves to "self-police." As Mollena puts it: "When you play like that [do edge play], you take that risk, so you have to police yourself to a certain extent." This resentment is of a neoliberal form of governmentality that shifts responsibility onto practitioners even as it demands that they master themselves in relation to an evaluative community.

In this way, personal responsibility merges self-cultivation (a governing of the self) with personal rationality (individual autonomy). Lemke argues, following Foucault, that "the key feature of the neo-liberal rationality is the congruence it endeavors to achieve between a responsible and moral individual and an economic-rational actor. It aspires to construct prudent subjects whose moral quality is based on the fact that they rationally assess the costs and benefits of a certain act as opposed to other alternative acts. As the choice for action is, or so the neo-liberal notion of rationality would have it, the expression of free will on the basis of a self-determined decision, the consequences of the action are borne by the subject alone, who is also solely responsible for them" (2001, 201). This is part of a neoliberal configuration that encourages practitioners to negotiate with *informed*—properly educated—consent and take responsibility for their risky SM practice. But it also imbues this new community with ambivalence, highlighting the tension between self-mastery and community norms, between individual and collective responsibility.

This tension is rendered most dramatically in the Dungeon Monitors Association. Some people speculate that the reason Jerome Bambrick founded the DMA was to reduce SMOdyssey's liability and play party insurance costs—he also runs SMOdyssey's parties in the South Bay. But today the DMA must contend with a broad-based community perception of paternalism, the social price of the requirement to master the self. I attended an all-day "Beginning Dungeon Monitor Training Course" in January 2003. The course's prerequisites were one year of active involvement in the scene, attendance at no fewer than twenty semipublic play parties, and having a basic understanding of common play techniques (in addition to being over eighteen, interested in "continuing education" on play styles, and being able to deal with emergencies). The bulk of the all-day class was devoted to safety (especially safer-sex procedures and issues of contamination and disease management—for example, what to do if a flogger gets bloody, or how long hepatitis A takes to die in the air) and judgment (for example, what to do if you are uncomfortable with some form of play, or how to deal with a difficult player), as we were expected to already have basic knowledge of SM and dungeon equipment. At least an hour of the class was devoted to etiquette—proper ways of handling various hypothetical situations, such as when barrier protection is not being used (this case also included practical instructions in how to check for the presence of a condom, dam, or glove without being overly intrusive), when prohibited play is taking place, or when the scene is too loud and disturbing other party guests. Phil and Domina, our teachers, stressed that at all times, we should smile, be calm and polite, and facilitate the guests' enjoyment of and safety at the party.

This etiquette training was combined with instructions about assembling a DM kit (a personal bag of safety and emergency items such as latex gloves, a flashlight, EMT scissors designed to cut through all materials, Band-Aids, and condoms), what to check before beginning our shift (the location of emergency exits, fire extinguishers, and phone), what information to pass on to our replacement at the end of the shift, how to file an incident report (a description of any potential conflict), and what to do in various emergencies (power outage, earthquake, and fire). We learned how to operate a fire extinguisher and how to remove latex gloves without getting "blood" (in this case, ketchup) on our hands. We also learned how to catch a person who falls off a cross. All this led up to the final portion of the class, the test: twenty-five multiple-choice questions on basic safety, the etiquette training we had learned, fundamentals of SM play, and "what should you do if" questions, like the epigraph to this chapter. If we passed the test, we were accepted as DMA trainees; we joined the group's e-mail list and were expected to begin further training.

During the lunch break, Phil came over to talk to me about the DMA. Although he was now on the group's board, he remained ambivalent about the DMA: the safety training is important, he said, but he wasn't sure how to counter community perception that the DMs at parties are power mad and taking themselves too seriously. Almost everyone I spoke to had at least one story about an overzealous DM who stopped a scene because it was too edgy, went too far, seemed unsafe, or—most galling of all—was an approved play style with which the DM was uncomfortable or unfamiliar. In response to this criticism, the DMA is trying very hard to train DMs to be objective, calm arbiters of safety and not, as Phil and Domina said over and over during our training, policemen: "A good DM is a lifeguard, not the police, the host, or the security"; "DMs facilitate play; they are not police and they do not interrupt a scene unless absolutely necessary!"; "you are there to help and to take care of people"; "you need to be flexible within the rules; be a facilitator"; "you are not a cop."

In spite of the DMA's best efforts, there is still a community perception of DMs as homegrown, deputized police. It is the monitoring of safety, safe play, and safe sex, combined with the insistence on party—and community—rules, that make DMs into police, no matter how much they smile. Lady Hilary, for example, argues that simply teaching people how to be dungeon monitors involves a quantification of play and play styles that alienates her. She comments: "I play hard [and] I can't play hard in public anymore" because the "dungeon monitor police . . . [are] going after me." Bailey, who is supportive of the DMA, explains: "I've been to DM training, I've DMed at parties, [and] I decided that was not something I really wanted to do" because "I just didn't want to be part of the condom police." Tom, a white, bisexual switch in his fifties, says: "What's happening now is that there is actually an attempt to formalize becoming a dungeon monitor . . . and so as part of this formalization there will be two levels of dungeon master—they're even talking about the first level having to go and get this first-aid training and man, I got enough regulations! I got enough law in my life; I don't need to go into what is a fringe sort of outlaw community to be told I have to qualify to be under another law to be a DM!" Tom's anxiety about the "rules and regulations" stems from his concern that requiring first-aid training would "legally obligate you to offer assistance." He explains: "As somebody who is an old-time player, it's an absolutely horrific concept that somebody would bring into BDSM a hurdle or a loop . . . that would require you to be subservient to government intervention. I mean, that would [have been] . . . anathema five years ago." If first-aid training legally obligates DMs to offer assistance, this would involve the state in BDSM and thus leave DMs open to liability if someone got hurt.

Further, the debate over DMs as police crystallizes the tensions between a vision of the individual as rational agent and a social absorption of risk. This is why Preston mockingly writes that SM politics are organized around a "plea for social acceptance" (1991, 212), "asking to be let in [to polite society] as exemplars of good citizenship" (215; see also Weiss 2008). Being a good citizen of the SM community means several things in this analysis: the proper management of sexual bodies (especially bodily barriers and risk avoidance), the proper management of relationships (being SSC and friendly, and maintaining etiquette), and the proper management of oneself (modes of self-regulation and cultivation). In addition, a good SM citizen is professional (and implicitly white), responsible, free-thinking, and agentic. It is not so much state interference that is the problem here, but the BDSM community's taking on the responsibility for SM practitioners and their health and safety.

Each of these developments—the class structure; the emphasis on negotiation, safewords, and SSC play; the definitions of edge play; the prohibitions on certain forms of play; and the development of formal party rules—are ways in which the SM community has canonized and codified rules for play, transforming itself into a risk community. By producing, regulating, and controlling the meanings of safety, risk, vulnerability, and security, the community also enables the production of particular SM practitioners: new SM practitioners become practitioners in relation to these rules. Yet rather than simply internalizing the rules, practitioners are asked to make the rules their own, to cultivate their own rules of conduct. This practice of the self requires self-mastery in the Foucauldian sense: SM practitioners who are subjects of themselves. But it also requires self-mastery in the neoliberal sense: SM practitioners who are responsible for themselves, and who thus operate within discourses of consent, choice, agency, and personal freedom that legitimate and reproduce social hierarchies. Practitioners reproduce neoliberal cultural formations that sustain certain social stratifications: the social privilege of the "more-educated, more-knowledgeable, and more-affluent people" that Bailey, and many others, seek out when they join the SM community. Here, community responsibility stands in ambivalent opposition to the project of self-control that the community requires, pitting self-cultivation and autonomy against social control.

THE PLEASURE OF THE RULES

This practice of the self contrasts with the way Karmen MacKendrick theorizes SM as a form of subjective rupturing or unmaking.[30] MacKendrick's work—inspired by readings of Nietzsche, Bataille, Barthes, and Foucault—is one of the few philosophical treatments of SM practice and subjectivity. She theorizes SM pleasure as *jouissance*, as "destabilizing and threatening not only to the political and cultural orders but to all manner of orders" (1999, 6). Practices of restraint (bondage) and pain, she argues, "throw the subject outside itself" and "break the limits of subjection" (156). This is the case because these practices give a subject a barrier or limit "against which to push herself past herself" (107); opening the possibility for the "pleasurable abandon of the subject, in which the subject freely breaks its own limits and is lost in pleasure" (121). SM practice, for MacKendrick, allows us to "surpass our subjectivity" (108); SM "breaks the subject" (111) and "implode[s] subjectivity" (115).

This argument relies on Foucault's understanding of "desexualization," a concept based in part on his reading of San Francisco's 1970s leather scene as heralding a "real creation of new possibilities of pleasure" ([1984] 1996, 384). Desexualization, for Foucault, is pleasure beyond sexuality: pleasure that spreads beyond the genitals to other parts of the body. As Foucault famously, if controversially, argues at the end of the first volume of the *History of Sexuality*: "It is the agency of sex that we must break away from, if we aim—through a tactical reversal of the various mechanisms of sexuality—to counter the grips of power with the claims of bodies, pleasures, and knowledges, in their multiplicity and their possibility of resistance. The rallying point for the counterattack against the deployment of sexuality ought not to be sex-desire, but bodies and pleasures" ([1976] 1990, 157). For MacKendrick and Foucault, unlike sexual pleasure mediated through disciplinary regimes ("sex-desire"), SM's pleasure is bodily pleasure, a disruptive or disorderly pleasure that might open the possibility for desubjectification (Foucault [1983] 1996, 378).

However, elsewhere Foucault claims that SM is an "art of sexual practice" devoted to exploring "all the internal possibilities of sexual conduct" ([1982] 1996, 330). This emphasis parallels his work on practices and care of the self, a technique fundamentally about subjectification—the self as subject—rather than desubjectification; about techniques of the self rather than techniques of domination. Interestingly, however, the pleasure of such work is also, for Foucault, opposed to disciplinary "sex-desire." Instead, it is biopolitical: the pleasure one can take in oneself, in the self as an object, in the care of the self. Such self-subjectification produces "pleasure without desire" (Foucault [1984] 1988, 66). This is, in short, the pleasure of the rules: not pleasure in rules externally imposed by fiat, but pleasure in inhabiting, embodying, cultivating, elaborating, and individualizing the rules (see also Mahmood 2004).

The new guard SM scene is, of course, quite different from the scene that Foucault experienced in the 1970s, and I suspect he might have agreed with Baldwin that today's scene is "oversupervised," "sanitized," and "flat."[31] However, practitioners' nostalgia, a longing for the past of authentic intimacies, also signifies the desire for pleasure to rupture, desexualize, or desubjectify—or, in practitioners' terms, to be raw, edgy, and real. In parallel to Miranda Joseph's (2002) argument against the "romance" of community, which positions community outside of and in opposition to capitalism, this nostalgia for rule-less SM practice imagines the rules, or social norms, in opposition to the freedom and authentic intimacies of play. As I read it, however, rather than producing a break, pleasure works in concert with the rules to produce SM subjects. If SM is a form of desexualization, it achieves this state through the subject's self-mastery of the rules. Yet here the role of the community as the generator of social directives that compel such self-making projects is ambivalent. Rather than standing outside of power—or outside the law—BDSM is a form of incitement, urging practitioners to construct themselves as practitioners in relation to, if not through obedience to, the rules. In this way, the very establishment of the new SM scene produces, together with these practitioners, their sense of autonomy—a circuit that consolidates social power and class privilege and simultaneously illuminates the deep tensions between such self-mastering projects and collective social norms.

THREE 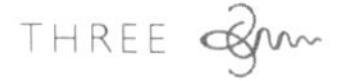

THE TOY BAG

Exchange Economies and the Body at Play

S/M is high-technology sex.—PAT CALIFIA, *Public Sex*

It's a Saturday night, and I am going to a pansexual play party at the Castlebar. I drive, since there is always lots of parking in the industrial neighborhood in which it's located, and walk through the light rain to the door. The door has no sign, just a large number on the square, frosted-glass window set into solid metal. I knock; a head peeks out and asks, "Are you here for the play party?" "Yes," I answer, wondering as usual if my outfit is all right.[1] The door opens, and I squeeze into a short hallway. There are four or five people in the hall, queued up before the pay station—a folding table staffed by a party volunteer. The men and women in front of me are wearing jeans, black leather vests, and black leather jackets. We are tightly packed in the hallway, out of the rain; as I press against the man in front of me to close the door, I almost trip over the large, black wheeled luggage he has on the floor behind him.

The luggage is a toy bag, filled with personal BDSM toys: a couple of floggers, rope, clamps and clips, leather restraints, cuffs, a cane or two, crops, a paddle, a blindfold, lube and safer-sex supplies, an emergency pouch with first-aid supplies, and perhaps a vibrator or dildos, or toys for medical, piercing, or electrical play. It's a lot of stuff to cart around. And, although some people have stylish toy bags (like a man who does a lot of medical play and carries a scary black doctor's bag), most have basic black duffel bags and, increasingly, black wheeled luggage. Some also carry black plastic tubes with straps, made for carrying architectural plans or other large documents, that hold canes and crops. As Hailstorm tells me: "When people come in [to a party], they come in with luggage. There's carry-on luggage, they've got backpacks, and there's stuff they're pulling on wheels and . . . [it's] like their recreational vehicle opens up and it's full of stuff."

Toys are an integral part of contemporary SM. In concert with the development of a more formalized, professional, and rule-oriented scene, there has been a tremendous expansion in the market for SM paraphernalia and the techniques that these new toys engender. And in the same ways that this new scene produces SM practitioners and communities in accordance with classed and racialized understandings of risk, safety, and subjectivity, buying and using SM toys produces certain kinds of subjects in accordance with larger social, political, and economic relations. The "tyranny of techniques" and proliferation of SM toys—combined with the codification and regulation of the body, its boundaries, and its mobilization—has transformed the subjectivity and sociality of SM practitioners. As I showed in the previous chapter, the contours of the new pansexual SM scene and the institutionalization of community rules produce SM practitioners in ways deeply resonant with late-capitalist forms of biopower. I continue this exploration here, taking up the development of a particular form of SM community and sociality—of intimacy—dependent on, but not defined exclusively by, commodity exchange.

Forms of subjectification are linked to forms of knowledge. Indeed, as Foucault argues in his seminar, "technologies of the self" are often combined with technologies of production, sign systems, and power (1988). For example, neoliberalism's emphasis on *responsible* and *rational* individuals brings together self-subjectification (self-care, personal responsibility) with *homo oeconomicus* (rational, agentic, economic [hu]man). As Thomas Lemke explains, summarizing the critical work that has been produced after the publication of Foucault's neoliberalism and biopower lectures, neoliberalism's economic rationality—and its emphasis on economic efficiency—has "colonized" domains previously understood as outside the economic, like leisure, the family, and the body (2001, 202; see also Brown 2005; Lowe 1995). So, for example, flexible work hours or performance reports are not only "intended to transform the organization of production" but are "aimed at the very relation between individuals and their labor," their "self-fulfillment." As he puts it, "the transformation of structures of production is possible only if individuals 'optimize' their relation to themselves and to work" (203). In these ways, neoliberalism functions as a "technique of power" in which "not only the individual body, but also collective bodies and institutions (public administrations, universities, etc.), corporations and states have to be 'lean,' 'fit,' 'flexible,' and 'autonomous.' "

Such an emphasis on flexibility, fitness, and efficiency echoes Emily Martin's analysis of the circuit between iterations of flexible late capitalism (such as just-in-time production, specialization, and flexible accumulation) and those of the body (such as immunology). As she argues, just as corporations must thrive and grow as if a biological organism, the human body must also become "a complex system that is in constant, anticipatory, flexibly adaptive change" (1994, 111). However, as Martin's analysis makes clear, there is a cost to workers required to be so flexible: the loss of stability, support, and security. She concludes: "It is no wonder that moving gracefully as an agile, dancing, flexible worker/person/body feels like a liberation, even if one is moving across a tightrope. But can we simultaneously realize that the new bodies are also highly constrained? They cannot stop moving, they cannot grow stiff and rigid, or they will fall off the 'tightrope' of life and die" (247–48). By calling attention to the circuits of exchange between the body and the subject, relations of production and signification, analysts like Martin and Lemke, via Foucault, point to the ways that late capitalism, together with neoliberal rationality, reconfigures the body's flexibility and adaptability, a shift that heightens the differentiation between "able" and nonproductive bodies. Indeed, productivity is a key way to understand these new demands on the subject-worker, as well as the relations of inequality they inscribe as embodiment. As Jon McKenzie (2001) argues, efficient performance is our dominant form of power/knowledge.

In this chapter, I consider the place of toys in these circuits between capitalism and embodiment. I explore the relationship between toys and consumer-players in terms of *technological prostheses*, broadening both terms to include not only technology but also the knowledge practices of techne, and not only literal prostheses but also changing forms of embodiment. I focus on the exchanges between bodies, subjects, techne, and toys, and I argue that these circuits produce a *body in play*: a body that is simultaneously divided into parts and extended through objects, both produced and transformed through consumption. Tracking the ways in which SM consumerism transforms subjectivities and produces relationality and community, I show how this sexual circuit creates multiple bodily potentials within social dynamics of privilege and inequality. In short, this chapter focuses on SM toys and their handlers in order to think through the biopolitics of consumerism.

"IT TAKES MONEY TO PLAY" THE MARKET IN BDSM

Several cultural critics have analyzed BDSM as a paradigmatic consumer sexuality because of its tremendous market appeal, its ever-expanding paraphernalia, its nonreproductive nature, and its affinity with the leisure demands of late capitalism (Brooks 2000; Ehrenreich 1986; Lowe 1995). Indeed, the growth of the BDSM scene is related to a more general proliferation of sexualities and sexual services, commodities, and purveyors (Hennessy 2000; Singer 1993). The proliferation of sex boutiques and stores—as well as online resources like stores, services, web pages, and chat rooms—has transformed the practice of SM. And although sexual services and technologies have increased throughout the United States, in the Bay Area, the high concentration of Internet jobs and workers, combined with San Francisco's general support for alternative sexualities, make the region an epicenter of the sexual commerce industry. SM in San Francisco, then, magnifies these bodily and social transformations—technological and commodified intimacies—just as it does the high price of belonging to such communities.

The cooperative, feminist sex toy store Good Vibrations now has four stores in the Bay Area (three in San Francisco and one in Berkeley), as well as an online and print catalog; they also hold classes and workshops, publish books, and produce and package some of their own sex toys. Several sex-related presses are located in the Bay Area, including, until its sale in 2010, Greenery Press, which has published many of the nationally known SM books. Online bondage photography and SM porn and other online sites also thrive: paintoy.com, CyberNet Entertainment, beautybound.com, and seriousbondage.com are just a few located in the Bay Area and run by practitioners.[2] And SM and leather stores of various kinds are scattered throughout the city, as well as in the East and South Bay. For example, Mr. S, the gold standard of pricey, customized, well-crafted bondage and SM toys, equipment, and clothing, has been in the South of Market neighborhood since 1979. Run by Richard Hunter and his son, Mr. S opened a women's and pansexual store, Madam S, across the street in 2001.

One day in March 2002, I went to Mr. S to meet Mark, the bondage aficionado described in the introduction, and some of his friends. They were late, so I walked into the store alone. Entering Mr. S is overwhelming: there is a huge, room-size cage immediately to the left, with body bags, harnesses, slings, gags, hoods, black boots, manacles, and spreader bars in black leather or metal strung up on the cage and the back walls. In the back of the store, a larger room contains gay and SM porn (including a vintage *Drummer* display) and some assorted sex toys (plugs, dildos, and cock rings), but mostly clothes: leather, vinyl, lots of latex, even wetsuits, and a small collection of polar fleece sweatshirts carrying the Mr. S logo. When Mark arrived, he showed me around, pointing out the bondage equipment and telling me how it is used. He asked Jess, one of his friends, if she wanted to demonstrate a body bag, and we all stepped into the cage. Mark laid out a large black leather bag with a double zipper and laces running across the front. Jess wriggled in and put her arms in the sleeves inside the bag. Mark zipped her up, cinched the laces, and then fetched six long leather straps to tighten the bag further. He added a black leather hood with pinprick eye holes, a collar that attached the hood to the body bag, and a blindfold. The bag itself cost $1,395; adding the straps, hood, collar, and blindfold meant that Jess was in bondage gear worth about $2,700. As he added the straps, Mark told me: "If you're going to spend this much, you might as well get the custom bag," since a customized body bag costs only 30 percent more and, obviously, fits the body perfectly. Mr. S prides itself on manufacturing and selling the highest quality toys and equipment, and much of its business is custom leatherwork.

The wide availability of SM and leather toys, clothes, and equipment has transformed the community. The ease of browsing in stores, online or through catalogs, has meant that many practitioners have large collections of toys and clothing; items that they might not have searched out or made themselves are now easy to find. Although SM has its imagined roots in a gay motorcycle scene—a decidedly working-class scene in both origin and image—today the community is, as Annalee puts it, "a middle-class preoccupation, because it's all about acquiring stuff. It's a consumer sexuality." Teramis tells me: "When I was coming out . . . there were no expensive toys. People were using clothespins from the laundry bag and laundry line for bondage and making their own floggers out of five dollars of stuff from Tandy Leather. People weren't precluded from playing because of economic issue[s]." But now, as Annalee observes, "if you wanted to be part of the fetish community, it would be extremely difficult to do without money . . . the BDSM community puts such a premium on your clothes."

Most of the practitioners I spoke with were professionals who had disposable income to spend on SM. Those who were not acquired what Annalee called "access to middle-class money" in a variety of ways: receiving support from friends, being "adopted" into a leather family, buying items on sale, working at SM stores, or doing sex work. For example, Bonnie—an Asian American, heterosexual masochist in her mid-twenties—worked at Madam S; she used the "funny money"—store coupons—she earned as part of her pay to buy fetish clothing. Meg'gan had been adopted as a houseboy by a large leather family in the South Bay, and they provided for her. But although most of my interviewees were at first quite adamant that the scene was open to all, many later conceded that, as Carrie—a white, bisexual bottom/submissive in her mid-forties—put it, "it takes money to play."

When I asked interviewees to estimate how much money they spend on BDSM during a year, many were surprised and horrified as they began to add up their expenses. Play parties (without doing work shifts in exchange for reduced or free admission) cost $25; classes cost between $3 and $25, depending on the location and one's membership status; and munches cost between $15 and $25—the price of lunch, dinner, or drinks. Since many people attend several events each week, it is not unusual for a practitioner to spend $100 to $150 a week attending events. And almost all of the practitioners I interviewed spent far more on their toys, clothing, and, in some cases, play spaces (or home dungeons) than they did attending events. Hailstorm notes:

> There are organizations you can join and pay $20 a year and all the parties are free. That's not very expensive for the participants. The

other places you go like PE [the Power Exchange], and you're going to drop forty, fifty, sixty bucks per person just to go there . . . The expense comes in the clothes, obviously, the toys, and that's where you can drop some big bucks. I went out and I bought a leather jacket from Harley Davidson, two hundred bucks; leather vest, a hundred bucks; set of floggers, two to three hundred bucks. You have hundreds and hundreds and hundreds of dollars, sometimes thousands of dollars, if you shop at Stormy Leather, if you want to dress you and your partner up and look nice. And leather's expensive and the toys are expensive . . . It's important . . . that you arrive in fetish attire. If you come in street clothes, it's like "You're an amateur. What are you doing here?"

Spending hundreds and hundreds, or even thousands, of dollars on toys is not unusual. Don, a white, straightish service top in his early forties, told me that he has spent $2,500 to $3,000 on his toy bag. Bailey told me she "may have spent $5,000 or $10,000 over the last five years" on clothes, floggers, canes, paddles, and piercing needles, among other items. Floggers, especially desirable handcrafted ones, cost between $150 and $300, depending on their size, number of tails, and material or type of leather.[3] Leather or wooden paddles are between $30 and $150. Other toys are less expensive; one can purchase rattan (to make canes) in bulk at garden-supply stores for $1 a foot. Clothing also ranges in price, but leather pants, vests, and jackets; corsets; and fetish clothing, made of vinyl, latex, or rubber are uniformly expensive. Madam S, for example, carries latex dresses in a range of colors and styles for between $200 and $1,000. Dark Garden, a corset store, will make a customized leather corset for between $500 and $600. The de rigueur black leather jacket can be a gift, scrounged from an area thrift store, or purchased at one of the "lower-quality" leather emporiums in the Bay Area, but, as in most matters of style, clothing of high quality—rendered in price—is much more desirable. Carrie comments: "When you add it up like that, it really does take money to play. I don't think that a lot of people who are wondering where they're going to buy their next milk and bread from are going to do that . . . It takes money to play, a certain amount anyway, and you think about the toys, the clothes, the social events and all that—it really does."

People buy their toys and clothes online, through mail order, at local leather stores, at the kinky flea market held four times a year, and at various leather fairs, especially the Folsom Street Fair. Estrella has a larger-than-average collection because she works as a prodomme.

ESTRELLA: I have thousands of dollars worth of toys, and I still don't have everything I want . . . There are definitely things I'd like to have that I can't afford, like a vacuum bed [vac sack], a cage—some of those things I don't have space for. I mean, I could theoretically put them on a credit card, but where would I put them? My daughter's room? "Honey, can I store this in here while I'm not using it?" But yeah, all the other toys—I have fifteen floggers and fifteen canes, maybe twenty canes, paddles, electrical equipment. I have some big leather [items] like bondage toys, miles of rope, corsets, fetish wear, shoes and all that . . . I always go to Folsom [Street Fair] with a budget and a list of things I definitely want.

MARGOT: What's your budget?

ESTRELLA: For Folsom, at least $300. I've spent as much as $800. But yeah, $300, that's a couple floggers, or a flogger and a couple of toys.

Some items can be found at specialized stores: tack and crops for pony play at saddle shops, or medical-play equipment at medical supply stores. Some people make their own toys; Domina, for example, makes and sells canes, and Panther does leather work. Organizations in the Bay Area also offer classes in do-it-yourself (DIY) toys, usually on leather working and "Make Your Own Folsom Unit," an electrical-play toy.

Although nearly everyone I interviewed insisted that one could get by without pricey toys, there are certain toys considered standard for toy bags and players. Annalee told me that she doesn't collect "expensive Mr. S–type toys," but she does have the "basic implements that you're supposed to have in order to participate in BDSM." I asked her what that included, and she listed a flogger, "spanky toy," riding crop, nipple clamps, canes, restraining devices, wrist and ankle cuffs, chains, hooks, and nylon rope. This is a pretty abbreviated list, but even so, Annalee commented that if she were to "put all my toys together, [she] probably would have quite an assembly." In *The Topping Book*, Dossie Easton and Catherine Liszt list the following toys as a "basic starter set": rope (four or more twelve-foot lengths, plus shorter pieces), restraints (wrist and ankle cuffs), a blindfold, a collar, clips or clamps, candles (for hot wax play), a soft flogger, a slapper (a stiff, folded leather paddle) or jockey bat (short riding crop), sex toys (vibrators, dildos, and butt plugs), safe-sex supplies (condoms, gloves, dams, and lube), and emergency supplies (shears and a flashlight; 1998b, 103–9).

Many practitioners' toy bags evolve from this "starter set." Lady Thendara describes this as she complains:

> If I go somewhere [to play], then we have to plan. I have to decide what I'm going to put in the toy bag . . . I used to be able to put everything in the toy bag [when I had] . . . three or four floggers and a couple of canes and a couple of paddles and some rope, and that was it. I could easily fit all that in the toy bag and not get a backache. But we've got like three body bags and . . .
>
> LATEX MUSTANG: . . . twenty floggers and fifteen canes, and it goes on and on and on.

This is by no means unusual. As Bailey remembers, "For a while there, I was buying shit every month. Or if I see something at a dungeon, I'm like, 'I want to try that!'" Gretchen tells me that a novice "can start to play without having expensive toys at all." But then, of course, "if you really decide that you like the lifestyle and you like playing, so it's a commitment for you, then you can start to put money aside for buying that really special flogger and that latex body suit or whatever you're into."

Gretchen's comments reveal how buying (one's own) toys signifies one's commitment to, or deepening involvement with, the scene. In addition to spending much of their discretionary income on toys, practitioners also spend a tremendous amount of time being SM practitioners. In a half-joking, anxious exchange, Stephanie tells me she devotes fifty hours a week to SM or SM-related activities. Anthony, her husband, says: "I spend at least forty hours a week doing scene-related stuff." Stephanie laughs and says: "Oh my God, honey . . . do you get health benefits with that? You should get a raise. You'll be employee of the month!" For many practitioners, fifteen hours a week is typical if they attend one munch and one class or organizational meeting, and play once or twice. In addition to these organized events, practitioners spend time online (looking at online magazines and web pages of stores, personal ads, and political groups); follow the latest news on SM in the media; read and watch (and, in some cases, write and produce) books, magazines, and videos on BDSM; and go to local BDSM stores. Participants who are officers of various clubs spend time performing their volunteer tasks as well: updating the online calendar of events, collecting money at the door, or making calls to arrange rental spaces for workshops. Mark, for example, is developing a bondage website and spends at least sixty hours a week on that alone. Dylan—a white, bisexual/lesbian submissive in her mid-thirties—estimated spending eight to fifteen hours a week, then added a few more hours to account for the pornographic writing she does. Hailstorm estimated three hours a day, every day; Don estimated between ten and fifteen hours a week. I suspect, based on the sheer size and volume of several very active local e-mail discussion lists, that my interviewees underestimated the time they devote to reading and responding to e-mail.

Finally, for many participants, most of their friends and social circle are people involved in the scene, so time spent going to movies, celebrating events, or having friends over for dinner is part of BDSM sociality. Gretchen, for example, estimates that 80 percent of her friends are in the scene; she is not at all unusual. SM sociality is certainly not confined to the bedroom; it includes attending classes and workshops, meeting scene friends for a drink, volunteering as membership secretary for an SM organization, and planning yearly trips to BDSM conferences or retreats, as well as having SM sex.

It should be clear by now that SM practitioners spend much of their time, money, and energy being—and becoming—practitioners. The time and energy that they devote to SM is connected to the understanding that BDSM is—or should be—a form of work or labor. As Jezzie put it: "I don't like people trying to convince us that what we're doing is play and fun because we put so much work into it, so much work. It's not easy." When I asked Jezzie and her husband, Anton, what they meant by "work," he answered: "Emotional, intellectual, also just thinking day-to-day, how do you do it? . . . How does one set up your life so that it's—so that it will work? You know, we do a lot." He went on to describe the kind of "work" he meant: talking, being honest, self-examination, organization, planning, and perseverance, even though "there's a lot of times when you just don't feel like putting forth the effort." As I explored in the previous chapter, this "work" is work on the self, a form of self-mastery and self-knowledge that produces SM subjectivities and communities in deeply class- and race-inflected ways. For these practitioners, BDSM practice is a biopolitical project: a time-consuming, expensive, formalized mode of working at sex, gaining expertise, learning skills and techniques, and mastering the self in relation to a community. And one primary way in which SM produces both subjects and communities is through practice—not only SM techniques, but also consumer practices.

PRODUCING CONSUMER-SUBJECTS THROUGH BODILY KNOWLEDGE

Much recent work on consumerism suggests that in new forms of capitalism, the increased distance between sites of production and those of consumption, the rise of service and knowledge work, and the spread of insecure, temporary labor, has, as Jean and John Comaroff argue, resulted in an "eclipse of production" (2000, 295; see also Harvey 1997). This is not to claim that production no longer matters, or that global capitalism itself depends more on consumption than production. Instead, these critics draw attention to the increased importance of consumption in identity formation, especially in places like the United States.[4] As the Comaroffs write, such global shifts produce a "culture that re-visions persons not as producers from a particular community, but as consumers in a planetary marketplace: persons as ensembles of identity" (2000, 304). Daniel Miller writes: "To be a 'consumer' as opposed to being a producer implies that we have only a secondary relationship to goods. This secondary relationship occurs when people have to live with and through services and goods that they did not themselves create. The consumer society exists when, as in industrial societies today, most people have a minimal relationship to production and distribution such that consumption provides the only arena left to us through which we might potentially forge a relationship with the world" (1995, 16). Taken together, these critics point to the increased significance of consumerism and commodities in the production of identity, community, and attendant social relations; as Debra Curtis argues, consumption practices are a form of self-production, a "means by which individuals construct their own lives" (2004, 120). In this way, buying practices solidify social belonging and create community.

It is for this reason that most practitioners have their own pricey toy bag, since toys serve as both emblem and means of achieving status, identity, and community belonging. Gretchen, for example, tells me that after her divorce, she went out and bought her own toys: "a couple of leather floggers and a horsetail flogger and a rubber flogger, and some canes and paddles, and my own needle kit." Although she is primarily a bottom, having her own set of toys helped her assert her independence and reclaim her identity in the scene. Toys are also a shared ritual of belonging. Like mastering the rules, buying one's own toy bag produces the self in relation to community ideas about growing expertise, mastery, and technique. Panther told me that he thought many couples start off in the scene by spanking: a simple OTK (over the knee), open-hand spanking, "no equipment needed! No toys, didn't have to wear leather, didn't have to do anything, just bend 'em over and spank 'em!" But because "BDSM is so open here, it's easy to get sucked in and start finding out about other things . . . All of a sudden, they see somebody with a really cool paddle, and they say they got it at Mr. S, and so you go there, and pretty soon you graduate." In this way, toys are also an entry into the scene, or into increasingly advanced scenes and scenarios.

Toys convey status and seriousness; they are concrete signs of the skill and expertise of the top (and, sometimes, the bottom). Hailstorm explains that there is a "pecking order where the doms will try to achieve a certain status within the community . . . Their technique with their toys and the way that they perform is a way of demonstrating to other people that they're competent." The toys themselves, combined with one's technique, become useful tools. As Estrella tells me: "There's a lot of stuff I know how to do . . . I'm good with a flogger, I can throw a singletail, I'm good with a cane, I know about safety, I know how to brand, I know how to cut, I know how to slap, pull hair, punch . . . It gives me a lot of tools at my disposal." This combination of knowledge of technique, combined with consumerism, produces an educated, informed SM practitioner. Consuming, in other words, is crucial to the identity formation of SM practitioners, in relation to community standards.

The value of toys has as much to do with the toy's quality and craftsmanship as it does with the "discursivity of the commodity"—a signified value based on the labor of the consumer (Joseph 2002, 41). Being a discerning consumer is linked directly to the production of oneself as a skilled and knowledgeable SM practitioner. Don, for example, describes himself as a "tech casualty" of the "dot bomb"; he was having a hard time finding enough consulting work to stay afloat. When he is "financially solvent again," he tells me, there are several floggers he will buy immediately: "I've gotten to the point where now the specific nature and quality and design and materials and everything all matter to me because I can tell the difference with what I'm trying to accomplish." Similarly, Gretchen asserts: "There's a big difference between a leather flogger made by Happy Tails and a leather flogger made by some other people . . . it's almost like the piece itself has an artistic value or an intrinsic value in being so well made. And people will swear by certain singletails . . . It *does* matter whether you buy something quality or not because otherwise the tails won't go where you want them to go, no matter how hard you practice." Crucial here is customization: the possibility for perfect technique or practice based on the synchronization of a toy and the body. For example, the customized body bag produces more intense sensations than a body bag a bit too large or too small for a user. Hailstorm boasts that he "didn't pick [his] floggers, they were made for [him]" by a friend: "We went down and we picked out this deerskin hide at the hide shop," and then "I went to his home and saw him make it. He custom-sized it for me in weight and balance." This is critical, of course, since Hailstorm wants properly balanced floggers both to perfect his throw and because he is known in the scene as a master of a difficult double-flogging technique (called "Florentine flogging")—this is the origin of his scene name. Dependent for their value in part on the skilled and educated consumer, toys enable social belonging through technique and training—in short, knowledge.

These kinds of exchanges rely on what Arjun Appadurai calls "consumer knowledge": "the knowledge that goes into appropriately consuming the commodity" (1988, 41). In a discussion of the "prestige economies of the modern West" (such as the art market), Appadurai—drawing on Baudrillard and Bourdieu—writes that these forms of consumption rely on "good taste, expert knowledge, 'originality,' and social distinction" (45). Consumer knowledge enables people to construct themselves as active subjects through differentiated consumption: by buying a Happy Tails whip *and* knowing how to use it. For it is not enough to simply buy toys; the production of SM subjects as educated and masterful consumers relies on their appropriate and skilled use of these commodities.

Consumer knowledge in BDSM is both a repertoire of technique and bodily knowledge. One of the critical functions of SM toys (and the techniques that go along with them) is to expand and reconfigure bodies, making novel sensations, positions, and relations possible. SM toys are carefully designed to amplify, prolong, or expand bodily sensations; toys are cataloged as stingy, thuddy, sharp, soft, cutting, surface, deep, intense, and so forth. The web page of Heartwood Whips, a highly respected purveyor, reads: "A whip which excites us is elegantly crafted. The passion which we feel for the erotic consensual exchange of power is translated into our creations. Beautiful leather feels wonderful not only in our hands as we work with it, but also in your hand when you play with it . . . each whip will express the unique power, and love of its owner." Their catalog of floggers is organized by material: deerskin, lightweight cowhide, elk, horsehair, rubber, regular cowhide, oil-tanned cowhide, bison, bull hide, lightweight buffalo, moose, and rabbit fur. Each material is capable of a different sensation. Deerskin floggers, for instance, are described as the softest: "This light velvety hide makes a perfect warm-up whip. It makes lots of noise but delivers a limited amount of impact. Deerskin is ideal for caressing the body like many erotic fingers." Bull hide is described as "the leather for whips with solid thud. It is a superior top-grain hide with an even surface texture. It is heavy, supple, and consistent in thickness."

In addition to materials, Heartwood floggers come in varying sizes (length of tails), densities (number of tails), colors, and styles of handle (which vary by length, thickness, color, braid pattern, type of knot, and type of loop).[5] Each of these variables determines the kinds of sensations a flogger can deliver; of course, the technique of the person throwing the flogger also makes a difference. About the length of the whip, Heartwood notes: "If you usually play in confined spaces, or like to whip in close proximity to your subject, then the short length whips will work best. If you like to whip with maximum impact, then the longer tail whips will deliver more force because of their additional weight and the fact that the ends of the tails will be traveling in a longer and, therefore, faster arc. But remember, if you are a heavy player, upper body strength and conditioning will play a part in how the bottom experiences your impact. Each type of whip has potential to deliver a specific kind of feeling, within a given range of intensity. For example, no matter how heavily you apply a deerskin whip, you will never turn it into a heavyweight flogger." Similar contrasts apply to the density or number of tails in a flogger, and the tail lengths; the tails of a particular flogger may be good for dragging over bodies, good for tall people, or good for people with less upper-body strength.

All major categories of toys—floggers, whips, canes and rods, paddles, and spankers—have their own specifications and sensation ranges.[6] They are designed to impart particular sensations to the skin of the bottom; they are also designed with the top's body in mind. A paddle, for example, allows a top to prolong a spanking without the top's hand getting sore. A cane produces sharp, stingy, cutting sensations and straight-lined marks or welts, all with minimal effort from the top since the cane is so light. Other categories of paraphernalia—clamps and clips, ropes, restraining devices, electricity, bondage devices, sex toys, gags, and hoods—are also designed to convey certain sensations to the body, amplifying or altering a top's capacity. Some sensations are possible using only the body, but they can be easier, stronger, more intense, or of longer duration using toys (compare, for instance, a strong pinch and the use of a clamp); some sensations are not possible with the body alone (for example, the shock of an electrical current). Either way, toys have a dramatic impact on the body at play, relying on and also rezoning and producing new knowledge of the body's range and potential.

In this way, SM is a body of knowledge about techniques and skills, mediated through toys. Easton and Liszt describe the toys that a top who has already acquired the beginning toy bag might want to consider. Their categories—helplessness toys, toys for hitting, toys for pinching, toys for poking, toys that heat or cool, toys that zap, toys for turning on and getting off, toys for role-playing, and toys for the road (1998b, 109–18)—are notable in that they rely both on knowledge of technique and attention to the body. For example, under "toys for hitting," Easton and Liszt write: "Long stiff rods fall under the category of canes. Bottoms mostly either love canes fanatically or hate them passionately—they hurt a lot, and the pain comes in two waves, one when the cane strikes, and another a few moments later when the tissue decompresses" (112). This begins to show the ways that SM relies on, and produces, particular bodily knowledge. To do SM, Atheris—a white dominant in her mid-thirties—tells me, "you just have to know a lot about the body": basic anatomy; the location of bones, organs, nerves, muscles, and fat; the way bruising and other skin damage works; blood flow; and other bodily systems. This knowledge of the body—about its organs, muscles, skin, and tissues—is one way SM functions as a form of biopower, operating through technique, cultivation, and education.

Vince described asking a lesbian friend for more information on how to flog his partner Pam's breasts or play with her labia: "As I learn to play with it [Pam's female body] more, part of it is anatomy . . . The first time I ever beat her tits I had to call up one of my friends and go 'Okay, so I heard this rumor . . . you know fibroid breasts'[7] . . . so I had to go get information . . . because [gesturing to Pam] your anatomy is different . . . The first time that I had your labia spread, it was only because I talked to someone and I found out that . . . it's really tough down there and you're not really going to tear it off, 'cause I really thought, okay it's thin, it's going to tear off!" Although Vince consulted a friend, classes on technique and SM skills always include a discussion of the body and anatomy as they bear on the topic at hand. Binding, suspension, flogging, and piercing require a repertoire of bodily knowledge about blood flow, body temperature, weight and pressure, tendons and connective tissue, organ tenderness, and skin depth. At a Janus caning class in April 2003, Brian, the instructor, explained that canes can do a lot of bodily damage, from welting, bruising, and breaking skin to breaking bones. Focusing on the skin, he said: "You can't hit someone very hard on places that are bony, but you can pretty much whale away on someone's ass. The skin is tight on the backs of the thighs, so it's easy to split the skin with a very hard hit . . . Be careful of the tip of the cane; the greater force can break the skin." "Also," he told us, "people with more melanin in their skin mark more, so be careful about that if you don't want to leave marks" (Brian was demonstrating with his African American partner, Charlotte).

Although it might be obvious that techniques for using toys, discussions of positions, and health and safety issues involved in different forms of play rely on explicit bodily knowledge, it is also true that less-technical training also invokes this anatomized body. Negotiation, for example, covers not only desires and limits but also specific bodily issues, problems, and needs. Both players are expected to know enough about bodies to know how weaknesses (for example, an old knee injury) might affect play. Aftercare, too, although frequently presented in psychological or affectual terms, is also about the body. Aftercare includes eating (most often some protein), drinking water, and resting the body, both immediately after a scene and for days afterward. From negotiation to aftercare, SM practice relies on and constructs various forms of bodily knowledge. This scientific, anatomical-physical knowledge constructs the body as a set of parts, each with its own needs, uses, and potential injuries.

Take, for example, the ass. Even a technique as simple and introductory as spanking requires a tremendous amount of bodily knowledge. Lady Green, a local expert, taught an Exiles spanking class I attended; she is also the author of *The Compleat Spanker* (1996). In her class, she covered such issues as how to safely support various body weights, problems people might have bending over, and how to protect the top's wrist when spanking.[8] Different techniques and positions for spanking (over the knee, bent over, lying face down, or standing), as well as the flow or rhythm of the spanking itself (warming up, varying blows, and pacing), are integrated into knowledge about the body and its skin, muscles, organs, and strong and weak spots.

Lady Green devotes a chapter of her book to anatomy. The pelvis and the femur, she tells us, are "large, sturdy bones" that are "buried in fat and muscle," so "unless you are spanking someone extremely elderly, you don't need to worry about injuring" them (18). However the coccyx (tailbone) is "fragile and quite sensitive to pain"; Lady Green recommends various techniques to ensure that the top is not spanking the coccyx. In the Exiles class, she suggested cupping the nonswatting hand around the bottom's tailbone, just to be safe. Moving on to the nerves, Lady Green explained that the body's largest nerve, the sciatic nerve, can be damaged from heavy paddling. Reminding us that the nerve is least protected when the person being spanked is bent over, she recommended a flat position (standing or lying down) for heavy paddling and, if the bottom is bent over, restricting the toys to lighter, "stingier implements." The large muscles of the ass (the gluteus maximus) and the thigh muscles are fair game, she writes: "Most people of normal size and fitness have very strong muscles in this area, that do an excellent job of protecting underlying structures" (21). However, one should avoid striking the lower backs of the thighs and knees, where the tendons, ligaments, and blood vessels are too delicate, as well as the kidneys, which are easily damaged. Finally, Lady Green discusses the skin: marking (caused by breaking tiny capillaries, and more likely when the bottom is using blood-thinning drugs), welting, bruising, blistering, and abrasion (more likely with rougher toys) are usually undesirable, whereas warming (increasing the circulation of blood to the ass area) is desirable; both entail careful technique.

This ass is subject to such anatomizing, clinical scrutiny that it nearly becomes a free-standing object. In *Beyond Vanilla*, Claes Lilja's 2001 documentary on BDSM, a man explains to the camera where one should aim when flogging a bottom's ass. He divides the ass in question into "quadrants" and tells us that we should focus most of the force on the lower, inside quadrant, an area commonly called the "sweet spot." Lady Green also recommends hitting the sweet spot: "The lower inner portion of the butt is fed by a nerve group called the 'posterior S4 dermatome,'" which is "shared by the genitals. Many spanking fans refer to this 'low and inside' area as the 'sweet spot' because being spanked there feels so good" (1996, 20). Combining toys and technique, bodily and technical knowledge, these practices divide the body in play into parts, pieces, and zones of pleasure and potential. These divisional zones apply to parts of the body, but also to the body as a whole: there are commonly agreed-upon red (unsafe), green (safe), and yellow (use caution) zones of the body. The red zone is out of bounds; it includes bony or unprotected areas like the spine, feet, and head, or areas with sensitive organs like the kidneys. The green zone is almost always safe: fatty or especially muscular areas—the upper back, ass, and thighs. The yellow zone includes legs and arms, locations that are safe for certain things but not others. These zones or parts are objectified, detached from the whole body through this medicalized gaze. The goal of this anatomical knowledge is twofold: to minimize bodily damage (inciting the management of risk) and to maximize bodily pleasure or sensation across these zones of play.

This body bears a striking similarity to the body that Foucault describes as "desexualized," the counterattack (to "sex-desire") that concludes the first volume of his *History of Sexuality* ([1976] 1990, 157). For Foucault, desexualization diffuses sensuality and pleasure across the entire surface of the body, so that desire does not adhere in genital pockets. In his interviews, Foucault suggests that SM, in particular, can create this sort of diffusion: "It's a question of multiplying and burgeoning of the body, an exaltation, in some way autonomous, of its least

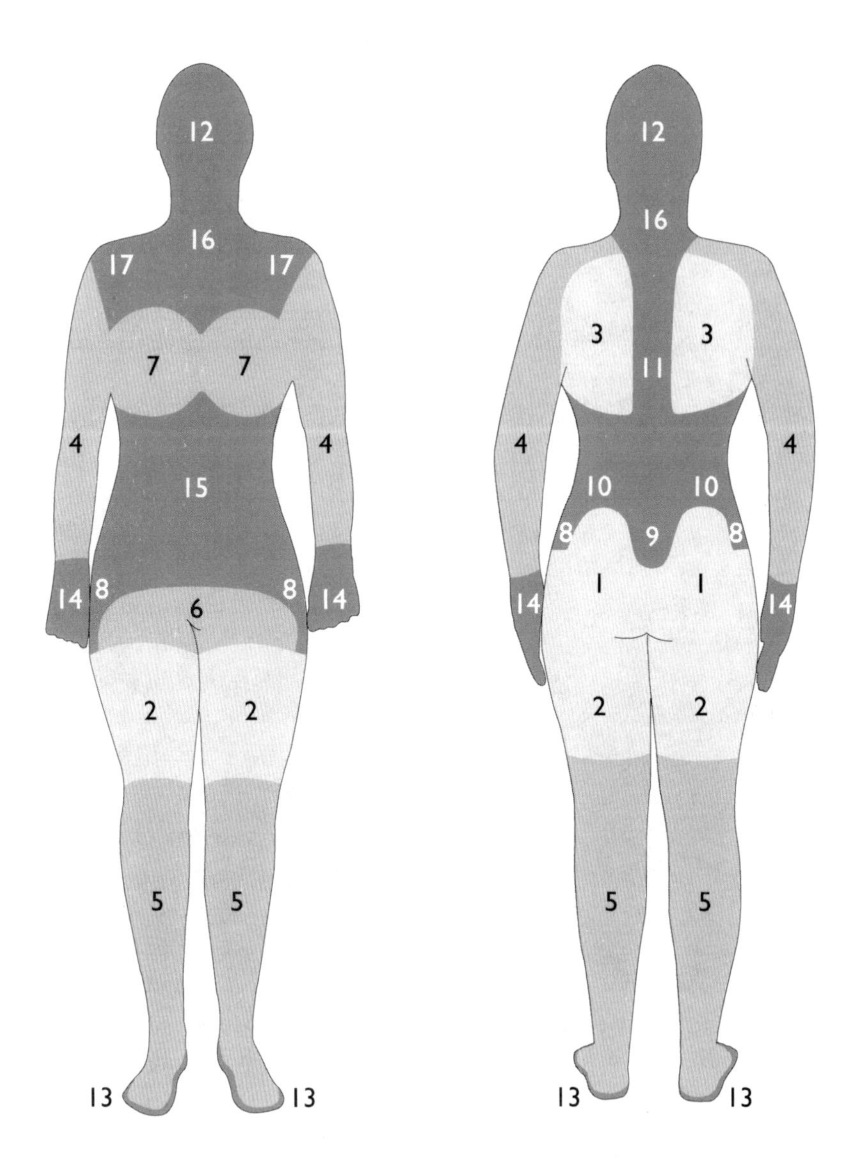

The safe zone is (1) butt cheeks, (2) thighs, and (3) upper back. The caution zone is (4) arms, (5) calves, (6) genitals and pelvis, and (7) breasts. The unsafe zone is (8) hips, (9) tailbone, (10) kidney area, (11) spine, (12) head, (13) soles of the feet, (14) hands, (15) abdomen, (16) neck and throat, and (17) shoulders.

parts, of the least possibilities of a body fragment . . . It's the body made entirely malleable by pleasure: something that opens itself, tightens, palpitates, beats, gapes" ([1975–76] 1996, 186–87; see also [1982] 1996, 331; [1983] 1996; [1984] 1996). For Foucault, such experiences require both the generalization of sensation across the body and the fragmentation of the body.

Yet this body also depends on consumption and knowledge practices. As Miranda Joseph argues, capitalism and community have a supplementary relationship: each depends on the other for completion and coherence (2002, 2). Yet, as Joseph notes, this relationship is obscured through a romantic discourse of community, in which community is imagined to humanize the social relations lost with capitalism. There is a similar relationship between toys and subjectivity: SM subjectivity produces and is produced by the market for SM toys and paraphernalia. Here, as Miller argues, there is a tendency to oppose consumption to authentic sociality or culture (1995, 30). Instead, capitalism, and consumption in particular, is productive; people become practitioners with a sense of collective belonging to the SM community by developing such technical and bodily knowledge and buying and using toys.

The ever-expanding market for toys and other SM accouterments means that SM practice and, critically, SM desire are also proliferating. This is acknowledged via a joke in the SM community: "never say never" is a common warning, and one not infrequently directed at me, that refers to the ways in which exposure to new toys or techniques might produce new desires. Yet like flexibility, proliferation is double-edged: it opens possibilities for subjects (new pleasures, desires, sexualities) but it is dependent on commodity exchange. I am not simply arguing that commodity exchange generates inauthentic desires (desires that cannot be satisfied, desires that drive consumption as opposed to more-authentic desires). Desires—demands or needs in an exchange relation—are socially produced. Rather, such desires are produced within hierarchical social relations where some have much more access than others to these commodities, education, and, thus, pleasures. What is being produced in BDSM is both new forms of pleasure and new forms of social privilege. That desire endlessly proliferates means that new pleasures are continuously made possible through new knowledge, toys, and techniques. That these proliferating desires are dependent on toys, however, gives practitioners differential community access to such pleasures.

The development of SM subjectivity and belonging as a practice of consumption is experienced within a cultural formation of neoliberal rationality. This means that the dependence on commodities is seen less as a social problem and more as a reinforcement of neoliberal ideas of freedom, where "freedom is reduced to choice: choice of commodities, of lifeways, and, most of all, of identities" (Comaroff and Comaroff 2004, 190). In this exchange of freedom to consume for other forms of freedom, social regulation and hierarchy—based on race, gender, class, and sexuality—are reinvigorated and enforced. As I will describe in more depth in the following two chapters, the neoliberal rationality that pervades the Bay Area also justifies these social hierarchies, enabling practitioners to imagine that racial, classed, and gendered inequalities are, instead, freely chosen positionalities for which one must take personal responsibility. The belief in the "free," unfettered market, and more flexible and mobile forms of capitalism, locates autonomy in consumption.

But not for all: these changes have not gone uncontested within the SM community. Indeed, with nostalgia that parallels the criticism of the rules, many in the SM community imagine the past—the old guard scene—as a lost space of social belonging that was not mediated through commodities. In this telling of the unregulated old guard days, a time before "more people, more money, and more commercialization," toys were, instead, tools.[9] Community historian david stein writes that the rise of the new SM scene "occurred during the same period that S/M activity came to be almost universally referred to as 'play' [instead of 'work'], S/M practitioners as 'players,' and the tools we use as 'toys.'" He continues, sarcastically: "The same revolution that decoupled heterosex from procreation and gave us sport-fucking has turned S/M into a sex-optional form of recreation . . . Less hazardous than football but almost as strenuous, it even has aerobic benefits" (2002, 5; see also Magister 1991, 98). Toys are commodities, always threatening to fall into an inauthentic, because too easily purchased, "Stand & Model" S&M. Tools, on the other hand, are valued for what they can do. Turning now to community debates about what has been lost in the transition to a more commodified scene, I explore how toys, and toy consumption, produce subjectivity and community in complex and contradictory ways, generating belonging but also social anxiety.

Community anxiety centers around lost social connections, the shift from an SM based on passion to an SM based on purchasing ability. In a dialogue on class in the now-defunct SM zine *Brat Attack*, Toni notes: "A lot of the 'stars' are people who have—they have a dungeon, they have toys . . . there's this whole movement to have the newest, strangest toy, or the strangest talent. I think it's really sad sometimes, because you can take someone out there with your hands and a belt. Or just your hands . . . It seems like as it becomes more chi-chi to be a pervert, we are also becoming more commodified, and consumerized. And that offends me because I find a lot of things that are spiritually important to me about SM getting lost."[10] In addition to the loss of authentic connection, Toni's comments suggest that, although "cheaper" leathers and toys are available, the inability to buy the latest or best toy relegates one to a second-tier belonging in the community. In the same discussion, Christine argues: "There's something about work exchange [working at a play party in exchange for door fees] that's humiliating. Why do I have to give up some time and do this work exchange to get in—'cause I'm not good enough, I don't have enough money to just pay and not think about it. So I think about it long and hard and then go, ok ok, it's worth it to me, I'm going to pay the money so I don't have to deal with that. And that's considering that I even have the money to do it." For Christine, it is "worth it" to pay for the party to become a good enough practitioner: a person who belongs at the party. Jeneieve points out the practical downside of work exchange: "It's tiring, too. If I go and I work a [party] shift at six o'clock that means I've got to be dressed and I'm going to figure out if I'm going to play, like all the stuff that I play with, I've got to bring all that. So we're talking an all-day thing, right, then I've got to get there at six and work there for three hours if I want to play. Otherwise if you try to play around eleven o'clock there's no way you'll get any dungeon space. And then you're tired by then, and I'm a top, so . . . you know, it's like I've got to have energy." Even if one accepts this exchange of work for "free" play as a reasonable accommodation (and not a way that the community creates tiers of classed belonging), this discussion shows that belonging to the SM community and being a recognized practitioner is bound to income: the assumption that one has the money to play.

Of course, some practitioners contest this. Teramis, for example, is adamant that "SM itself doesn't cost jack shit . . . A tone of voice and a hand is more than sufficient for a scene that can last for days, and clothespins from the laundry bag. SM doesn't have to be expensive." But, she notes, "if you're new and that's your introduction to the community, you're going to be inclined to [say,] 'Oh, I want leather cuffs just like that!' You could also use a bandana tied correctly, but you don't think about that when everybody around you has leather cuffs." Edward—a white, heterosexual dominant in his mid-thirties—tells me he has between $600 and $700 in toys and equipment, a comparatively low number (most practitioners estimated owning between $1,500 and $3,000 worth of toys), in part because he is willing and able to make his own furniture (like his homemade St. Andrew's cross), and in part because he likes what are called "pervertables," vanilla items that can be converted into an SM toy.[11] He explains: "You can spend $150 on a custom-made paddle, but why, when a $5 paddle does the same thing? I'm not in it for the looks. I'm not in it for a fashion show. [If] a $5 paddle does the same thing as a $200 paddle, I'm happy."

Yet, as I discussed above, many people believe that a $5 paddle does not do the same thing as a $200, customized paddle. This drives a kind of toy collecting in which, as Annalee puts it, people can "really get into the technicality of" SM toys: " 'How many size canes do you have?' 'Well, I have size three, size five-inch, and size twelve-inch, and each one has its own special properties' . . . that [relentless consumerism] appeals to the middle-class person who has six kinds of frying pans—they also have six kinds of cat-o'-nine tails."[12] Some of my interviewees had the room for a serious home dungeon; during my interviews, Lady Thendara, Mark, and Mark F., a white, gay top in his late forties, each took me on a tour of their home dungeons. I left the tape running during my tour of Lady Thendara and Latex Mustang's space; the transcribed tour is twenty-pages long. Throughout the tour, Thendara made comments like "This is really embarrassing . . . that we would have this much stuff!" and "You *can* have too many toys!"—comments that betray a familiarly anxious stance toward consumerism. But at the same time, they showed her pleasure: her toys and furniture were obviously loved and cared-for objects, carefully cataloged and arranged.

One wall was mostly taken up with clear plastic storage boxes filled with color-coordinated goods, the boxes neatly labeled: "clamps," "gags," "latex," "pain," "crops." As she narrated the tour of her home dungeon, she gave each object a story, explaining how she likes to use it, where she got it, and what it means for her play:

> Here's some different floggers. . . . This is actually a Happy Tails one . . . This is a Sarah Lashes—you know how when you shop you can say this is Donna Karan's? [Well], this is a Sarah Lashes, this is a Happy Tails, this one we got at a Taste of Leather and I don't know who makes it . . . This is a horsehair flogger. It's very light—if you used it very hard, it would cut skin. I've never used it that hard . . . This is a natural rattan cane. This I got at Cost Plus ages ago, it's really good, it's really stingy . . . This is a very mean cane. It's very stingy, carbon fiber . . . We've got a couple of these long whips . . . This is a buggy whip . . . and then this is my very favorite flogger. This is called Butter. I don't usually name my toys, but that one gets a name 'cause it's so soft . . . This is one of his [Mustang's] favorite collars, especially 'cause it locks on . . . This is stuff that we were playing with the other night, so I like to keep it all nice and neat. It's a really good blindfold, it's a $30 blindfold. Most of them are about ten bucks, but it really blocks out all the light and it's very comfortable to wear for long periods of time . . .

Thendara told me that she and Mustang have never done the same scene twice; part of the appeal of SM for them is novelty and variability. This couple has more disposable income than most, and their dungeon and toys reflect this. In addition to standard toys, Thendara and Mustang have an assortment of very expensive toys: a vac sack, body bags, a variety of bondage and restraining equipment, and the specialized paraphernalia for pony play (hooves, saddles, reins, knee pads, tails, Thendara's riding outfits, curry brushes, headdresses, and even a cart that Thendara sits in and Mustang pulls). Mustang explains that they typically spend between $1,500 and $2,000 a year on toys, but, he points out: "It's no different than owning a boat. It is my major interest in my life and I have very specific and very unique interests, not only to play with certain things but to collect them . . . I have disposable income and it's one of the things I've decided to spend it on."

The consumption that drives this collecting is not, of course, unique to SM. Paul, like many, told me that SM is more about "emotional connection and intensity" than toys, but then flippantly remarked: "You know, I'm a hetero guy, I like collecting things."[13] When I asked him about the size of his collection, he said: "It's never large enough! Jesus my Lord, what are you saying? For God's sake, woman! We live in a consumer economy; there's never enough. There's no such thing as enough!" Paul, here, is mocking the compulsion to buy, collect, pack, display, and organize toys (and, to a lesser extent, clothing); he is also pointing to the compulsory nature of such consumer practices. Consuming is a primary mechanism through which SM practitioners solidify their identities and their belonging within the SM community.

Yet both Paul and Thendara also highlight the anxiety that such reliance on toys engenders. For example, Don admits that "it gets really expensive if you decide you want to get esoteric about it," buying specialty floggers, or tools for electricity play. But he continues: "I guess I'm just a toy whore. I like sensation and I like having a broad palette to work with. In just floggers alone, I probably have six or seven, all different sizes, different materials, and there's a couple more that I want 'cause they're unique." A comment like this one points to the ways in which the desire for newness and diverse sensations fuels consumerism, while at the same time, the joking disavowal of "I guess I'm just a toy whore" shows Don's discomfort or unease.

Part of this anxiety stems from a concern with being *just* a consumer, where consuming is understood as an inauthentic social relation. Like the rules that are seen as eroding authentic connections between practitioners, toys produce some anxiety about a possible overreliance on commodities and the concomitant forsaking of social ties. Participants in the *Brat Attack* roundtable discuss this in terms of the ability to "purchase an identity" or buy the lifestyle, instead of doing the necessary labor to become a practitioner:

> TONI: I have a real hard time not getting pissy about that, especially when I see people who can just walk out and buy it. Like someone I know who has a lot of money . . . she decided she was a pervert one day and she [snap] had the pants, had the jacket—
>
> JENEIEVE: Just went out and bought everything, right? . . .
>
> TONI: And I was so annoyed . . . I think, "This doesn't mean anything spiritual to you!" And who am I to judge that—but of course I do. I think, "Ok—you've been a perv for 8 hours."

ROE: But even if they go out and they have all their stuff custom made, I know that I can tell. It's the way they wear it, the way they conduct themselves. They can put everything on, they can have it all custom made, they could posture, they can have the whole array of toys, and not really have a clue in a sense . . . I'm sorry, but they just don't have a clue. Because it's not coming as an intrinsic part of their personality.

This discussion suggests that the ability to purchase SM paraphernalia so easily, and have these purchases signify one's SM identity or community belonging, will destroy the spiritual center, heart, or something else *authentic* about SM relationality. If people can simply buy into this community, then a community of practitioners with authentic desire and identity is in jeopardy. The anxiety is that class status gives one an unearned, free (from labor) ticket into social belonging via toys: BDSM as "Stand & Model."

As Lady Hilary explained, when she first came out, you had to work to earn your boots, vest, chaps, and jacket, and now you just "go out and buy it. And there's nothing wrong with that but there's nothing special about it either . . . It meant something, and now people just show up. It's good that people can show up and see that they have choices, but the ritual or the sacredness of it is gone." She continues, describing the new scene in contrast to the old guard rituals: "It's no longer a private club. It's no longer a secret. It's no longer sacred . . . anyone can walk in . . . Do I want new people to learn? Yes. Is it a good venue for them to learn? Sure. But it still has watered down the intensity that you found when you had to search for the answers . . . It's too accessible, it's too easy, no one has to work for it anymore, you're not expected to work for anything." This emphasis on "work" focuses attention on the ways practitioners want other people to "earn" their identity as practitioners, not just buy it from a store; toys might short-circuit the necessary labor involved in becoming a practitioner.[14] At the same time, however, Hilary explained that although she could live without toys, she wouldn't want to: "Toys, for me, are about giving in to the moment . . . [it's] part of the ritual. It moves my head space into finding and focusing intensity." There is a fine line between becoming a practitioner through the (tainted, inauthentic) buying of an identity versus the (skillful, masterful) use of toys to create scenes.

One way to read this anxiety explores the toy as a fetish, a reading that corresponds to some of the ways practitioners relate to their objects. Vick—a white, lesbian daddy/top in her mid-forties—explains why leather is appealing: "Some of this stuff is just really pretty to look at and nice to play with. I mean, I saw a guy wearing a bondage suit and . . . your mind starts going off on what you can do with it, 'cause it's really cool. But you could just take Saran Wrap, too. I mean, it doesn't quite have that black leather look to it or smell, but it works. I think part of the intensity, part of why people are into leather, is the smell of it. There's something about the feel of it; it's very sensual." Hailstorm expresses similar feelings when he describes how he gets ready to play: "You open up your toy bag with all of your implements, and then you take out your toys and you line them all up . . . You have restraints, so you might have leather restraints, they might be fleece lined, and then you might have little locks on them . . . And then you have the other paraphernalia, which I love and I don't know why—you have the snap hooks and the chains and the quick release, and I just love all that kind of stuff. The shininess and the sound it makes when it clicks together, it just—there's something about it I really like." Chris comments: "There's almost a fetish around the toys themselves, and switching among the toys, and the anticipation of the toy or the threat of a toy. That's pretty big, that's hot." For these practitioners, it is not only the use of toys but the toys themselves—their material, feel, smell, look, and sound—that matters.

Taking Chris literally, then, toys are a kind of fetish, a way to plan or prepare for a scene, to mark one's intentionality, and to transport players out of mundane reality. Anne McClintock argues that imbuing objects with fetishistic power enables such a transformation; it also enables a production of the scene as safe and separate. She writes: "By scripting and controlling the frame of representation . . . the player stages the delirious loss of control within a situation of extreme control" (1995, 147). As I will discuss in the following chapters, toys along with the rules help to produce this controlled scene, figuring the SM scene as a "safe space" through the bracketing function of the SM play frame. The toy as fetish is one reason why pervertables like Saran Wrap aren't as desirable as leather cuffs and metal chains: toys enable and produce an SM scene that is imagined as safely outside real social relations.

But thinking of the toy as fetish also allows us to parse some of the practitioners' anxieties about the role of toys in the scene. Loosely following both Freud's and Marx's understanding of the fetish, we can see toys as stand-ins or substitutes for missing social relations—sexual relations for Freud[15] and social relations (of production) for Marx[16]—in such a way as to produce social relationships between people and things, or things and things, instead of between people and people. Linda Williams argues that "for both [Freud and Marx], fetishization involves the construction of a substitute object to evade the complex realities of social or psychic relations" (1989, 105; see also Allison 2000; Appadurai 1988; Apter and Pietz 1993).[17] The saturation of BDSM communities with things seeming to stand in for authentic relationships between practitioners occasions both pleasure and anxiety.

I attended a Janus class in September 2002, right before the Folsom Street Fair, called "Shopping at Folsom." The class was intended to help people find quality toys and not get too caught up in a "buying frenzy" at the fair. The presenters reminded us: "There will be other opportunities to buy toys!" As one put it: "When you're surrounded by all those vendors, your wallet is burning a hole in your pants!" They provided tips on differentiating a hobbyist toy seller from a reputable one, on determining whether something is a reasonable price, on negotiating a discount, and on how to judge the quality of toys. In his presentation, Charles told us: "You have to remember you are buying the item, not the fantasy. You are buying a ball gag, not the pretty girl in the catalog [modeling the gag]." He was reminding us that the slippage between ball gag and girl means that the gag is standing in for both the desired girl and a shared social relationship; he was simultaneously pointing to and distancing himself from the social relations imagined to be eclipsed in a consumer's "frenzy" for an object.

Eroticizing the smell or look of leather, the sound of restraints or whips, or the knife rather than the hand that wields it provokes both pleasure and anxiety, which must be read culturally and historically. Following McClintock, we can read the fetish as the "historical enactment of ambiguity itself," where social contradictions—in the organization of race, sexuality, and gender; between the private or domestic and the public or market; and between the personal and the socioeconomic and historical—are displaced onto an object (1995, 184; 1992). She notes, however, that such a displacement does not resolve these contradictions or crises of meaning, but rather imbues the object with those tensions. In this way, we might see this displaced ambiguity as enabling both the fetishization of objects within SM and the dense pleasure/anxiety nexus that such displacements perpetually generate. Toys, in this reading, function as a fetish as long as they are imbued with the displaced contradictions of contemporary social relations. It is not surprising, then, that practitioners are ambivalent about the saturation of commodities in the scene, or that they express this concern by simultaneously celebrating consumerism (along with connoisseurship) and expressing anxieties about its effect on social and sexual relations.

This reading, emphasizing the ambivalence of the toy as fetish, allows us to depart from the more one-sided understanding of bodily commodification as necessarily alienating, or productive of a violent dehumanization. In anthropological work on, for example, the global market in human organs, the divisibility of a body into parts detached from a whole person not only objectifies the body, but, as Leslie Sharp writes, can also "dehumanize individuals and categories of persons in the name of profit" (2000, 293; see also Scheper-Hughes 2002b, 78, and 2002a). For Sharp, bodily fragmentation disrupts an organic wholeness or an integrated, noncommodifiable person. Of course, the kinds of divisions that these authors discuss entail very different power inequalities and ethics than those at work in the SM scene. Taking this comparative risk, however, I do want to argue that, to think through SM play, we must avoid a critique of technology undergirded by a desire for an authentic wholeness of the person or the body. One can see this technophobic reading in Sharp, who writes: "Especially unsettling is the now routine use of a host of artificial, mechanical prostheses that extend life and enhance bodies. Heart valves, pace makers, artificial hip joints, prosthetic arms and legs . . . are now regularly implanted in human bodies. Furthermore, the monster now has a legitimate (and unstigmatized) medical label: 'chimera'" (2000, 311). Like the romance of community and the nostalgia for the old guard past, such imaginings fail to see that the circuits between technology and techniques produce new possibilities for the production of subjects and communities, even as these possibilities are constrained through such knowledge practices.

SM bodily knowledge can be understood as part of the ongoing cyborgification of human bodies. The wired, technicalized body is bisected with biotechnological knowledge; this produces the body in play as a cyborg body (Haraway 1991).[18] Driven as they are by SM toys and the techniques to use them, as well as the formalization of SM knowledge practices, these bodies are deeply embedded in flexible late capitalism. But the risks of such hybridization lie less in the creation of a monstrous, artificial, enhanced body, and more in the reentrenchment of the class inequalities that enable such transformative experiences to begin with. Donna Haraway calls on us to recognize both the risks and the potentials of technological relationality; she insists that we must refuse the dream of wholeness as we take responsibility for new networks of domination. This is the biopolitics of capitalism; SM's bodily knowledge is produced, in part, by new biotechnological knowledge (see also E. Martin 1994; Rose 2007). These knowledges receive careful attention as practitioners augment and analyze their own bodies and bodily techniques in the service of ever-better play. As new toys and techniques are developed, practitioner knowledge about the body and its parts grows, and this cycle of commodity-body-knowledge is transformative—and productive. The body in parts is also a body in play. It is at once a commoditized and an objectified body, opened to diverse sensations and pleasures that are enabled, if not bound, by toys: Foucault's desexualized body as a consuming subject. In this way, these flexible, agile bodies are reconstituted in fragments, open to pleasures provided by new techniques and new commodities.

Technophobic readings obscure the ways in which forms of exchange (including the objectification and commodification of the body) produce social relations, along with new forms of subjectivity, embodiment, and community. Paying attention to technological prostheses, we can see the social relationships produced by toys: buying and collecting toys produces good capitalist citizens—consumer-subjects—a position coercively normalized as well as anxiety-generating and pleasurable. Belonging to the SM community and being a real SM practitioner are deeply tied to practices of consumption, while the class basis of leisure time and money enable some more than others to take on this identity (leaving others to "work harder" for it). In this way, exploring the pleasure and anxiety discursively produced at this nexus illuminates the social fetishization of the toy: toys are necessary for SM social connection and, at the same time, toys might deprive us of social connection—a contradictory relationship that requires us to broaden our understanding of exchange to account for both commodity and power exchange.

CONNECTION

DYNAMICS OF EXCHANGE AND THE TOY AS PROSTHETIC

If the toy refigures the body as an object of knowledge but also of pleasure through techniques, what about the actual playing? For one does not only collect, smell, fondle, buy, choose, label, and lay out one's toys; one also plays with them. And it is here, in the playing, that toys reveal a different relationality. The body in play—divisible in pleasure—points to the circuits between person and object, body and subject; each version connects the flesh to exchanges of commodities, knowledge, and power. The interconnectivity of toys and bodies in play requires and produces productive, flexible subjects but also possibilities for connection and intimacy.

The social connectivity of SM play is an interesting object of community debate, since "connection" is one of the primary motivations for SM play. Many people I spoke with described SM as producing a special kind of intimacy or connection; some modified this with "energy" or "spiritual."[19] Larry explains: "About half the people come into the leather scene looking for sex . . . [but] generally what they find, the longer time they spend in a true SM dungeon, their reason for being in the dungeon isn't sexuality, it's spirituality and the exchange of energy with other play partners. The longer they're in the scene, the closer that becomes to truth with every visit they make, because they soon learn that there's a lot more to power exchange than just having sex with a bunch of different people. You can go to an orgy for sex. That's not what a dungeon's about. A dungeon's about power exchange, the spirituality of power exchange and the spirituality of energy that resides within us and how to exchange that energy with other people." Larry's comments make it clear that real SM is not about "sex" (Foucault's "sex-desire"), nor is it about commodities; real SM is about "energy" or "power exchange."

In her Exiles class "Setting the Scene," Cal told us that an emphasis on toys can be distracting: you can't get to your erotic center if you're too busy fussing with toys. So, she said, "even though I work at Mr. S, you should reduce your toy bag" and focus instead on giving your energy to the moment. This critique of toy fetishism was echoed in Doris's class on sensual domination, called "Bringing Them to Their Knees." At one point in the class, Doris, seated at the front of the room, slowly and sensually fed strawberries to an audience member, who knelt at her feet. "These are just strawberries, not fancy toys from Mr. S," she told us. "When shared with passion, things that might seem boring are transformed into something exciting and special." SM, she said, is about closeness, intimacy, pleasure, and seduction, not about the toys themselves: "It's not about your skills with a flogger, or how many knots you know; it's about caring and crafting a scene." When you play, she continued, make sure that your bottom is subbing to *you*, not to the music or to your flogger. Doris and Cal emphasized that SM play requires practitioners to be in the moment, to care, and to create intimacy, forms of exchange that might be blocked when you are "fussing" with toys or expecting toys to do the work of connection for you.

Like the concern that toys provide an unearned, class-based shortcut for the labor of becoming a practitioner, the concern here is that imagining that SM requires nothing more than technique and a toy bag places too little emphasis on authentic connection. As Stephanie notes, there are some people, especially newcomers, who think: "Oh, if I had the technical skill, that's really all I need. If I learn how to use a singletail, if I learn how to wield a knife . . . that's what this [SM] is." They are wrong, of course; SM is "about confidence and it's about respect and it's about understanding people . . . It's such an important thing, it's such a deep, profound connection to people." Similarly, Paul tells me: "things have an appeal for me. But, you know, my ideal isn't to have lots and lots of toys and lots and lots of beautiful girls to put in the toys . . . I really want to be in love with someone."[20] Of course, and importantly, very few of the people I interviewed felt that *their own* use of toys distracted them from their partners. Skillful players use toys (thus, toys become tools), as well as techniques and bodily knowledge, to create a connection between players.

These concerns show how the toy contains multiple social contradictions, including those between objects and people, and between inauthentic and authentic intimacies or social relations. In part, this is because the toy is also a prosthesis. In an essay on how the Guatemalan nation—as a body politic—uses the *mujer Maya* (Mayan women) to prop itself up, Diane Nelson argues for something she calls "prosthetic relationality": the ways the body "changes through its articulation with the prosthetic which must be *incorporated* by the body that relies on it" (2001, 305; italics in original).[21] Nelson is building on Elizabeth Grosz's argument in *Volatile Bodies*, where Grosz writes: "Anything that comes into contact with the surface of the body and remains there long enough will be incorporated into the body image—clothing, jewelry, other bodies, objects . . . External objects, implements, and instruments with which the subject continuously interacts become, while they are being used, intimate, vital, even libidinously cathected parts of the body image" (1994, 80). The prosthetic mediates across binaries (especially mind/body, self/other, and public/private) but also connects disparate parts. It challenges an articulation of the liberal subject as independent and autonomous by stressing the connections between bodies, and between bodies and machines via incorporation.

In a discussion of body image and phantom limbs, Grosz quotes Paul Schilder: "The body image can shrink or expand; it can give parts to the outside world and can take other parts into itself. When we take a stick in our hands and touch an object with the end of it, we feel a sensation at the end of the stick. The stick has, in fact, become part of the body image . . . it then becomes part of the bony system of the body" (quoted in Grosz 1994, 80). Similarly, SM tools, clothing, objects, and instruments become attached to the body, become a part of the body when they are used. Sometimes this is exceedingly obvious, as is the case with Panther and his fangs. Panther has a set of fangs that were "custom-made specifically for my mouth and the shape of my teeth." He was wearing them during our interview but took them off to eat, explaining that he didn't want to risk breaking them and have to go through the time and expense of replacement (there is only one man who makes them, and they cost $170). But he wore them to meet me because he was breaking them in: "I want to get to the point where I'm totally comfortable with them in. I'll probably wear them for a month or so, until my mouth is really comfortable with them." His fangs, which are a key part of his SM identity, are also a part of his body. Jewelry such as collars and piercings (along with brandings, scars, and tattoos) are also relatively clear cases of bodily transformation. I met many submissives and slaves who wore collars all the time; sometimes the collars were decorative (they looked more like vanilla necklaces), but sometimes they were not. In either case, the collar becomes a part of the body in much the same way that a tattoo does: it transforms one's body in the image of one's desire. Similarly, wearing piercings, handkerchiefs, or rings on the left side of the body signifies one is a top, while wearing them on the right side signifies one is a bottom. Wearing markers like this is yet another way that clothes, jewelry, or accessories might become part of the body, thus transforming an unmarked body into a particular SM body (a top, a bottom, a slave, a panther) as part of a process of identity making via the incorporation of objects.

Like Schilder's stick, toys can also become a part of the body through their use, and this use transforms the body. A flogger can be incorporated into a top's body through rhythms, sensations, and muscle movements. As a prosthetic, toys do not fill a gap or lack but rather work as an extension: they allow the top to reach out two or more feet beyond the end of the hand; they give the top access to a wide range of sensations—scratching, biting, cutting, petting, and belting—that may not be possible to inflict with the body alone; they transform the bodies of both top and bottom. In this use, toys—detached objects—become tools. Grosz notes: "It is only insofar as the object ceases to remain an object and becomes a medium, a vehicle for impressions and expression, that it can be used as an instrument or tool" (1994, 80).

In this way, tools convey and carry the intentionality of their users; they are inalienable. Doris's strawberries are "not fancy toys from Mr. S," but, "shared with passion," they are "transformed into something exciting and special"; Heartwood's whips "express the unique power and love of its owner" because the whip maker's "passion" is "translated into our creations." This language of translation and transformation suggests that these tools contain and express their users and their makers. We could read this in terms of the fetish, where floggers are imagined to contain the identities of their consumers—their passion or desire. We could also read this in terms of the gift or the tool, where floggers serve as an inalienable medium for the users' and makers' (and, perhaps, recipients') desire. But reading toys as prostheses does more than blur or transfer the site of relationality from objects to people; it also shows that when toys become tools, incorporated into bodies, they become vehicles for connection.

This kind of exchange—the community definition of power exchange—relies on commodity exchange to produce something practitioners call "connection." Here, Appadurai's emphasis on the social dynamics of exchange relationships encourages us to see these exchanges as densely, and complexly, social (1988, 48). Appadurai argues that "consumption is eminently social, relational, and active, rather than private, atomic, or passive"; it is not based on universalized or naturalized needs, but on culturally specific processes of negotiation, an active location of "sending" and "receiving" "social messages" (31). Thinking culturally about this exchange encourages us to see that what is being exchanged varies; my interviewees used words like "control," "trust," "respect," "energy," "love," "safety," "protection," "sensation," "pain," "authority," and "responsibility" (see also Moser and Madeson 1996, 27–30). But it is through this exchange that practitioners feel connection when they play. Hailstorm tells me: "When I hit somebody, I feel it . . . I can relate to where they are if I'm feeling their pain, if I'm up there with them, then I can do a better job at what I'm doing. I don't believe in standing back and whaling on somebody. I'm always up there and I'm always touching." Feeling through the flogger—or, more precisely, incorporating the flogger into his body's nervous system—Hailstorm is describing the density of connections in a circuit between top, flogger, and bottom. There is an exchange at work in SM: toys became a medium not only of sensation, but of intimate connection to others. Similarly, Francesca tells me, when her partner is flogging her, "I'm working with my partner . . . it's like wanting to plow through something . . . together." Mediated through commodities, such play creates intimate connections between people; the toy as prosthetic becomes a social prosthesis—a way to produce connection and intimacy.

Indeed, at these moments, there is little differentiation among the top, toy, and bottom—the skin surface does not contain the body. Instead the body is desexualized, transformed into a medium or receptacle of sensation that is often not sexual or genital. In her autoethnographic account of San Francisco's LINKS SM parties in the early 1990s, Susan Stryker writes of taking over for another top during a flogging scene:

> Something serene and paradoxically solitary can be found in the experience of giving oneself over to the inhabitation and enactment of a shared pattern of motion—a contemplative solitude born of one's ecstatic displacement into a space where the body actively receives and transmits the movements of others . . . a whip strikes flesh with sufficient force to blossom the creature's skin red and welt it back toward the leather. The young thing moans a low moan, transforming the kinetic energy of the blow into an audible frequency by passing breath over

> slack vocal chords, and my attention is drawn toward the physicality of the assemblage we cohabit . . . this is not, for me, primarily a sexual experience. (2008, 41)

Instead, as Stryker reflects on this space of embodied exchange, she writes: "I envision my body as a meeting point, a node, where external lines of force and social determination thicken into meat and circulate as a movement back into the world . . . [in] proprioceptic awareness, as I flog, of the role of my body as a medium in the circuit of transmissions, and of the material efficiency I process in my subjective ability [to pattern, to flog, to choreograph]" (42). The body in play is attuned to its own motion. But it is also connective, through the flogging: Stryker flogs; the whip meets flesh, which welts "back toward the leather"; a moan draws attention to "the assemblage we cohabit." This circuit, in Stryker's lyrical writing, enacts—produces—a shared space of embodiment; the exchange of motion, pain, and sound is embodied as well as productive. Stryker concludes: "S/M had become for me . . . a technology for the production of (trans)gendered embodiment, a mechanism for dismembering and disarticulating received patterns of identification, affect, sensation and appearance, and for reconfiguring, coordinating and remapping them in bodily space" (43).

That this exchange isn't "sexual" draws attention, again, to the Foucauldian distinction between what Jeremy Carrette terms "pleasure-intensity" and "sexuality-desire." In an essay on theology and SM, Carrette argues that, because pleasure is nonproductive, SM "becomes a site of resistance because it seeks to reconfigure pleasure in its intensity of exchange rather than through its productive or commercial value" (2005, 23). This exchange, which Carrette opposes to capitalist exchange, is nonproductive because it requires "a pleasure generated through an exchange of deep trust and intense intimacy" (23): love rather than labor. For Carrette, SM's exchange (pleasure and intensity) is not only a form of Foucauldian desexualization, but it is also opposed to capitalism, commodity exchange, and "economies of lifestyle" (21).

But if SM play is not about "sex-desire," genitally focused, or oriented toward orgasm, it is productive of more than love. For example, Maxx—a white, bisexual switch/bottom in his mid-twenties—compares SM play to marathon running or lifting weights, telling me: "A lot of the S&M stuff isn't really sexual, just more like an endorphin high. Pain doesn't arouse me sexually . . . I just have a very high pain tolerance, and I've found that the more I could take the better I feel." Similarly, Bonnie explains: "Play for me does not necessarily have to be sexual. Play for me can be a number of different things . . . I like to learn about technique and I like to feel how the different techniques feel and I enjoy the sensations, but it's not necessarily always sexual for me." She continues: "It becomes meditative for me just as a test to see how much I can handle, how much I can take, what hurts, what doesn't, how much it takes to mark, and so it becomes for me an exploration of my body: its tolerances, its abilities to not be injured, what positions I can get into, how long I can stay there, how I can be dommed." For Bonnie and Maxx, SM practice is not (strictly) about sex-desire—orgasm or genital sensation—but a way to craft a new relationship with the body, a relationship that for Maxx is about an endorphin rush (see also Mains 1991), and for Bonnie is a way to experiment with technique and sensation, a test of the flexibility and limits of the body.

This kind of pleasure cannot be opposed to commodity exchange. Instead, we need to see these forms of exchange as operating together: the exchange of commodities and the exchange of intimacies, together producing forms of identity, subjectivity, pleasure, relationality, and community. Consider the circuit created through pain. Teramis describes an intense flogging: "She put me in a chair and started to flog me and flogged the skin off my back . . . We channel energy on purpose . . . I don't like to play with someone who can't get energy connected. So there was actually a feedback, consciously flying between us. I need that so I can process that level of pain. I'm grounding a lot of it . . . I'll be in certain positions with my palms flat to the ground, and I'm running energy through my body [and] breathing and [finding] the rhythmic way to flow with it." In Karmen MacKendrick's argument, pain (along with bondage) is one way that SM practice enables practitioners to surpass or break subjectivity through the "*useless* and *excessive* nature of deliberately invoked pain and restraint" (1999, 110; italics in original). Further, for MacKendrick, these dynamics are profoundly anti-economic: subversive of a libidinal economy, unproductive and inefficient, an "absurd expenditure of energy" with no gratification (114). She writes: "Pain's play with pleasure can explode our exchange-oriented economic sensibility" (121). Instead, as I read it, SM exchange is both social and material, productive and technological: it enables intimacy, connecting bodies through the incorporation of toys, relying on differentiating techniques, and producing both—as Stryker writes—"embodied knowledges and knowledges of embodiment" (2008, 38).

In a class titled "Spirituality in the Scene," which Dossie Easton and Janet Hardy held to gather material for their book, *Radical Ecstasy: SM Journeys to Transcendence* (2004), they began by talking about how it was almost impossible to find words to describe the mysterious connection or intensity of SM, especially because Janet is not a fan of "spirituality talk." People in the audience began volunteering descriptions and terms: it's "what makes me real," "it's about being a part of something larger than yourself," "it's unfiltered," "it's being present, in the moment," or it's "about a heart connection." Everyone who spoke agreed on the basic terrain: love, energy, ecstasy. "It's the radical potential for connection," someone said. Hayden—a white, lesbian masochist/slave in her late twenties—notes: "If you're with someone that you connect with, it's not—I'm not going to say it doesn't hurt, but it doesn't hurt as much because there's this energy going on . . . Some people describe it as connecting. I don't know, I don't have words for it. It just works." This kind of connective body is transformed through a medium of social connection called "energy." Or, in less new-age-y language, a prosthetic relationship develops between partners in SM through a toy-mediated exchange.

These kinds of connections are complex: reliant on toys, they create both commodity and energy exchange. Rather than being inefficient, they rely on, as Stryker puts it, a "proprioceptic awareness" of the "material efficiency I possess in my subjective ability" (2008, 42)—in other words, on skill, technique, and education. And rather than being useless or nonproductive, they produce forms of bodily knowledge, techniques, and the kinds of players, bodies, and communities to use them. Such energy is interpersonally connective; toys forge a pathway through feedback, connection, and channeling energy between bodies newly connected with such circuitry. This play is effective when it connects bodies to other bodies, creating an assemblage—a circuit. Lady Hilary explains: "I don't like to see just a body being beaten when there is no emotion attached to it . . . I like to see things that . . . show passion and the wow-ness of it, the excitement and the joy of it, and not sort of this strange boredom." There are several jokes in the scene to describe this; bottoms can, for example, view tops as the "life-support system for the whip" or "the pain delivery device." But this "strange boredom," the boredom of commodity fetishism, is not because of the saturation of toys but rather because of the ways toys have taken on, as a fetish, the contradictions within broader social relationships—contradictions between authentic and inauthentic, intimacy and commodification, human and object. Focusing on the body at play, then, reveals two important effects: toys divide, remapping the body as object of knowledge; and they also connect, serving as prosthetic extensions that reach out, and fill, spaces between players or bodies. This accounts for the pleasure and anxiety generated around toys and their handlers in relation to a desired social connection.

Thus, although the objectification of the body, its divisibility into parts, and the commodification of BDSM all herald new forms of power and knowledge—of technique—they also suggest new possibilities for connection. For players, this happens when a toy can be transformed into a prosthetic tool, incorporated into the body in order to create connection. Yet this is an unstable and anxious endeavor; in the pleasure/anxiety nexus, the very solidification of SM community and identity through commodities—toys—also enables those same toys, transformed into tools, to prosthetically bridge and reconfigure the bodies and relationships of the players in ways that are deeply connective. It does so, however, not by transgressing the social relations that demand efficiency and productivity from worker-subjects, but by embracing these demands—producing bodies in line with new technologies of knowledge and power.

PLEASURABLE BODIES OF SILICON VALLEY

In this way, I am arguing against the most common reading of SM practice as transgressive. As I have discussed above, this perspective sees in SM the loss of or an escape from individuated selves, rigid identities, knowable subjects, fixed Freudian aims, and economies of exploitation. It is the perspective of MacKendrick, writing of the ways that pain and bondage rupture subjectivity: "pain and restraint . . . throw the subject outside itself . . . break the limits of subjection" (1999, 156). For MacKendrick, "freedom from subjectivity is freedom from the forces of subjection, and the body knows such things are possible" (120). This knowing body is aligned against a more fixed subjectivity, just as SM's desexualized pleasures are aligned against the rigid normalization of "sex-desire."

Moreover, Carrette and MacKendrick position SM pleasure against capitalism. Carrette, for example, writes that SM practice can "bring about the fracturing of hegemonic capitalist sexuality" (2005, 26) and "free our gendered bodies from the market of global exploitation" (27). MacKendrick writes: "The counterpleasures [such as SM] are conspicuously resistant to absorption by exchange value" (1999, 11). She continues: "In our time, with subjectivity constructed by the orderly divisions and controlling gaze that strive to make us both more efficient and more knowable—the subjectivity of individuating discipline in the market demographics of late capitalism—sadomasochistic pleasure plays with the control, movement, sensations, and possibilities of the body to turn carnality to its full, postsubjective power" (20). It should be clear by now that, although SM "plays with the control, movement, sensations, and possibilities of the body," it does *not* do this through desubjectification, inefficiency, unknowability, or uselessness. The pleasurable body in SM is not, it is true, a genitalized body. But at the same time, these bodily experiments, while not genitally focused, rely on technique and knowledge of the body, which have everything to do with self-mastery and community production, rather than transcendence; pleasures that come from taking one's self (and body) as an object of knowledge and cultivation, rather than desubjectification. This is an "efficient" body, as McKenzie would put it, the body made into a useful and technical thing.[22] And rather than transgressing economic rationality—the demand that one be productive and efficient in one's labors and one's pleasures—this body is produced in and through the demands of late-capitalist production. Indeed, this is precisely the flexible body available to and required for the computer, service, and informational workers who swell the ranks of the new guard BDSM scene; a laboring body, not a body that can overthrow or move beyond subjectivity.

These bodies and pleasures are based on exchange: circuits of commodities and of energy, both of which produce forms of subjectivity, embodiment, and community in accordance with the flexible and adaptable subjects of late capitalism. As Emily Martin (1992) argues, the body in late capitalism is no longer the Fordist body (regimented, steady, and regulated) that corresponds to Foucault's disciplined, ordered modes of production and identity, but rather a flexible body that corresponds to flexible capitalism. We can see the tremendous flexibility of the SM body, open and adaptable to new toys, tools, and techniques as they are marketed. These are also able bodies: able to expand and contract along with the demands of new economies, based on relations of both production and consumption. These subjects, the new service and knowledge workers, as Rosemary Hennessy argues, are required to have "habitual mobility, adaptability in every undertaking, the ability to navigate among possible alternatives and spaces, and a cultivation of ambivalence as a structure of feeling" (2000, 108). It is therefore not surprising that, as Hennessy puts it, these subjects experience their sexualities in ways that are mobile, unfixed, open, fluid, and ambivalent. This sort of subject goes along with the flexibility and adaptability required of both workers and consumers today. Yet, as both Emily Martin and Robert McRuer (2006) caution, these dynamics produce—and require—flexibility for some bodies and inflexibility—exclusion—for others. These demands, as well as their proliferating possibilities, reproduce and solidify some forms of social hierarchy: freedom as freedom to consume; belonging mediated through consumption. As Hennessy summarizes: "Postmodern sexualities participate in the logic of the commodity and help support neoliberalism's mystifications" (109).

Late capitalism doesn't so much discipline or exile erotics as strategically use pleasure for market proliferation and subject differentiation. This dynamic relies on, as Linda Singer puts it, "the market's way of producing a 'revolutionary' development and sustaining a sense of apparent freedom through the proliferation of a range of erotic options, styles and scenes" (1993, 48). In this way, sexualities like SM "function as . . . compensatory indulgences, selective circumscribed sites of transgression" (39). In SM, commodity and power exchange links together social norms and social hierarchies as differential economies within social relations of class: agile and flexible bodies, coding in the South Bay by day and practicing elaborate suspension bondage in the dungeon by night.[23] These new intimacies, socialities, and knowledges are unevenly accessible. Sufficient leisure time and money are, if not prerequisites, ideals, making it easier for some people to become practitioners, to participate in this community, and to experience the new connections made possible through these exchanges. Practitioners negotiate such exchanges with ambivalence and anxiety. Indeed, unpacking the toy bag as a social fetish focuses attention on the contested ways that consumption relies on and produces social relations. In this way, *production* does not simply stand in for relations of production but rather opens out to encompass the biopolitical formation of subjects and communities. SM sexuality requires reading the relationships between capitalism and community, consumerism and subjectivity, and flexibility and bodily pleasures as ambivalent and anxious: capable of both creating and limiting possibilities for new bodies and new relationships. I see ambivalence as a location of conflict, but conflict in terms of both social norms and social relations (of production and consumption), where the constraints are simultaneously the potentials. This contradiction, like that around the rules, is itself a crucial aspect of contemporary SM; it reflects and provides some relief from the bodily demands of contemporary capitalism. In the end, these moments of cultural ambivalence reveal the fetishistic displacement—onto people, objects, and toys—of the social contradictions of late-capitalist social relations. In other words, even as we see commodity exchange and bodily objectification as more than lack or asocial destruction, we must also recognize that these bodily and relational potentials are produced within social dynamics of privilege, exclusion, and power.

FOUR

BEYOND VANILLA

Public Politics and Private Selves

> Calling an S/M person sexist is like calling someone who plays Monopoly a capitalist.
> —DEAR AUNT SADIE, *Coming to Power*

> For a lot of people, BDSM is not about whips and chains, it's about control, it's about power exchange. I think there are a lot of people who can relate to the power exchange: losing control, who holds the remote, who holds the checkbook, who chooses the radio station, who is driving, who decides where we're eating, where we're going on vacation. It's like the classic joke: "we know who wears the pants in that family" or "she knows her place."
> —PANTHER

On a Sunday evening in mid-September 2002, I showed up at Paul's house for what we were half-facetiously calling a "focus group." At the San Francisco munch the day before, Paul, a former graduate student, key informant, and friend, had asked me if he could do anything to help me with my research and proposed organizing a group interview at his house. We had been sitting with several noted Bay Area SM authors, various community leaders, and other participants in the upstairs room of a tapas restaurant as the munch was clearing out; when they seemed willing to go over to Paul's for cocktails and conversation, I was thrilled. So, at 5:30 p.m. the next day, I showed up with my mini tape recorder in hand.

When Jeff, Malc, and Rachel arrived, we ordered pizza. As Paul fixed drinks for everyone at the tiki bar in his living room, Jeff looked around the room. "Not much diversity here," he remarked, in the semi-embarrassed tone that I recognized from the standing introductions at munches across the Bay Area. When men there rise and say some version of "Hi! I'm Bill, and I'm a het male dom," their tone anticipates their audience's knowing, slightly mocking amusement; it betrays a half-joking discomfort with being a heterosexual, male dominant. Tonight, the three men were all "het male doms," or "HMDs" for short (Rachel is a white, bisexual pain fetishist/submissive in her early twenties who lives with Jeff and his wife as their submissive). That they were also all white is a lack of diversity unremarked upon, but one I will return to below. Throughout the four-hour group interview, as well as in other interviews with HMDs, the men seemed painfully aware of, and almost embarrassed by, their sexual/SM orientation. They seemed to think that—in what is supposed to be a subversive, alternative, and underground sex community—some might find their orientations clichéd, conservative, the very opposite of transgressive.

Why Paul, Jeff, and Malc want to be transgressive, and what they want to transgress, are the subjects of this chapter. These quasi-joking comments point to a desire for sex to be transgressive—not only, as I discussed in the previous chapter, of capitalism, but of social norms more broadly. As Linda Singer argues, sexuality is imagined as "a mechanism for resistance, transgression, opposition to the sphere of demand . . . Sexuality functions in a late-capitalist economy as a prototype or emblem . . . of freedom, and that in the name of which demands can be made of an alienating social system" (1993, 36–37). Of course, sex is not oppositional to capitalism, as the preceding chapters have made clear. Indeed, as Singer notes, capitalism produces sex as liberatory; inciting and managing "excessive" pleasures is central to profit making in late capitalism. But sex is also positioned in opposition to social normativity: to both the private/reproductive and the public/productive spheres.

In this construction, SM, despite its obvious commercial value, comes to stand in for authentic pleasures and freedom from vanilla social norms. But the very desire for SM as transgression produces the fantasy of sex as outside of or in opposition to economic and hierarchical social relations. This both guarantees profit (especially through the proliferation of commodities) and strengthens some forms of social normativity by differentiating legitimate vanilla sexuality from policed and demonized SM. Singer notes: "Regulation works through the installation of a set of binary relations that entail the legalization and normalization of some practices at the same time that others are criminalized. This binary system of regulation functions to fetishize and target specific institutional forms for regulation by leaving the larger structures of power to circulate and proliferate" (1993, 42). Not only are social norms and the market intertwined, but the very production of a split between sexual norms and sexual labor, private and public, simultaneously generates the fantasy of sex as liberatory and bolsters the supplementary relations between profit and social normativity.

Thus, the desire to transgress social norms through SM practice—the quasi-joke of the HMDs—sets up a complicated circuit. On the one hand, SM is figured as outlaw: as transgressive of normative sexual values. On the other hand, SM is dependent on social norms: practitioners draw on social hierarchies to produce SM scenes, just as such norms performatively produce subjects. BDSM scenes "play with" real power to produce legible scenes; dungeon parties commonly feature scenes based on police interrogation, rape, slavery, teacher-student relationships, and race or cultural trauma dynamics. These scenes draw on socially meaningful, and powerful, historical relations of inequality, the same "regulatory ideals" that performatively produce subjects and, at the same time, reproduce social norms (Butler 1993, 1; Foucault [1976] 1990, 155–56).

This chapter takes up the desire for SM sex to stand outside of social relations by focusing on cases of a resemblance between an in-scene role and the social reality of gendered, racial, and sexual inequality. For heterosexual male dominants and female submissives, the fact that their BDSM seems to replicate normative constellations of sex-gender-sexuality appears problematic; that this normalized gender is also racialized and classed does not. Exploring the imagined connections between "real-world" social norms and the "safe" world of the scene, I contrast the two most common analyses of SM play: the radical feminist anti-SM position, and the queer pro-sex position. In the radical feminist argument, this seeming replication means that the politics of SM roles and play scenes are the same as the social relations of domination (patriarchy, racism) that give them form. In the queer argument, SM scenes flout hetero- and vanilla-normative conventions and thus transgress or subvert social norms. This debate, stated baldly, is the SM version of the familiar dichotomy between replication/reenactment and subversion/transgression.

Yet the ambivalence voiced by these HMDs suggests another reading, in which the desire to be transgressive relies on the construction of a boundary between the "real world" (of capitalism, exploitation, unequal social relations, and social norms) and the "SM scene" (a pretend space of fantasy, performance, or game). Unpacking this boundary-making project, we can see the ways in which gendered performativity produces subjects who view their SM practice as private and individual, as a form of self-cultivation and self-mastery. However, this sense of personal autonomy, agency, and choice also relies on liberal (sometimes inflected as libertarian or neoliberal) ideologies of agentic individualism and freedom, formulations that are complexly bound to both material and discursive formations. Thus, the fantasy of sex outside material relations, the desire to transgress social norms of gender, produces a split between the public space of the law and the private space of desire that simultaneously creates opportunities to transgress social norms and restricts those opportunities to those with privilege. The ambivalence of practitioners whose SM desires seem to match up with their social locations, then, illuminates a complex and contradictory social field in which the topography of social power, the justifications of social hierarchy, and the dense interconnections between gender, race, sexuality, and class are produced, reproduced, disavowed, and embodied.

REENACTMENT LOCATING THE SM REAL

In my joint interview with Stephanie and Anthony, Anthony gave me an example of SM "reenactment":

> ANTHONY: There's a woman that I play with who has a terrible traumatic history. Her father started having sex with her when she was ten. It was all in the family and the mother used to send her to the basement after dinner, and it's a big fucking horrible story. Her thing in the scene is daddy rape.

STEPHANIE: Basically reenacting.

ANTHONY: Kind of reenacting that whole scene. Well, what I do is: I go—in my mind, I can hold that as something horrible, and I can go, "Okay, fine. That was horrible. What a fucking shit low life her dad is. Her mom, what the hell was she thinking?" And then place that somewhere else, and go, "Okay, I'm daddy. What do I do? And what is it about doing the daddy thing with her that's going to get her where she lives?" Somewhere in that scene, I hit on, "Your daddy spoiled you." And that was the trigger. And I went, "Daddy spoiled you all night," and that was the hot thing for her all night, and that scene went places from there that it couldn't have gone [otherwise]. But just one little line was the hook that turned that scene into something that was really fabulous. So that's what I look for . . .

STEPHANIE: And at that point it is not play.

ANTHONY: Yeah . . . [to find out] what is it she wants from me in that, and beyond that, where is the big button for me to push? I know there's a big button there for me to push; where is it?

I want to pause at this story—even though raising the specter of child abuse among SM practitioners is dangerous for its potential to replay SM stereotypes—because here Anthony articulates some of the connections between repetition and transformation that guide this chapter and the next. First, for Stephanie and Anthony, "reenactment" means mimicking an originary trauma. Second, in order to do this, Anthony has to separate the trauma from the SM scene; he has to put his horror over this woman's real incestuous rape "somewhere else" in his mind. Third, he needs to find the "button"—the hook, line, or trigger—that "get[s] her where she lives," that accesses her desire to do, and her eroticization of, this scene. Fourth, when this "big button" is pushed, the scene ceases to be "play" and instead becomes "fabulous," somehow real.

Many practitioners who play with trauma such as rape understand their play as recoding or remaking a traumatic experience into a pleasurable one; indeed, this is the reading of SM as therapy proffered by many (for example, Baumeister 1988; cf. Hart 1998 and Barker, Gupta, and Iantaffi 2007). Mollena explains that she doesn't "want to have to deal with horrible racists." "I don't really ever want to be abducted and gang raped by ten guys." But she does want to do rape and race play to "tap into" the feelings of helplessness, loss of control, and terror that these experiences produce (experiences, I should note, that she hasn't had, disrupting any simplistic reading of SM as essentially repetitive). As she explains, such play might help people "get past the guilt over the fact that perhaps they had a level of eroticism" about such scenes, or might turn something horrible "into something that's erotic"; both, she thinks, might enable practitioners to gain control over trauma by eroticizing it.

The relationship between what is understood as an originary trauma and SM's replication of trauma in an erotic scene has occupied a central place in feminist debates about sexuality and power since the late 1970s. It is, of course, precisely this realness that raises ethical and political questions about SM play. Does SM, as some radical feminists would have it, simply reproduce real-world relations of inequality, particularly racism and patriarchy? Or does SM enable the transgression of such social hierarchies through their staging or dramatization—does it matter that SM is consensual, fictional, just pretend?

Published in 1982, at the height of the feminist sex wars, *Against Sadomasochism* still stands as the major radical feminist critique of SM.[1] As Robin Ruth Linden writes in her introduction: "Throughout *Against Sadomasochism* it is argued that lesbian sadomasochism is firmly rooted in patriarchal sexual ideology . . . There can be no doubt that none of us is exempt from the sphere of influence of patriarchal conceptions of sexuality and intimacy . . . Sadomasochism is as much an irreducible condition of society as it is an individual 'sexual preference' or lifestyle: indeed, sadomasochism reflects the power asymmetries embedded in most of our social relationships" (1982, 4). Linden further specifies that "sadomasochistic roles and practices attempt to replicate the phenomenology of oppression through role playing," an oppression that is "always received rather than chosen" (7).

The authors in the collection argue that such "replication" means that SM is morally wrong, that it strengthens these inequalities—or, even more reductively, that it is actually the same as rape, torture, slavery, or Nazi concentration camps. For example, Bat-Ami Bar On writes: "The eroticization of violence or domination, and of pain or powerlessness, is at the core of sadomasochism, and consequently . . . the practice of sadomasochism embodies the same values as heterosexual practices of sexual domination in general and sexually violent practices like rape in particular" (1982, 75). Marissa Jonel argues plainly: "I know that sm is very dangerous . . . The danger is that our society puts women in the kind of space where we respond sexually to being second-class, less than good. There's something wrong with a woman who has an orgasm while beating or fist-fucking another woman. There's something wrong with pleasure derived from degrading nicknames like 'stupid cunt' and 'fucking whore'" (1982, 19). For these radical feminists, SM is the product of internalized oppression wrought by patriarchy, one place where individual desires express and reproduce the fundamental oppression of women.

It is not only that SM is "a conditioned response to the sexual imagery that barrages women in the society," but also that this is true "whether a woman identifies with the dominant or submissive figure in the fantasy." Either way, "she is still responding to a model of sexual interaction that has been drummed into us throughout our lives," a model, of course, we should be committed to eradicating (Nichols, Pagano, and Rossoff 1982, 139). Making explicit the connection between male/female, butch/femme, and top/bottom, Jeanette Nichols, Darlene Pagano, and Margaret Rossoff argue that "sexual polarization justifies passivity and glamorizes domination, reinforcing the legitimacy of power imbalances outside the bedroom" (140). Or, as almost all of the contributors argue, by replicating toxic patriarchal heterosexism, lesbian SM strengthens it: "By replicating the dominant patriarchal model of heterosexuality, lesbian-feminists are . . . practicing and validating the system in which one person has power over another, which is the basis of patriarchy. Why don't they see this behavior as contrary to feminism?" (Wagner 1982, 34). Thus, it is not only that SM is the expression of internalized oppression but that the replaying of these roles actually reproduces patriarchy. These are strong claims; the performance of SM power exchange, for these writers, is the performative production of racism, sexism, fascism, and inequality—not just its internalization.[2]

These claims have been refuted by a number of feminists in the last twenty-five years, but, as Patrick Hopkins argues, many of these refutations take essentially libertarian positions, arguing that sex is primarily a private issue, divorced from political considerations. This line of argumentation cannot respond to the radical feminist claim that sex practices, under patriarchal conditions, are a primary cause—and a primary effect—of domination. Instead, Hopkins argues that SM does not (or cannot be assumed to) "replicate" patriarchy; it "simulates" it: "Replication implies that SM encounters merely reproduce patriarchal activity in a different physical area. Simulation implies that SM selectively replays surface patriarchal behaviors onto a different contextual field. That contextual field makes all the difference" (1994, 123). In Hopkins's work, a rape scene, for example, is desirable because of the social context of the scene, whereas real rape is not; such conditions as "negotiation, safe words, [and] mutual definition" produce a "self-defined community," and it is this context of community that makes the rape scene a *scene* (124).

Yet, as Melinda Vadas notes in her radical feminist reply to Hopkins, SM scenes remain dependent on the violent referents that give them form. The pleasure of SM, she argues, "is a direct function of the actual, historical occurrence or existence of the death camps, rapes, and racist enslavements they simulate. If these historical events had never occurred or could not occur . . . the simulation would not only not be thrilling to the SMer, there would be no simulation at all because there would be nothing to simulate" (1995, 160). In other words, a reliance on "context" is unstable: Hopkins's defense relies on a distinction between the "real world" (where the "source-event" occurs) and a "scene world" (where the event is simulated, but "in no way replicates any of the injustice of the source-event") (Hopkins 1995, 166). In contrast, Vadas argues that a new, SM context cannot sever historical inequalities from their simulations. This debate on the ethics of SM play from various feminist positions takes two opposing stances regarding the relationship between the scene and social systems of domination. In the radical feminist argument, these "spaces" turn out to be fundamentally linked, even the same; in the defense of SM, these spaces are held apart, separated, through social mechanisms such as consent, community formation, simulation, and performance.

This latter understanding was shared by many people I spoke with in the SM scene. For example, Annalee and I discussed the politics of race play. She explained that she thinks "it's healthy to have a scene where you obviously step into a role, you're playacting, there's an end to it, and it's contained." This bracketing, for Annalee, is like "going to the movies": "There's a space that you go into where you suspend [dis]belief and then you leave." Annalee understands these more limited scenes as allowing a "critical perspective," without which a scene becomes "just a reenactment of slavery or historical traumas like women being subjugated by men." The difference for Annalee between "just a reenactment" and a scene that is "play" has to do with the ways in which practitioners are enabled to bracket, or fail to bracket, the scene from the everyday, the "play" self from the "real" self, the space of fantasy from reality (see also Stear 2009).

For many practitioners, SM play happens inside what Gregory Bateson calls the play frame. Bateson's example of the play frame is this: "the playful nip denotes the bite, but it does not denote what would be denoted by the bite" (1955, 41). In SM, bracketing or framing play as inside a play frame can become an alibi or a cover that allows participants to play with race or gender in ways that would be impossible outside of the frame. In this analysis, play with Mr. S–brand shackles denotes slave shackles, but it does not denote what would be denoted, in a nonplay frame, by the shackles: slavery. At the same time, like the nip and bite, the Mr. S shackles might "really evoke that terror which would have been evoked by a real"—slave—shackle (Bateson 1955, 43). Hence the effectiveness of these objects and dynamics: the shackle, slave auction, or flogging simultaneously incites and denies the *real*ness of these historical or socially meaningful scenes of power (a point I take up again in the next chapter).

It is this tension that distinguishes BDSM. In SM, the play frame—SM as a safe space—can function as an alibi, allowing practitioners to recode or experiment with familiar experiences of power in new ways. Because the scene is "just play," play with these forms of social power is possible. This construction produces the scene as a bracketed space, inside of which there are no outside social hierarchies. Patricia Duncan summarizes her analysis of lesbian SM: "The respondents were very aware of s/m as play. Although they recognized the way power differentials are based in reality and in our culture, they also made it very clear to me that power, in their s/m practices, is a dynamic process, exchanged between two or more partners within the parameters of a scene" (1996, 102). For the women Duncan interviewed, SM practices are "sites of transformation," a way to play with real, structural inequalities in safe and pleasurable ways: in ways that make such play *play* (103). Similarly, the dyke/trans BDSM practitioners in the United States and Western Europe whom Robin Bauer interviewed emphasized that SM play happens within a "safe space," a "playground," defined by BDSM community standards such as negotiation, consensuality, and rules (2007, 179; 2008, 233). This frame promises, as Anne McClintock notes, symbolic mastery over the social hierarchies from which SM objects, props, and scenes are borrowed (1995, 147); in this way, the production of a safe space can also serve as a phantasmatic mastery over social inequality.

This is not to say that SM play doesn't feel real to practitioners. The SM persona, even in different clothes, is, of course, real. And conversely, as Lynda Hart argues, "the controversy about whether s/m is 'real' or performed is naive, since we are always already in representation even when we are enacting our seemingly most private fantasies." She continues: "The extent to which we recognize the presence of the edge of the stage may determine what kind of performance we are enacting, but willing ourselves to forget the stage altogether is not to return to the real, as s/m opponents would have it" (1998, 91).[3] In this complicated dynamic, all sex and subjectivity—not just SM—is performative; at the same time, such performances are real, in the sense of being social, compelling, authentic, and material. For example, many practitioners distinguished the serious play that they did from "fantasy role-playing" or "acting." Jezzie explains: "I'm really turned off by fantasy role play . . . because to me that detracts from the reality of what's going on . . . If you're pretending that he's a pirate and I'm a captured whatever, then might not the power also be pretend? If he has to pretend to be a pirate in order to have control over me, then the control is pretend." Bailey also feels that thinking of SM as a performance diminishes the "reality" of the scene: "I've never been much into role play, you know, 'you're the pirate and I'm the captain.' I am just into down and dirty emotional and sensation exchange with my partners . . . It all becomes real to me. It's not a fantasy."

For these practitioners, the "scene world" is very real—sometimes even more real (in the sense of authentic) than the "real world"—and the majority of my interviewees described SM as a deep, almost innate, part of themselves. Hailstorm puts it this way:

> The reality is, that's [SM's] your reality. This is the fantasy out here, this is where we put the mask on and go battle the world. This is where you follow the rules. This is a trite fantasy world where you conceal who you are, where you conceal your feelings, where you conceal the truth because you have to get along with people. And the fantasy world, that's the reality because that's where people come out, that's where you see who people are and people see who you are. And you live for that world, you live for those few hours that you play in the evening. That's what drives you if you're a player, if you're a part of the community, that's the serious part of it. Everything else is paying the rent, getting by, but that's where you live. That's where the masks come off. That's where you become yourself, and that's why it's important to people to play—because that's their reality.

Gretchen feels the same way: "The real me is the life outside of work versus the one that goes to the engineering office and solves complex engineering problems."

However, both the real and scene world are bound together; SM works more as a circuit than a stage, more as an exchange than a toggle. Carrie explains: "What I'm doing when I'm playing is acting out a role. Even though it feels like it is coming from inside of me, it's still a play, it's still an act. I am an actress playing this role. And so it's not real . . . But let me tell you, when I do it, it sure feels real then. When I'm deep in the middle of it, there's no acting, it's definitely so intense and it's so good. It just makes me feel so complete." Bracketed from the real (just for play) but also based on and reconnecting to the real (in order to be effective), SM play creates a circuit in which the scene is first set apart and marked as safe, not real—and then, in play, becomes real, in the sense of authentic and transforming. Indeed, as what Sherry Ortner calls a "serious game," SM pretends to be "only a game," even as it—and social life in general, in her argument—is a game played for extraordinarily high stakes (1996, 12–13). Following Clifford Geertz's (1973) analysis of the Balinese cockfight, this tension between only a game and more than a game, or just play and for real, enables practitioners to play games with higher stakes through the alibi-setting production of the scene as a safe and separate space.[4]

This is one place to begin to answer the questions of why the HMDs with whom I opened the chapter want to be transgressive and what they want to transgress. These men, and many others in the scene, want to transgress normative social power, and they are aided in this by imagining that the SM scene is a space outside social norms and structures of inequality, a safe and separate space, bracketed from the real. This boundary-producing work creates anxiety, since keeping the scene separate from the social real of male dominance, white privilege, and heteronormativity can only ever be a partial—even failed—endeavor. Here, then, is the radical feminist insight that I will retain, while jettisoning the anti-SM rest: the understanding that SM is produced through social power, that sexuality (scenes, erotics, desire, and fantasy) is always social, and that "none of us is exempt" from this condition. In this, SM sexuality is like all sexuality: it is not possible to sever sexuality from power; sexuality is a social relation within an already existing social world. At the same time, the spectacularity of SM's play with social power makes its politics more visibly problematic; such a crowded social field demands ethnographic consideration. The radical feminist argument can begin to reveal how the construction of the scene as a safe or bracketed space is itself a way of pushing aside the social relations of power that form SM desires, and that SM communities and scenes produce.

TRANSGRESSION AND SOCIAL NORMS

For radical feminists, SM is politically and ethically wrong because the reenactment of social inequality produces it. Whereas radical feminists conceptualize social norms as patriarchal (and SM as reflecting or reproducing sexism), for most pro-SM feminist and queer theorists, SM is, rather, transgressive of the norms of vanilla heterosexuality. This divergence is illustrated clearly in *Coming to Power: Writings and Graphics on Lesbian S/M* (Samois [1981] 1987), the first widely read anthology of lesbian SM. For Samois, the San Francisco leatherdyke organization that put together the volume, *Coming to Power* represented not only an attempt to provide more information for leatherwomen, but also a "feminist examination" of the politics of sexuality in response to feminist "anti-S/M attitudes" like those in *Against Sadomasochism* (Davis 1987, 8). The writers in *Coming to Power* understood lesbian SM as transgressive: writers described practitioners as "radical perverts," "erotic dissidents," "heretics," and "sexual outlaws" (Califia 1987, 253, 277; Davis

1987, 8; Rubin 1987, 226). This transgression, for many of the essayists, was a response to the vilification of SM practice in both mainstream and feminist—especially radical feminist—views. For example, Samois's statement of purpose read, in part: "We believe that sadomasochists are an oppressed sexual minority. Our struggle serves the recognition and support of other sexual minorities and oppressed groups" (quoted in Rubin 2004, 4). As Ann Ferguson argues, writing in 1984, the "anti-prude" or "libertarian" feminist position (she cites Rubin and Califia as examples) celebrates SM as "oppositional practices" that transgress "socially respectable categories of sexuality" (1984, 109). In this argument, SM is seen to transgress heteronormative, vanilla sexuality as well as the normative lesbian-feminist sexuality endorsed by anti-SM radical feminists.

This position is neatly articulated in Gayle Rubin's classic essay "Thinking Sex." She writes of the "charmed circle": "According to this system, sexuality that is 'good,' 'normal,' and 'natural' should ideally be heterosexual, marital, monogamous, reproductive, and non-commercial. It should be coupled, relational, within the same generation, and occur at home. It should not involve pornography, fetish objects, sex toys of any sort, or roles other than male or female. Any sex that violates these rules is 'bad,' 'abnormal,' or 'unnatural' " (1984, 280–81). These rules legitimize some sexualities and delegitimize others; the circle—linking SM with sex for money, same-sex sex, and cross-generational sex—reflects a series of binary oppositions that position some sexualities as good and moral, and others as hated, feared, and policed (SM, here, is opposed to "vanilla sex"). Rather than tolerating or accepting "benign sexual variation" (278), Rubin argues that the social control of sexuality makes sex and sexual practice "a vector of oppression" (293). Or, as she argues in her essay in *Coming to Power*, "contrary to much of what is said about straight SM in the feminist press, heterosexual SM is not standard heterosexuality" because SM practitioners are "stigmatized" and "persecuted" as "perverts" (1987, 221).

Many queer and sexuality studies scholars following Rubin have argued that SM practice flouts or even subverts gendered norms; others have argued that SM's public performances transgress heteronormative sociosexual relations (Bauer 2008; Day 1994; Langdridge and Butt 2005; MacKendrick 1999; Reynolds 2007). In the first argument, SM is understood to disrupt the heterosexual logic that animates sex-gender-sexuality binaries because roles are chosen, rather than naturalized (based on sexed bodies). This allows practitioners, as Karmen MacKendrick puts it, to "destabilize rigidly identified subjectivities" because SM is not limited by gender (as in object choice or sexual identity) but is instead fluid (1999, 96). Writers drawing on this argument emphasize SM's play with gender norms, the way it can create a space that appears to avoid "*predefined* power relations in regard to gender and sexuality" (Bauer 2008, 234; italics in original).

These theorists see SM as subverting gender roles not only through play but also through reversal; SM "reverses and transmutes the social meanings it borrows" (McClintock 1993, 89). For McClintock, this reversal is based on SM's particular "economy of conversion: slave to master, adult to baby, pain to pleasure, man to woman, and back again" (87). In "playing the world backwards" (87, quoting Weinberg and Kamel 1995), SM, McClintock argues, "inhabits the anomalous, perilous border between the Platonic theory of catharsis and the Aristotelian theory of mimesis, neither replicating social power, nor finally subverting it, veering between polarities, converting scenes of disempowerment into a staged excess of pleasure, caricaturing social edicts in a sumptuous display of irreverence" (112). Thus, although SM cannot, in the end, disrupt the social order, or "finally [step] outside the enchantment of its magic circle" (89), the work it does do—conversion, caricature, transmutation—comes from the mobilization of crossings, roles that are decoupled from a sexed (or otherwise imposed) body and instead performed and enacted. Foucault's comments are similar: "the S/M game is very interesting because it is a strategic relation, but it is always fluid. Of course, there are roles, but everyone knows very well that those roles can be reversed. Sometimes the scene begins with the master and slave, and at the end, the slave has become the master" ([1984] 1996, 387–88). Although this perilous border between the real and a role is, indeed, precisely the problem of SM, these theorists emphasize oppositionality: role reversals of slave to master, man to woman, and so on.

This analysis is fitting for the heterosexual prodommes and businessmen submissives who are the subjects of McClintock's essay. Like much queer work on gender transgression based on Judith Butler (especially her analysis of drag [1990]), the ability to reverse social power—in play—is critical to the celebration of such play as transgressive.[5] So, for example, in some work on butch-femme, butches can seem more transgressive than femmes because a butch exposes the noncontinuity of sex and gender (cf. Halberstam 1998; Hollibaugh and Moraga 1992; Lapovsky-Kennedy and Davis 1993; B. Martin 1994b; Nestle 1992). This kind of analysis locates the transgression of binary gender roles (and the system of opposite-sexed bodies—heterosexuality—that animates these forms) in the figure that most clearly represents the split between the sexed body and performative gender. In SM, this would apply to the businessman in bondage or the female top—roles in which real power and scene power are discordant. And, although important, this focus can lead to an analysis in which it is the fact of this seeming discord that produces a political reading—in which crossing itself is transgressive, irrespective of its material context, audience, or effect (see also Glick 2000).

I am not arguing that such counternormative scenes are absent from SM. For example, the First Annual Iron Dom contest that I attended in March 2003 featured a competition based on the television show *Iron Chef*. The organizers gave each top a grab bag containing a two-liter bottle, a belt, plastic forks, a scrubbing pad, dowels, two potatoes, a child's tambourine, an inner tube, socks, a zucchini, tongue depressors, a lemon reamer, a piece of leather, and a plastic chair mat (with sharp little prongs on one side).[6] Contestants had two hours to turn the items into toys; they were then matched with a bottom and given ten minutes to demonstrate their toys in a scene in front of the large crowd. The tops (four men and five women) drew the names of their bottoms (four men and five women) from a hat; the rules specified that "you do not get to choose your sub (what if the only sub on the Island were of a non-appropriate gender?"). The final couplings included one male top with a female bottom, one female top with a male bottom, and four all-female and three all-male couples. The pairs performed very different scenes—some rough and grunting, some cool and detached, others sly and erotic.

At the end of one scene between a female top and female bottom, the top, dressed in a girdle, had the naked bottom suck her "cock": a zucchini penis and two potato balls, held together with a dowel. One judge noted that it was "great to see a lady in a girdle doing cock worship!" The scene was sexy and cruel; the top had placed the plastic fork on the bottom's clavicle, prongs nestled under the woman's jaw, so that the bottom couldn't lower her head during the zucchini fellatio. Displacing both the fleshly penis and phallic mastery, it is not difficult to analyze these scenes in terms of gender transgression. Taking Butler's famous question in *Gender Trouble*—which possibilities of doing gender "repeat and displace through hyperbole, dissonance, internal confusion, and proliferation the very constructs by which they are mobilized?" (1990, 31)—we can read these scenes as displacing gender through reiteration, illustrating how subjectivity, identity, sex, and gender come together by performing their coming apart.

But what about a submissive woman, bound and flogged by a male master? What about SM play that does not entail such oppositional reversals? A political analysis of SM scenes must be based on the conditions of a performance—its performers, audience, and ideological and material effects—not its abstracted or formal structure. Otherwise, such a reading necessarily bifurcates the real (of oppression) and the performance (of a role). This follows from Foucault's analysis of SM politics: "Even when the roles are stabilized, you know very well that it is always a game. Either the rules are transgressed, or there is an agreement, either explicit or tacit, that makes [the participants] aware of certain boundaries" ([1984] 1996, 388; see also Plant 2007). These boundaries produce, for the practitioners I interviewed, the SM space as a bounded site of personal desire and freely chosen roles. Through its boundaries, rules, and constructions of consent, the SM community produces an understanding of SM as a marked-off, delineated space of play oppositional to and outside of real power—in short, a queer counterpublic.[7]

This is the second queer reading of SM: as subversive of—through public performance or counterpublics—hetero- or vanilla normativity. For example, Lauren Berlant and Michael Warner conclude their "Sex in Public" essay with a description of an "erotic vomiting" performance at a "garden-variety leather bar" (1998, 564). In this performance, they suggest, "sex appears more sublime than narration itself, neither redemptive nor transgressive, moral nor immoral, hetero nor homo, nor sutured to any axis of social legitimation." Instead, they write,

> in these cases . . . paths through publicity led to the production of nonheteronormative bodily contexts. They intended nonheteronormative worlds because they refused to pretend that privacy was their ground; because they were forms of sociability that un-linked money and family from the scene of the good life; because they made sex the consequence

> of public mediations and collective self-activity in a way that made for unpredicted pleasures; because, in turn, they attempted to make a context of support for their practices; because their pleasures were not purchased by a redemptive pastoralism of sex, nor by mandatory amnesia about failure, shame, and aversion. (565–66)

The oppositionality to heteronormativity is based on a queer counterpublic, a queer world-making project that develops, fosters, and elaborates collective, nonprivatized (publicly accessible), and nonheteronormative intimacies and relations (Berlant and Warner 1998, 558; see also Muñoz 1999; Rudy 1998; Warner 2002).[8] For these theorists, queer sex, in combination with the community developed around it, can produce a sexual and social world that opposes the "majoritarian public sphere" and its gendered and raced relations of heterosexuality (Muñoz 1999).

Before the erotic vomiting scene, however, Berlant and Warner describe "riding with a young straight couple we know, in their station wagon," a couple whose "reproductivity governs their lives, their aspirations, and their relations to money and entailment, mediating their relations to everyone and everything else" (1998, 564). This couple, it turns out, has begun experimenting with vibrators, an experiment that Berlant and Warner describe as "queer sex practices": when they begin using sex toys, their bodies "become disorganized and exciting to them" (564). I detail these two examples because they show how work on queer counterpublics can reaffirm a static hierarchy of sex practices based on oppositionality. In Berlant and Warner's essay, the conflict between a reading of the couple as straight (defined by and through their heteroreproductivity) versus as queer (via their use of sex toys) solidifies both the "queer" and the "counter" in this public through a series of comparative oppositions: erotic vomiting versus hetero-reproductive penis-vagina sex versus using vibrators; male-male BDSM practice versus straight couples; leather bars versus station wagons. Through such condensations, internal differentiation within the categories of hetero and queer—and, most important, the differential relationships to power held by variously positioned people within these categories—drops out of the analysis (see also Cohen 1997; R. Ferguson 2004; Schlichter 2004).

As Biddy Martin argues, this kind of analysis can produce "superficial accounts" in which "to be radical is to locate oneself outside or in a transgressive relation to kinship or community" (1994a, 123), a queer counterpublic opposed to a rather undifferentiated mainstream public. For Martin, this "radical anti-normativity and a romantic celebration of queerness or homo-ness" posits "the very demise of current forms of societalization" (123)—a constitutive outside seen, in different ways, in queer antisocial arguments (Bersani 1995 and 1987; Edelman 2004).[9] Beyond the "romance" in this construction, however, is a tautological argument in which both queer (as oppositional to heteronormative) and counterpublic (as oppositional to normative public) function with prior political designations: we know what heteronormative is, and thus its opposite queer; and thus all queer sex practices are oppositional to heteronormative social institutions.

In this analysis, as Tom Boellstorff notes, queer studies can veer into "a self-congratulatory exercise where the cast of characters is settled and the conclusion known in advance" (2007, 15). These analyses risk this a priori politicization precisely where they contrast an almost impossibly straight world—the mainstream public and its social norms and institutions—with an expanding set of queer counterpublics produced through sexual practice. As Warner, for example, writes, sexual practice produces some heterosexual people as queer; prostitutes and leatherfolk are his key examples, although "fairly conventional heterosexual married couples" who "find they enjoy anal play, sex toys, sex in public places, sadomasochism, etcetera" are also included (1999, 37). Categorizing sexual practices in this way both requires and produces an oppositional relationship between queer and heteronormative, resistant and consolidating, counterpublics and straight society.

This oppositionality is more challenging to sustain when there is no clear discordance between SM and "standard" heterosexuality, as, indeed, is often the case in the pansexual community. For example, among the practitioners I interviewed, the majority of heterosexual couples were male dominant/female submissive.[10] Although most people I spoke with insisted that there is no necessary relationship between gender and SM role—that anyone can be submissive or dominant—Hailstorm explains: "The typical breakdown is male top and female bottom; that's mostly what you see. You do see some female top/male bottom. It's out there, but it's not as common. Male subs do not have a lot of respect in the community, for whatever reason." Although almost everyone will immediately point out that so-and-so is a female dominant, or so-and-so is a male submissive, my observation in the pansexual SM scene supported this generalization: most male/female couples are male dominant/female submissive.[11]

Furthermore, rather than reporting a scene free of gendered assumptions, many practitioners complained about sexism in the scene. Some explained that male submissives are sometimes treated with scorn; women of all SM orientations reported that some men assume they must be submissive. Lenora and Gretchen both told me that others have accused them of not being "real submissives," or have expressed surprise about their SM orientation because they have strong opinions and are articulate and socially assertive—or, as Lenora puts it, "basically because I'm not a doormat." These assumptions are also racialized; Bonnie explained: "[As an Asian American,] I get a lot of men talking to me as if I'm supposed to be quiet and submissive, and I'm not necessarily quiet nor submissive; that can be really frustrating. Or people brushing me off because I happen to be female, even." These assumptions rest on a supposed congruence between the sexed body and the SM role—on naturalized gender. For example, Don, simultaneously distancing himself from and endorsing the assumption that women are naturally submissive and men naturally dominant, told me that "if you walk[ed] into the Castlebar on the night of a party and you stripped everybody naked so nobody had collars on or wore their floggers . . . the vast majority of the people there would assume that men are tops and women are bottoms. It's just the way it usually plays out. There are notable exceptions on both sides, lots of beautiful bottom boys, lots of really interesting top women. But, you know, stereotypes and generalizations exist for some purpose. So the sexism itself might come . . . if a woman walked in clothed but not wearing a collar and a stereotypical heterosexual dominant male were to notice her: he would probably assume she was submissive because she was female." It is not only that the SM scene reflects—especially for heterogendered couples—normative gendered arrangements, but also that sexism is not a phenomenon located safely outside the scene. Rather, SM both requires and reproduces these social relations of inequality.

This analysis relies on Butler's reading of the productivity of social norms, with one crucial departure. Butler argues: "The category of 'sex' is, from the start, normative; it is what Foucault has called a 'regulatory ideal.' In this sense, then, 'sex' not only functions as a norm, but is part of a regulatory practice that produces the bodies it governs, whose regulatory force is made clear as a kind of productive power, the power to produce—demarcate, circulate, differentiate—the bodies it controls. Thus, 'sex' is a regulatory ideal whose materialization is compelled, and this materialization takes place (or fails to take place) through certain highly regulated practices" (1993, 1). "Sex" has, as Butler puts it, "the power to produce" bodies and subjects through social regulation—somewhat rigid ideological structures that compel recognizable performances of sexed body/gender/sexuality, which then form the basis for subjectivity. In this way, these practices are densely social. In Butler's work, intelligibility provides a horizon of recognition for subjectivity itself, within which all subjects are either recognizable or unrecognizable as subjects (2005, 17–18). These norms are contextual, social, variable; even as sex-gender-sexuality assumes structural force and coherence through heteronormativity, it is only in particular performances that these norms are produced and reproduced. In this way, social norms are critical to subjectification: subjects are produced by social norms, and the performativity of this production reproduces social norms.

This understanding provides one way to think about the coherence and productive intelligibility of social norms within the SM scene. Yet, as Saba Mahmood points out in her graceful critique of Butler, within much feminist and queer work following *Gender Trouble* (1990) and *Bodies That Matter* (1993), performances are read as either solidifying or eroding social norms. Mahmood observes that Butler not only privileges those moments when norms are resignified or subverted (a point also made by Glick 2000; McKenzie 2001; and Morris 1995), but also that Butler's "analysis of the power of norms remains grounded in an agonistic framework, one in which norms suppress and/or are subverted, are reiterated and/or resignified" (Mahmood 2004, 22).[12] The focus on discord between the sexed body and performed gender not only reproduces a politics of oppositionality based on visibility or discordance between figure and ground, but it also requires and produces an opposition between the safe/queer/counterpublic and the hegemonic/heteronormative/public, the SSC scene world and the oppressive real world.

Instead, and following Mahmood's turn to Foucault's techniques of the self, I explore the much more mundane, and more common, work of normative embodiment. This kind of work on the self—the cultivation, monitoring, and transformation of the self as an "object of knowledge and a field of action" (Foucault [1984] 1988, 42)—focuses attention on performance less as a subversion of social norms and more as the norm's embodiment: the ways social norms are "lived and inhabited, aspired to, reached for, and consummated" (Mahmood 2004, 23). Embodiment, as Mahmood argues, does not take the body as a "signifying medium," but rather "as a tool or developable means through which certain kinds of ethical and moral capabilities are attained . . . the process by which an experienced body is produced and an embodied subject is formed" (2001, 844). This analysis extends Butler's understanding of social norms as the necessary ground for the production of the subject toward the lived embodiment of social norms themselves.

This is not, to be sure, the radical feminist argument: that there is nothing but social power endlessly replicated, internalized, and reproduced.[13] Nor does it rely on the creation of a safe, bracketed space of play, a space where real-world inequality can be set aside, played with, rebelled against, or parodied. Instead, rather than continue this binary debate between the performative transgression and the performative production of material inequality, I turn to other relationships between privilege and social power produced in these scenes. An emphasis on the anxiety and ambivalence with which many of my interviewees expressed the overly close resemblance between their scene role and their "real life" role shows how neoliberal ideologies actively encourage practitioners to position themselves vis-à-vis community and social norms, at the same time that such performances produce community. The debates over the generative role of oppression or power in SM begin to reveal how the SM community imagines a split between real power and play power along private and public lines, and how this split further produces the ambivalent politics of SM play.

EMBODYING SOCIAL NORMS FREEDOM, CHOICE, AND GENDER

The political problem of SM—whether it is feminist or antifeminist, how or whether to politicize sexuality, how to describe the relationship between the personal and the social—has received the most attention from feminist theory. But this problem is not only theoretical; for SM practitioners of all (political and sexual) orientations, these questions remain vital. Many people with whom I spoke—male-, female-, and trans-identified—experienced difficulty trying to reconcile their (often feminist) politics and their SM practice. And, as they narrated stories of reconciliation, they relied on, and simultaneously constructed, the concepts of *choice* and *freedom* as freedom from social norms. As I will show, this tension between public politics and private practice is often resolved through a fantasized split between the "real world" of power and SM as a pretend game. Critically interrogating the creation of these divisions between inside and outside the scene illuminates the way the SM community stands within and in relation to—not magically or romantically outside—social inequality and hierarchy. Indeed, it is precisely the ways in which practitioners navigate and produce a split between real and fantasy, coerced and freely chosen, and replication and subversion that reproduces the divide between compelled social norms and performative, consensual selves—public and private—that lies at the heart of neoliberal cultural formations.

Critical to contemporary SM, as I have discussed above, is the concept of consent, with its liberal understanding of free choice. Guides, essays, and analysis intended for the pansexual community emphasize that SM is a consensual fantasy. For example, William Henkin and Sybil Holiday begin the "Myths, Fears and Stereotypes" section of *Consensual Sadomasochism: How to Talk about It and How to Do It Safely* by explaining that "SM does not necessarily replicate reality" (1996, 33). They go on to discuss the nature of consent, stressing that consensuality is one of the fundamental principles of SM. Similarly, the majority of my interviewees resolved any potential conflict between feminism and BDSM with a liberal analysis, arguing that SM is consensual, that SM practices and roles are freely chosen, and that SM is empowering, and thus compatible with feminism. Teramis, for example, tells me:

> I see no conflict at all between being a slave and being a feminist. Slave is about choice. Feminism is about choice. That's what makes me happy, you know, that's that. So to me the whole issue boils down to something that's very simple in that regard, and I don't have to tear my hair over it and go through all the gyrations to come to terms with it. I feel sorry for women who do—for some people it seems to be a big hurdle. Also, I think it's easier when you're gay because in my little world paradigm, if somebody's beating someone else in a kinky scene, it's a woman beating on a woman. I don't [feel] I've sold out to the patriarchy because I'm

letting my husband beat me. It's a nonissue. We both chose to do the kinky thing: I like to be the catcher, you like to be the pitcher, and we're both happy.

Teramis's response is interesting in that she is simultaneously arguing for free choice (as the definition of feminism), and noting that this freedom to choose might be more of a problem for women in heterosexual SM relationships, where relations of inequality might be more fixed or rigid.

For women who play with men, however, choice was similarly foregrounded. Gretchen told me that, while she doesn't experience any personal anxiety over feminist politics and being a bottom, her best friend, a lesbian, wanted her to "turn the tables" and top the men with whom she was playing. She explained: "I was having all these really wonderful experiences and I was exactly where I wanted to be—which was on the bottom—and there didn't seem to be any conflict for me . . . but for her it was really important . . . not letting a man have power over you." Gretchen dismissed this concern: "If I have a choice about it, then it's not really about 'you're a man and I'm a woman' . . . [If] I'm choosing to do the submission thing, it's not that I'm making myself less powerful or less of a whole person." Similarly, Lenora compared her 24/7 (full-time) D/s relationship with her male partner to a "traditional fifties marriage," where the wife was "obedient" and the "roles were defined." When I asked for clarification, she replied: "The main difference would be the choosing. Nothing is happening because of society's prescribed roles. We have said we want this to be this way and that to be that way. I'm very big on choice and on personal accountability." "Choice" and "personal accountability" in these narratives operate to ensure that the fact that Lenora's and Gretchen's relationship dynamics appear to echo normative gender roles does not mean that their relationships are actually based on social norms of gender. For these women, and many others, SSC SM (based on consent and free choice) is enough to make SM feminist, or at least make SM—in particular, female submission—politically neutral.

Like choice, many practitioners understood freedom within a liberal framework: subjects as rational agents who exercise free will and free choice. Vicki—a white, lesbian dominant in her early fifties—explained when I asked her about consent: "I was taught to follow very closely the precepts that are in the Bill of Rights that formed this country. So, for example, there are people out there who do some really strange things in the BDSM world. My reaction to that is: I don't want to know, but everybody there agrees they are consenting, they are able to consent, [so] I'm happy, let them have fun." Later she said:

> Let's say I went over and tied a girl up on that table over there. These people [other people in the cafe] didn't consent, but my freedom of expression is protected in the Constitution. Let's pretend that this is a public place, not a private restaurant. Let's say it's out in a public street. I have the right to express myself. She has the right to be expressed on, whereas other people have a right not to know. As adults . . . the solution is very simple: the people who don't want to know, don't look. You're looking this way and go, "Oh, I don't want to see that." Don't look this way. Now, as adults, she and I should figure out we shouldn't do this every day at noon when people are going out to lunch. We need to be courteous toward people who don't want to see that but do want to go out to lunch.

This argument brings liberal humanist and free-market libertarian conceptions of personal responsibility, choice, freedom, and individual agency together with a strict opposition between public/political and private/domestic spheres.[14] For Vicki, consent must be negotiated between SM practitioners and an audience, each of whom is an independent stakeholder. This construction of a subject who makes free, individual choices relies on a separation between the private and public spheres—where all private (coded as consensual) decisions have no effect on others or on the social world, and where lone individuals make rational choices based on maximizing personal freedom. In other words, the emphasis on consent, negotiation, and free choice on which this defense of SM relies—in ideological opposition to the radical feminist critique—produces an unbreechable boundary between the private, consensual scene and the public, social world.

Further, this reconfiguring of the public and the private recasts the private as the space of authenticity, of freedom and choice, and the public as the space of control, of inauthenticity, of oppressive norms and values. Here again sexuality is critical, since, as Singer argues, sexuality "has already been constructed as that which is or belongs to the realm of the private, i.e., opposed to the social" (1993, 59). Singer links this situation—in which desire produces the individuation of pleasures; individuals expect fulfillment in the private, not the public, realm; and change or something like politics is grounded in the individual, not in social relations or institutions—to both neoliberalism and late capitalism. The construction of one's identity as a private matter works to ensure the reproduction of unequal social relations with "a minimum of capital or social investment" (59). Or, as Berlant and Warner argue, US "citizens have been led through heterosexual culture to identify both themselves and their politics with privacy. In the official public, this involves making sex private . . . replacing state mandates for social justice with a privatized ethics of responsibility, charity, atonement, and 'values'; and enforcing boundaries between moral persons and economic ones" (1998, 553–54; see also Berlant 1997; Duggan 2003). Conjoining social norms and capitalist social relations, this dynamic relies on neoliberal cultural conceptions of freedom, choice, and privacy to both justify and help reproduce this formation. Key to this is the figuration of the individual as free within that subject's private space—which also, as I will show, works to justify certain forms of privilege in the name of self-empowerment and self-improvement. In these narratives, reconciliation takes place when practitioners solidly locate BDSM practice in a private, apolitical, and asocial space of personal desire and use neoliberal rationalities to justify this retreat from a shared social and political landscape.

Other practitioners, however, found such reconciliations more difficult; this was especially true for those who strongly identified as feminist. For these practitioners, reconciliation took the form of an empowerment story; their narratives detailed how they came to terms with their identities and eventually arrived at personal freedom. Although this argument similarly emphasizes self-determination and liberal understandings of consent and personal freedom, it also understands sexuality as bound up in politics, sociality, and power. For example, Dylan argues against what she describes as the "lesbian-feminist nonpenetration, no sex" version of "good" sex: "It's so judgmental and oppressive in and of itself, and it's not allowing the person a choice." Dylan's complicated navigation of "choice" is instructive. She explains that she was able to wear lingerie and "be sexy in the bedroom" with her male partner only after she had dated women: "When I started dating women, it was my choice. I found out how much I liked it just for me and how much it was my thing. And so now I can come back to a relationship with a guy and wear lingerie and do things and not at all feel that kind of oppression." Dylan's narrative simultaneously relies on a construction of free choice and acknowledges that these choices are not free from gender as a social form. Describing how she plays differently with men than women, she explains that although Daddy/little girl play is her "favorite thing": "With a guy, there's a certain reality to it. So that is a lot more playing with fire, I think, but it's also less appealing. The whole Daddy/little girl thing with women has a different background to it than it does with men, and it has a different connotation."

This "different connotation" is the social force of gender norms and roles, the "reality" that Dylan simultaneously recognizes and would like to avoid. Her narration shows that gender and power permeate desire, identification, and power exchange in ways beyond the control of an individual, articulated most strongly at precisely the moments when the individual imagines herself to be free from these norms. Similarly, KB—a white, het/bi prodomme in her late fifties—tells me: "when I was in the het community, I felt ashamed to bottom." She "didn't like the certain rigid roles and stereotypes" about submissive women and dominant men. For KB, "a lot of the het men and het women . . . tend to have this one channel [tuned] to the heterosexual way to do it. Sometimes it pushed really horrible buttons: this is the heterosexual society, and its value system [sucks]." The homophobia, sexism, and ageism KB recounts is, as she comments, "what we all—what I was born into and wanted to walk out of," not re-experience in the BDSM scene. KB found "the het scene" of the Backdrop club "very limiting. It was like staying in kindergarten, whereas going into this other scene [the gay men's and pansexual early Janus scene] was like grades one through—it seemed endless," a "way to get out of" heteronormativity. These responses highlight the enmeshment of desire and erotics within social relations, even as they also cast individuals as navigating such norms with agency. Rather than deny that sexual desires are formed from social relations of inequality, these practitioners map out the complicated ways that SM both relies on and re-encodes relations between sex, gender, and sexuality.

Some women told me that it was much harder to "come to grips," as Gretchen puts it, with their submissiveness than it was with their masochism.[15] Masochism—a technique of the body—is, in some ways, safer (to norms of gender, at least) than explicit power play is. Gretchen explains that, when she began playing with submission, she wanted to do resistance or takedown play: "I think that there's something about projecting your desires on somebody else and letting them be responsible for them that's comfortable." Gretchen describes coming to terms with her submission as a "progression" and "part of a journey towards self-mastering" when she started to "admit that this is something that [she wanted] and that [she] could choose" for herself. This "journey," as I described in chapter 2, is part of the way SM practitioners become practitioners through techniques of the self, through modulating, refining, and developing their own sense of themselves as practitioners.

Chris, for example, a dominant man with a "strong feminist" submissive partner, told me that they both struggled with the sense that BDSM was politically wrong. He explains: "I think that she has some demons around that to get worked out and I have some demons around—I like hurting people, and how can somebody actually respect me when they know that about me? And she loves me completely with just an amazingly powerful love and yet I—there's still a part of me that can't quite figure it out. That is, I'm still conditioned to think that that part of me is wrong." Chris had what he describes as a "huge breakthrough" when he realized that "there's a way of holding this all, that you can kind of do some real alchemy and make it very empowering, very empowering and very pleasurable and fulfilling . . . of course, as long as it's consensual." For Chris, because the power dynamics in SM are consensual, they are freely chosen; SM can be empowering to individuals through self-actualization and cultivation with, not in opposition to, norms.

These subjects are forged and remake themselves through the embodiment of various social norms, not through their internalization (à la radical feminism) or their subversion (à la queer transgression). This kind of embodiment requires self-cultivation, but—especially for those whose SM roles match social norms of gender—navigating these norms produces anxiety. For example, Carrie also describes her difficulty "coming to grips" with her submission, because of the similarities between submission in the scene and vanilla femininity: "Part of me still thinks it's wrong . . . it still feels shameful . . . In my vanilla neighborhood life I am in charge of the house, I'm in charge of some of the school events. I'm in charge of my work, my massage therapy . . . I have to be very strong and independent and [a] businesswoman and all that. So reconciling that with . . . this other part of me who . . . doesn't want to be in control, who wants to have somebody else tell me what to do . . . I kept thinking to myself, 'How can I?' " Carrie's shame points to an anxiety that being submissive or bottoming to men reinforces the gendered roles and stereotypes that she spends much of her vanilla life combating. But rather than viewing Carrie as either a dupe of gender or, via her SM practice, as standing radically outside normative gendering, focusing on this anxiety or ambivalence reveals that social norms are performed, inhabited, and experienced in what are often politically ambivalent ways (Mahmood 2004; see also Muñoz's [1999] understanding of "disidentification").

Understanding sex as a form of biopower enables us to see how subjects form and work on themselves in relation to social norms of gender, race, and sexuality, while moments of ambivalence and anxiety show us some of the places where these constellations generate conflict. For the remainder of this chapter, I focus on two practitioners who do not appear immediately transgressive: two white, heterosexual, male dominants I interviewed, J. and Paul. Their narratives illuminate how, on the one hand, resisting social norms (of white privilege, heteronormativity, and sexism) can produce a narrative of self-empowerment and, on the other hand, how such freedom to sidestep or remake oppressive social norms relies on precisely these forms of privilege.

J. AND PAUL WHITENESS, MASCULINITY, HETEROSEXUALITY

J., a man who had been involved with left-wing politics in the 1970s, and Paul, a political theorist informed by feminist and postcolonial theory, both told me that they had difficulty resolving their feminism and their dominance. J. told me: "[I] had a lot of internalized values around the feminist critique and tried to live my life accordingly." In this analysis, polarized power dynamics were unacceptable, and so J.'s SM fantasies "went underground." When he met a woman who wanted him to dominate her, "it was a crisis of identity" as well as a "crisis between feminist values and my personal and internal values of wanting to play this role." In this relationship, J. explains how he felt: "externally I was this feminist man, but internally and in secret, I was playing with S&M."

Paul also described this sense of having a secret, unacceptable fantasy life. As he was coming out as an SM practitioner, Paul had "incredible guilt about trying to reconcile being a sadist and having been raised as a feminist man." Paul said: "[It took more than ten years] to make my politics and my libido fit together because in my mind for a long time, I felt like one or the other had to go. I couldn't reconcile being a dominant male sadist and being a feminist. It just seemed like I was living this lie." He continued: "I'm not asking for anyone to cry tears for us or anything, but there's a problem with being a sort of sensitive guy who nonetheless has very serious feelings of sexual dominance and sadism, yet being someone who's been raised . . . feminist and who doesn't want to sort of act like that. It's tricky."

For both J. and Paul, the conflict between feminism and dominance or sadism was cast in terms of a crisis between political commitments and personal desires, between a social good and individual pleasure. In these terms, being a male dominant feminist was impossible: the resolution of the conflict between the political/social and the personal/individual was to abandon either the political (feminism) or the personal (male dominance); otherwise, one had to "live a lie." Paul and J. resolved their crises differently.

Once J. found the SM community and began learning its values and norms, he started to reconfigure his feminism from a radical critique of patriarchy to a more liberal feminism that focuses on "liberating ourselves from our traditional ways of having sex . . . and allow[ing] women to choose their sexuality."[16] Critical to this shift was a valuation of the consciousness and consent of SM dynamics within the SSC community. J. explained: "Once I learned about the community, the community's values, the consciousness that goes into this, I came to a place where I can go, 'Oh, so if I have a partner who's consenting to this, who enjoys this, who finds it tantalizing, then I'm not violating her.' Then what I'm willing to do is engage in a sexual play, a role play that is comfortable for both of us. So we're pretending to be doing this rape thing, but what we're doing is we're connecting in a sexually particular way." Having established this redefinition of value and ethics, J. began to see SM as not only acceptable, but empowering for women:

> There's actually more equality and more consciousness brought to [BDSM] sexuality than most relationships ever have, because people are talking about what their needs are. They're talking about their desires. They're talking about their fantasies. They're talking about their limits, and they bring that all into the sexual or relationship experience and

that allows for [a] greater level of actual equality. Even if it's a traditional male top/female bottom, I think the female is still more empowered than she would be in a standard heterosexual relationship because her desires and wants are more clearly identified and talked about and expressed than her [non-SM] sexual relationships ever are, and because there's so much more consciousness brought to that process.

J.'s story points to anxiety about the interconnections between the social world and one's interior sexual/psychic world. Yet his reconciliation entailed a shift from a radical feminism to a liberal feminism, resolving this conflict through an emphasis on free choice, self-awareness, and self-empowerment in accordance with neoliberal rationalities.

This resolution recreates a binary between the social or political sphere and the private, personal sphere. Insisting on individual agency, self-mastering, and personal freedom, J.'s self-cultivation and political process entails severing the relationship between his SM play in the consensual community and larger social systems of inequality. For J., the fantasy of consensuality and freely chosen sexual roles is critical to an eventual resolution (even if only partial) between feminist politics and BDSM practices in the shift from radical to liberal feminism. In this, he is aided by community discourse on the scene as a safe space of consensual desires and private exploration, along with liberal feminism's emphasis on the personal rights of the individual (not the good of society), individual agency (not the structuring structure of patriarchy), and free choice (not false consciousness). In this way, liberal feminism corresponds to both a free-market ideology and a particularly American emphasis on individualism, personal agency, and freedom.

However, this resolution also depends on the coconstruction of gender with race, sexuality, and social power. Individualism and choice are not equally available across the social landscape, but rather are tied to the particular ways that masculinity and heterosexuality intersect with whiteness. In an era of what Howard Winant calls the "neoliberal racial project" (1997, 45), racial discourse focuses on individual agency and bars a consideration of larger social structures. As George Lipsitz notes, this project figures race as the "sum total of conscious and deliberative individual activities," as "individual manifestations of personal prejudice and hostility. Systematic, collective, and coordinated group behavior consequently drops out of sight" (2006, 20). The emphasis on individuality reinforces, by both justifying and concealing, an investment in whiteness as a material, structural, and economic advantage (see also Wiegman 1999; Winant 1997). In other words, neoliberalism as rationality guides practitioners in thinking about the SM community as a safe space unrelated to and disconnected from material reality or social norms—a space where, crucially, an individual's social location (as a white, heterosexual man) has nothing to do with racism, heteronormativity, or sexism as intersecting institutionalized systems of inequality.

These intersections create opportunities for some to feel empowered, to remake themselves, as precisely the normative subjects of BDSM community. Like a focus on the agentic individual, an emphasis on choice can obscure the larger social dynamics of racial inequality. During a dialogue about race and SM in *Against Sadomasochism*, Rose Mason notes that the ability to play with power inequality itself betrays racial privilege: "How dare you take the privilege at my expense. I've never had a choice as to whether I want to deal with power issues around my life. And there are white women in the movement who are very unaware that that's what it is, that it is a privilege that goes along with your skin color, being able to make that choice and then to make it in a decadent way is disgusting" (Sims and Mason 1982, 103). This resistance to liberal ideology suggests not only that social positionality matters ("choice" plays out differently for those with and without racial privilege), but that the construction of "race play" *as* choice itself relies on racial privilege. McClintock notes: "Privileged groups can, on occasion, display their privilege precisely by the extravagant display of their *right to ambiguity* . . . In short, the staging of symbolic disorder by the privileged can merely preempt challenges by those who do not possess the power to stage ambiguity with comparable license or authority" (1995, 68–69; italics in original). Here, the very rhetoric of choice not only displays privilege, it also allows people with privilege (of race, class, or gender) to sidestep the fact that they are beneficiaries of that privilege, to position themselves as lone individuals, outside of the material relations of power that give form to both privilege and oppression, opportunity and constraint.

In contrast, Paul's commitment to feminist theory precluded this resolution. Paul told me that when he read *Coming to Power* it was the first time he thought that there might be "ways that one can reconcile this kind of libido with that kind of politics," although he remained well aware that, as a white, male dominant, he was not in the same position as a leatherdyke. Paul also struggled with his attraction to "more darkly complected" women: not only did he want to dominate women, he wanted to dominate nonwhite women. He explained: "Of course, for me, it wasn't that I wanted to cause pain to someone who looked like that [wasn't white]; it was that I was attracted to these types of people and when I'm attracted to someone and get intimate with them, these are the sorts of things psychosexually that excite me." But Paul was also aware that "you can't just divorce your own desires" from a patriarchal, imperialist, racist history.

Paul's comments are provocative because they draw attention to the ways in which race and gender—whiteness and masculinity as forms of domination—structure our "private" desires. Further, they emphasize how this split between the outside of power and the inside of desire is produced. Paul explained:

> All my life as far back as I can remember . . . my primary attraction to women has always been to women who are more darkly complected than I am . . . It caused me years and years and years of very serious conflict . . . I have this part of my sexuality that—and I know I went to the capital of PCdom in the world, [UC] Santa Cruz in the eighties—it was really hard if you take feminism at all seriously as I do and did then, to reconcile. People in the scene are kind of quick, just like Americans everywhere, kind of quick to try and eliminate disturbing ambiguities and dichotomies and to resolve it into binary oppositions and choose the good one, right? And I went through this myself, for years and years—and I mean literally like ten years—I thought that I had to either choose my libido or my politics because they seemed to be antagonistic.

Paul first split apart what he calls his "guilt on the one hand and desire on the other"—politics and libido—and could not "choose the good one."

But, he continued, "it would be foolish for me and intellectually dishonest to deny there is something about the fact that I am a heterosexual white man [that] has something to do with my object choices," and further, that "my identity as a hetero white man is part of being able to fulfill that role [as 'the historical oppressor'] in the scene." Instead, he explained, "I think people in the scene are much too fast to wash that away and say 'Well, you know as long as everybody consents and as long as you've actually thought about it, then it's all okay.' No, it's really not because it's foolish . . . and dishonest to deny [that] the social identities of the people involved in an interaction like that are massively important and present, and I don't think—no matter what anybody says they can do—I just don't believe that you can wash that out. So I think it's always present when I'm playing with someone who is not white." As an antiracist white man, Paul is avoiding the kinds of moves facilitated by neoliberal whiteness. This is not to say that antiracist whites do not receive the material benefits of whiteness, but rather that Paul's words help us understand what Winant calls "white racial dualism": the "contradictory, as well as confused and anxiety-ridden" current situation of white identity, as a result of the continuing "deep structures of white privilege" combined with antiracist aspirations (1997, 41). This "dualism" is reflected in Paul's reference to "guilt" and "desire": a toggling between the social (site of oppression) and the individual (site of personal desire) that showcases some of the unresolved contradictions of whiteness as racialization. As Winant argues, the disavowal of white supremacy and concomitant commitment to formal equality is, itself, a product of neoliberal racial projects (see also Omi and Winant 1994).

The dualism and internal ambivalence of masculinity is also critical to these narratives. For example, Paul described "two archetypes of male dominance" in the scene: the "hairy caveman guy, the brute who will sort of grab you by the hair and just have his way with you, a sort of ravishment," and "the cold, steely, icy, controlling, domineering dom who is emotionally unavailable." He continued: "I've spoken with a number of other hetero men here in the San Francisco scene who feel like we don't really fit" because, for Paul, "that's never going to be [him]." Paul described himself as too "emotionally labile" to be properly dominant; he told me, "sometimes I feel like I'm pretending" when he claims he is a male dominant.

These models of heterosexual male dominance in the scene clearly reflect "real world" social norms of gender, norms that are racialized as well as thoroughly heterosexual. Paul went on: "A lot of derision is correctly heaped upon men who have a very narrow idea of what they are looking for in a submissive: 'I want a large-breasted blonde with an IQ measurable in the low double digits who calls me master and has dinner ready for me.' Those of us in the scene laugh at guys like that . . . they're jokes, they're pathetic. They're out there, but no one takes them seriously. I wish that there was the same kind of derision cast upon women who want to look at men in a similarly stereotyped way." For Paul, it is the heterosexual woman's demand for these types of men—types that are not only socially normative but erotic—that drives the reproduction of "narrow" ideas of masculinity. SM forms of white heterosexual male dominance promise the deep satisfaction of the fulfillment of these polarized roles—dashing men, strong men, cold men, withholding men—while simultaneously producing fantasies of masculinity that many—or even all—men could never embody. As Homi Bhabha argues, masculinity is mired in "compulsion and doubt" (1995, 59); its essence is an "ambivalent identification" with and against the universal and natural (58). For Bhabha, this is psychoanalytic; "anxiety," he reminds us, "is a 'sign' of a danger implicit in/on the threshold of identity, in between its claims to coherence and its fears of dissolution" (60). What Bhabha terms "anxious ambivalence" (60) is a product of masculinity's complicated relationship to both "personal and institutional power" (Berger, Wallis, and Watson 1995, 3), an ambivalence marked by the awkward—both desired and disavowed—relationship of masculinity to domination.

In this dynamic, the HMD is opposed to the white heterosexual submissive man, who, in some way, disavows his very masculinity. Stephanie and Anthony, both dominants, discuss prejudice toward submissives, Stephanie arguing that being submissive is "equated with weakness." Unlike the assumptions made about dominants (or in contrast to the lack of pathologizing assumptions made about dominants), people in the scene assume that there must be "some reason" for being submissive, reasons that Anthony elaborates as "you're fat or you were abused as a child . . . or there's something missing or there's something that's not quite right . . . or that you can't say no." Although Stephanie and Anthony intend their comments to refer to men and women, as Stephanie continues, her example is of a male submissive: "There are all sorts of—you're right—this pathologizing thing, 'Well, why would he want to do this? Why would he want to crawl around on his hands and knees and kiss the feet of this woman and have his dick chained or something? What kind of man would want to do that sort of thing?'" The implicit answer, of course, is that the kind of man who might be submissive isn't a real man, isn't a masculine man. There is nothing "wrong" with a woman who enjoys submission (and it is this that disturbs feminist, submissive women). However, a submissive man risks his masculinity.

In part, this assumption is based on the linking of the abject position —submissive—with women, although it also reflects the fear/disavowal of homosexuality that forms the basis of dominant masculinity; both of these mechanisms are policed by other men.[17] Tom explains: "there are party groups in which I'm marginally tolerated because I'm a sub." He blames this on the "Internet crowd," arguing that "starting in about '94, the web probably quadrupled the rate of influx and completely eliminated the mentoring process." Many practitioners agree with Tom that heterosexual men new to the scene—the Silicon Valley practitioners who entered the scene in the 1990s—are most likely to presume these kinds of parallel and naturalized gender roles. These men are "clueless male tops" who, lacking a more subtle appreciation of the art of SM, think SM is, as Tom put it, "slap, slap, 'down on your knees, bitch, and suck me off.'" The clueless men have an acronym in the scene: CHUDWAH—clueless het-dom wannabes. A CHUDWAH is a new het male dom who doesn't "get it"; high on the list of things he doesn't get is that not all women are submissive—and its far scarier corollary: not all men are dominant.

Phil explains that it is other men who act as the enforcers and arbiters of masculinity and of access to power:

PHIL: I was a 24/7 bottom to [his wife]: we had a monogamous relationship for three years, I was her slave and she was my mistress, and we had very formal things going on, like contracts . . . I enjoyed it a lot—that intensity of 24/7 . . . After I became known as a submissive, a lot of my male friends who were switches or tops didn't like me now. There's a lot of prejudice [on the part] of male tops—even gay male tops—against submissives. You don't see it unless it's right there in front of you . . . It was funny, I lost a lot of apparent respect as soon as they found out I was a male bottom. I still find that . . . I still find it a lot with the newbies, especially the het male tops, they can't even *conceive* of a woman being dominant . . .

MARGOT: I wondered about that.

PHIL: Well, it's true! Some of the closest people would suddenly walk right off from me. I lost some very good male friends. I tried to help them, "I'm not any different than I was a month ago" . . .

MARGOT: Do you think it's a gender thing?

PHIL: . . . Yeah, in a way, it's something that—men seem to have trouble with it, but I think it's because of the social station that society puts men at.

This masculine anxiety, gay or straight (or otherwise), is formed around the submissive male, showcasing the dense connections between heterosexuality (as ideology) and power. But at the same time, invisibility—what you see or don't see—is structured around dominant fictions of gender, which are exposed in their inversion; this helps to illuminate the slide from sexual submission to gender inversion hinted at in Phil's comments.

Submissive men—unlike dominant women—are not celebrated as transgressing gender norms. For Phil, this is because of men's "social station," their social power and privilege, which renders masculinity more fraught, more precarious, and more heavily policed than femininity. These issues show that gender in the scene is deeply connected to gender outside the scene, and to the ways in which heterosexuality, whiteness, and dominance produce possibilities for intelligible gendering. The male bottom, in other words, experiences a sort of double bind produced not through abstract gender roles, but through the particular meanings of masculinity bound to race and sexuality that are performatively produced in the scene.

Here, then, is another place where the relationship between social norms and SM performances cannot be reduced to internalization *or* subversion. Instead, unlike the anti-SM feminist version of heterosexual relations, gender is a source of conflict, tension, and anxiety over being, seeming like, performing, and resembling. Men do not walk into the role of dominant with phallocentric ease or comfort; similarly, submissive women take care to differentiate their in-scene submission from their intelligence, competence, assertiveness, and equality outside the scene. At the same time, although the discordant figure here—the male bottom—can, indeed, show us some of the obligations of masculinity, so too can the gender-normative HMD. It is he who reveals the ambivalence around the denial and enforcement of male privilege (founded on heterosexuality and whiteness), a privilege he is keen to resist (or at least deny) in this purportedly transgressive, nonnormative scene. The anxiety of the HMD is based on wanting to escape or break free from these oppressive social norms—to disidentify with the oppressor—while simultaneously recognizing yet disavowing that his very positionality, his role as a "strong, dominant man" (and hence his effectiveness in the scene), is based on these norms. In this way, HMDs show that the desire for transgression is not to transgress normative gender roles, but rather to transgress or disavow the social force of gender while at the same time maintaining a desired and desirable masculinity.

AMBIVALENCE, MIMESIS, AND MASTERY

Analyzing the ambivalence of the HMD is one way to track the "dualism" Winant describes in relation to whiteness, in which sexism is deemed irrelevant and the firm affixture of masculinity to structural inequality is denied. These forms of white, dominant, heterosexual masculinity produce ambivalence or dualism at precisely the moments when practitioners simultaneously consolidate gendered, racial, and sexualized positionalities and enact a barrier between these "roles" and "real life" power or oppression. Understandings of the scene as completely outside social reality, as not a part of gendered relations of inequality, help construct this barrier, which has as its corollary the idea that—because roles are freely chosen by free, agentic individuals—such burdensome contexts as gendered inequality have no bearing on the SM scene. The kinds of self-cultivation or techniques that SM practitioners enact—glossed as self-empowerment—work simultaneously to provide a (fantasized) out from privilege (and with this, the possibility of remaking gender roles into something perceived of as more free) and to justify certain forms of inequality.

This split itself is produced by a circuit between the body and the social body, a deeply productive exchange that both produces subjects with neoliberal ideas of agency and choice and creates anxiety around the social contradictions embedded, and not resolved, in these dynamics. In particular, these debates reveal that the tension between aspiration (to be antiracist, feminist, even queer—in short, transgressive)[18] and anxiety (over being white, male, dominant, heterosexual—in short, privileged) is critical to the ambivalence that these HMDs articulate. Focusing on these men's ambivalence is one way to think about places where neoliberalism as a cultural formation intertwines with forms of social dominance—whiteness, masculinity, and heterosexuality—to produce a contested relationship between social norms, social oppression, and social privilege.

For example, J. credited a form of feminist-inspired SM with "liberating [him] from the constraints of sexuality that society says you can have and expand that to a wide variety." "So if I wish to have vanilla sex, I can have vanilla sex. If I want to have kinky sex, I can have kinky sex. If I wanted to do role play one night, I do that. And if I want to be a bottom one night, I could be able to do that." For J., radical feminism limited his choices; it wasn't politically acceptable for him to be married to his ex-wife, a woman of color. He explained: "One of the things that I had to come to terms with was . . . to accept that I was a man and that I had male energy and male desires and [a] male use to the world and [that this wasn't] all bad." J. wanted to "question gender roles"; feminism, for him, means that "we should look at these things and we should allow women to be who they are in our society. And the other component of that is we need to liberate men from the social roles that [are inflicted upon them] by society and allow them to be who they are."

This new masculinity was enabled through SM in a way that made J. feel less trapped by social norms of gender. J. explains his SM desire: "[it] allows me to be a man or allows my sexual attraction to be present, but it also recognizes that she's a woman and she has rights and I should respect her and not objectify her." He told me that SM toys and scenarios enable "you to connect in a different way than we may be right now [gesturing to S.], holding hands and seated side by side talking to you." "For me it's more about [how] it allows the whole person to be present because SM allows things to be expressed that often you don't do or allow in relationships. You know, for her to struggle against me and for me to overpower her, it's not appropriate, it's not appropriate in the Hollywood version of lovemaking. But love allows us to do that." For J., SM permits the full person—including dominance and submission, or more aggressive forms of love and sex—to be present, a kind of authenticity denied in Hollywood movies. SM power exchange can enable this wholeness, however, only as long as it remains in the private space of desire, and not the social world of power.

A focus on ambivalence shows us that these categories are not monolithic by foregrounding the tension between transgressive aspirations and privileges: individuals resist the oppressive social norms from which they simultaneously benefit.[19] Such stagings or self-cultivations can produce a sense of freedom from oppressive social norms, especially for practitioners who occupy privileged social locations. But this authentic masculinity—men being "who they [really] are"—is always mediated through oppressive social relations, produced in the intersections of systems of social power and local and individual discourses, practices, and techniques of the self. This is a form of masculinity that feels free, but where freedom depends on a fantasized escape from social norms of gender, race, class, and sexuality. As Robyn Wiegman argues, developing Winant's concept of white racial dualism, even as it is "attuned to racial equality and justice," liberal whiteness is "self-empowering" by "aggressively solidifying its advantage" (Wiegman 1999, 121). This dualism creates the opportunity for self-empowerment narratives that echo a "national [American] narrative of democratic progress" based on transcending fixed, unequal social hierarchies through an alignment with the universal. Yet such purportedly universal subjects turn out to be quite particular: white, middle-class, heterosexual men. In SM, this dualism invigorates a supposedly neutral, authentic individual by requiring practitioners to distance themselves from their own performative investments in masculinity, whiteness, and heterosexuality, even as it is their recognizable—intelligible—white, male, heterosexual masculinity that makes them attractive play partners and effective tops.

The anxiety expressed by these practitioners shows us the fundamental impossibility of either embodying social norms or of living outside them, and reveals the performativity of social norms themselves—the mimetic structure of gender, race, and sexuality. Mimesis, as Michael Taussig argues, "sutures the real to the really made up" (1993, 86). By this charming phrasing, Taussig means that mimesis structures a relationship with reality in which we can pretend that gender or race are not social constructions or inventions, but rather are immutable, natural facts: it is via mimesis that we are able to pretend "that we live facts, not fictions" (xv–xvi). Moreover, Taussig emphasizes the transfer of power from the original to the copy, the way mimesis grants "the copy the character and power of the original, the representation the power of the represented" (xviii).[20] This conception of mimesis accounts, in part, for the effectiveness—the power and desire—of the HMD and other performative SM genders. At the same time, as Butler puts it, mimesis shows us the performative construction of the "so-called original": for example, "categories like butch and femme were not copies of a more originary heterosexuality, but they showed how the so-called originals, men and women within the heterosexual frame, are similarly constructed, performatively established" (2004, 209). Mimesis (or performativity) not only denaturalizes—by exposing the constructedness of—the original, it also undermines the binary and unidirectionally dependent relationship between original and copy. This conception of mimetic performance accounts, in part, for the anxiety—the disavowal and discomfort—of white, heterosexual masculinities inside (and outside) the scene.

In this dynamic, SM gender does not occupy the status of the original (as in the radical feminist version of these relations), nor is SM gender merely a copy of the original (as consented to, performed, and thus fully differentiated from "real" gender, in the liberal rejoinder). Rather, racialized and sexed gender is itself a mimetic performance, a copy that can only ever seek to replicate a phantasmatic original. Mimesis is always a flawed, incomplete, or partial repetition, "almost the same, but not quite" (Bhabha 1984, 127). In Bhabha's formulation, this marks colonial authority with profound ambivalence; authority "can neither be 'original'—by virtue of the act of repetition that constructs it—nor 'identical' by virtue of the difference that defines it. Consequently, the colonial presence is always ambivalent, split between its appearance as original and authoritative and its articulation as repetition and difference" (1985, 150). In the BDSM context, SM gender roles retain the ambivalence of all gender, in that it is impossible to faithfully replicate heterosexuality, masculinity, dominance, or whiteness as though these categories occupy the status of "real originals." Instead, repetition, a partial mimesis, marks every process of subjective embodiment.

At the same time, the need to stage a culturally recognizable performance relies on these originals—the originals that are themselves performatively produced through their repetition within the SM scene just as much as at work, in the club, driving the car, or in the bedroom, as Panther's epigraph highlights. Mimetic performance produces subjects who embody and cultivate social norms, even more than they subvert or consolidate them, at the same time that it produces the "regulatory ideal" of these norms themselves. In this way, SM's gendered and racialized performances participate in the forms of mimetic performativity that forge all subjects; it is only the fantasized break from the real of power—the scene as a safe space—that enables practitioners, and theorists, to imagine that in-scene gender is *only* a copy or a performance, that it has no social effects.

This contradiction—between gender as fundamentally mimetic and mimesis as that which makes gender real—is useful for thinking through how such performative roles produce social relations via social norms. The concept of mimesis accounts for the mimicry, the repetition, involved in gender play and at the same time points to at least one critical reason for my interviewees' ambivalence about this so-called imitation. Chris, another HMD, told me in our interview that, although he had been interested in SM since high school, he "basically thought that what [he] was doing was wrong." "I had it in my head that there was a way of interacting that was all right, and anything that didn't fit into that [feminist] form was wrong. And the idea that you could sort of do an 'as if' kind of interaction somehow never occurred to me." Echoing Bhabha, Chris was explaining that his male dominance can be read as mimetic of heterosexist gender relations, a copy that is "almost the same, but not quite." Here, mimesis structures an emotional relationship of ambivalence: the scene world of play as an imitation or copy of an impossible real. The impossibility of the real of gender (or race, or sexuality) is expressed in the language of anxiety, an anxiety that marks the desire for, and the impossibility of, actually subverting or transgressing these social norms: of mastering social power.

In this way, the production of the "seems-like" space of SM relies on the separation of public and private that cannot but replicate certain forms of privilege as it opens opportunities to cultivate new, seemingly nonoppressive, masculinities. Yet to return to Malc, Paul, and Jeff's "lack of diversity," the whiteness of these HMDs—and indeed of *vanilla* social power—is critical to this freedom; these performances empower some (men, whites) both materially and discursively, while at the same time strengthening cultural narratives that justify these unequal relations (such as the emphasis on personal responsibility or agency provided by neoliberalism). In these projects of self-cultivation, the SM community plays a critical role: the SSC scene enables this bracketing, relying on economic, cultural, and political rationalities to justify the reproduction of forms of inequality that are anything but safe, sane, and consensual.

THE POLITICS OF FREEDOM

As James Ferguson (2002) argues, an anthropologist reading the cultural performance of imitation can read it either as parody (and thus subversive rebellion) or appropriation (and thus covert resistance). Either way, we must celebrate the miming. Of course, "anthropology's disciplinary identification with powerless people" is more complicated in the case of SM practitioners, who are simultaneously excluded from the norm via sexual practice and privileged via race, gender, and class (Kulick 2006, 933). In this case, rather than valorize the queer or condemn the seemingly normative, we must locate BDSM within social categories of power, which I have done in this chapter by investigating the ways these performances produce ambivalence through mimesis. The mimetic performance of gender captures the crisis over the status of copies and originals that is the basis for arguments against SM, but also for the production of SM scenes themselves. This move gets us well beyond the either/or structure of transgression/consolidation, as well as beyond the twin poles of freedom/oppression produced by practitioners (freedom as freedom from social inequality) and by radical feminist analysis (oppression as the unbearable weight of patriarchy in structuring everyday lives), both limited forms of binary thinking that can't quite get at the ways that social relations structure and are structured by subjects. Instead, we must investigate the politics of race, gender, and sexuality as they are intertwined and embodied, enacted and practiced, lived and resisted by practitioners navigating social norms and political rationalities produced in simultaneously discursive and material ways.

As a circuit between the individual and social body, sexuality is a social relation produced by and bound up with other social relations of power, and it thus requires a reading that refuses the economic/material and performative/discursive split. If we can do this, we can start to understand the transgressive desires—the desire to transgress—of the HMD. The desire of these men to reconcile their politics with their desires is a way to make themselves politically acceptable, to defend SM against its critics, and to opt out of the social hierarchies of whiteness, heterosexuality, and masculinity that these progressive men fight in their non-SM lives. Though an understandable goal, this desire also produces an imaginary in which individual desires and actions can be separated from social systems and power. It re-encodes the safe, sane, and consensual scene as a playground of equality, SM play as "only a game," and racialized and sexualized gender as individually chosen and, thus, mastered. SSC SM locates players in social worlds at precisely the moment when it enables practitioners to fantasize about the break or gap between the SM scene and the real world.

At the same time, the ambivalent desires for and of white, heterosexual, dominant masculinity open up new horizons—for SM practitioners and for cultural analysis. Ambivalence should encourage us to examine more closely the dense interconnections between race, class, gender, and sexuality; the points of conflict between social norms and social relations; and the contradictions of normative constructions and performances as they are embodied and cultivated. In this way, the binary options for a cultural critic reading such scenes—Subversive or reenacting? Political or personal? Feminist or queer?—fails to consider the particular productivity of these relations. To understand SM play, we must instead pay more careful attention to what is being produced at such moments—a production that includes privilege and power, in addition to nonnormative self-cultivation and practice.

I will end this chapter with Paul's words, words that to me summarize the necessary, if painful, work of ambivalence and a refusal to "opt out" of either one's responsibilities for social relations of dominance or the ethnographic complexities of these on the ground:

> What I eventually came to was what should have been obvious to me in the beginning as a good poststructuralist, which was that trying to choose one or the other [BDSM or feminism, sexual or intellectual satisfaction] was a false choice. That the intellectual honesty consisted in living in the middle, living in the tension. I think that my position as a hetero white man has something to do with my sexuality. It has something to do with everything. It has something to do with my politics. It has something to do with my economic place in the world, the way I can speak, the privileges that I have, the abilities that I have, the choices that are open to me, and I think it's just crazy for people to try and

> pretend that sexuality is this magical realm that is somehow natural and is unaffected by anything social, economic, or political. You can see that I had tied myself up; the greatest act of bondage I was doing in those years was with myself in my own head.

We should take seriously the radical feminist contention that sexuality, desire, and fantasy are bound up in real-world structures of inequality, that we cannot separate the private/bedroom from the public/social world. Indeed, it is precisely the strain with which the private and public are held apart that reveals the ways in which subjects and communities—through practice and play—are bound ever more closely to the real world of power that makes subjects of us all.

FIVE 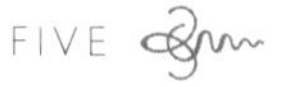

SEX PLAY AND SOCIAL POWER

Reading the Effective Circuit

I do not believe that sexuality is separate from living. As a minority woman, I know dominance and subordination are not bedroom issues . . . S/M is not about sex but about how we use power. If it were only about personal sexual exchange or private taste, why would it be presented as a political issue?
—AUDRE LORDE and SUSAN LEIGH STARR, "Interview with Audre Lorde"

I do not believe that sex has an inherent power to transform the world. I do not believe that pleasure is always an anarchic force for good. I do not believe that we can fuck our way to freedom.—PAT CALIFIA, *Macho Sluts*

The difficulties for nonsadomasochists have been primarily with sadism and with psychodrama that appears to make light not only of rape and incest but also of histories of oppression, such as American slavery and the Nazi Holocaust, drawing upon those histories to construct sex-games.
—CLAUDIA CARD, *Lesbian Choices*

S/M is more a parody of the hidden sexual nature of fascism than it is a worship or acquiescence to it. How many real Nazis, cops, priests or teachers would be involved in a kinky sexual scene?—PAT CALIFIA, *Public Sex*

As these four epigraphs make clear, SM play with social power, especially cultural—and national—trauma like slavery and the Holocaust, is contested and politically complex. Such play echoes and plays off traumatic histories; indeed, it is this dramatization of historical structures of exploitation in the guise of fantasized or performed display that makes SM play erotic. As I argued in the previous chapter, SM's play with such historical referents is a challenge to read without falling into one of two positions. In the first, SM play is a matter of private desires, just a consensual game or parody, and thus we might read these scenes as transgressive, as remaking the social world, as a form of resistance through reiteration. This reading relies on a fantasized split between the real (social inequality, norms, oppression, politics—the public) and the scene (radicalness, transgression, equality, desire—the private) that can serve to "excuse" some practitioners from their privilege while concealing the generative force of social norms on SM play. The second reading is the converse: SM is a public and political problem, a form of racism, sexism, or fascism, and thus we ought to read these scenes as the violent reinforcement or production of social inequality, or, at the very least, as appropriative of real human suffering. This reading, too, relies on a simplification of the social world, making the conditions of any particular performance—the social context, audience, or effect—irrelevant to analysis. The politics of such scenes are, in this reading, the same as that of their referents. Indeed, in both of these readings, it is an a priori determination—SM as an SSC scene or SM as a mimicry of social inequality—that determines a scene's politics.

Instead of this binary analysis, this chapter marshals the performative materialist methodology developed in this book to read the politics of BDSM scenes. This entails considering the material conditions of SM performance, alongside the material—although often discursive—effects of SM play. A political reading of SM must, as David Savran puts it, emphasize "the conditions of performance: the multiple social positionalities of the performer (rather than his or her intentions), the discursive strategies put into play by the performance, and the reception of said performance" (1998, 9). These conditions—social location, audience reception, and discursive and ideological production—are central to an analysis of any particular scene. But these particularities are also central to the way scenes *work*: the effects of a scene, political or otherwise. In this chapter, I focus on the performative efficacy of SM's play circuits, bringing Jon McKenzie's (2001) theorization of performance to the forefront. For McKenzie, performance draws attention to the efficiency or functionality of flexible circuits, to how subjects and scenes are linked through complex feedback loops and series of exchanges. Developing the concept of effectiveness, I explore when and why scenes work: when, as Anthony put it in the last chapter, players find the "button" or "trigger" that accesses the erotic power of a scene—and what happens when they do.

This form of efficacy is material as well as performative: SM scenes are cultural performances that reflect and produce larger social relations.[1] Although SM practitioners imagine a split between the scene and real life, I argue that effective SM scenes connect the real (the social) and the scene (the performance) via hot-button issues. This connection creates a circuit that not only produces hot SM sex but also possibilities for consolidating, reimagining, or responding to the national imaginaries of racialized, gendered, sexualized, and classed belonging from which SM draws both its scenes and its erotic power. Such imaginaries are unevenly accessible; as I have shown, the neoliberal rationality that pervades the SM scene functions to justify social inequality (based on race, class, and gender) through purportedly neutral subjectivity: the rational, autonomous, responsible, self-mastering individual. This circuit can create the opportunity for privileged subjects—subjects who correspond to the ideal SM practitioner—to imagine themselves free from oppressive social norms, a situation that reinforces their very privilege. But the circuit can also challenge the division of private desires and public politics, opening opportunities for recognizing, and responding to, these ideologies.

This chapter takes up the performative efficacy of the circuit by reading several scenes of what some call "taboo" or "cultural trauma" play—play with racial, ethnic, and national themes. Through ethnographic readings of the slave auction, Master/slave play, Nazi play, a black/Latino mugging scene, torture/interrogation play, and the "sadomasochistic" Abu Ghraib torture photographs, I argue that such effective circuits put into place complex workings: some, for example, enable the further disavowal of white privilege and racism, while others enable more ambivalent, open-ended readings of social power; some make visible, and thus available for reimagining, the normally invisible construction of racialized belonging, while others make spectacle, and thus detach the audience from such productions. Crucial here are the personal, social, and national imaginaries available for play; the social tensions—between the visible and invisible, known and unknown, and public and private—that animate SM dynamics; and the effect of affective involvement, an emotional attachment to particular scenes and dynamics, for players and audiences alike.

Juxtaposing and contrasting these scenes, this chapter invites you, the reader, into these readings, to ask what each circuit enables and disables, what social relations are produced (emotionally, politically, and discursively) in these exchanges, and what sorts of political claims can be made about SM play. For a political reading relies not on a purely discursive—nor a purely formal—analysis of social power, but instead on the mobile and contested performative circuits that produce national belonging alongside social, often racialized, difference; on the materiality of social relations that we call sexuality.

THE SLAVE AUCTION THE VISIBILITY OF RACE

Recall the auction stage at the Byzantine Bazaar and Slave Auction. Picture the effeminate Asian American man, gender humiliated in a complex racial performance; the Latina dyke resisting the audience's demand for feminine sexualization; the white HMD, mocked and objectified in his tighty whities; and the African American slave, displayed by her icy, controlled white male master. The performances I watched that day were uncomfortable and disturbing, but also funny and lighthearted. I laughed along with the audience; I was also profoundly troubled. This scene—the first of my real fieldwork—captivated and also frustrated my political readings; I could not account for the gap between the specificity of these particular bodies and the larger racial, gendered, and sexual implications of this display.

My first approach to the auction I saw that day came in the form of a conference paper in 2001—the first paper I gave at the annual American Anthropological Association meetings. In the paper, I read the scenes through Butlerian performativity; I analyzed the politics of the slave auction in terms of the uncontrollability of a performance's effects, and the instability of what is reiterated and what is excluded. So, the white top "one night only" bottom could be read, I argued, as a failed citation of the law of heteropatriarchy. Displayed in his underwear, sexualized, and mocked, this man stood as the absurd token of a masculinity, a heterosexuality, and a whiteness that must, to perform, exclude this very performance. I offered a similar reading of the butch Latina; the slave auction, I argued, offered the possibility for the displacement of racial, sexual, and gendered categories because of the inherent instability of social norms.

Of course, I was not alone in this analysis; this reiteration reading is common to most queer, feminist, and performance studies scholarship. It is also shared by some in the SM scene. In a presentation at a panel discussion and workshop on the experiences of people of color[2] in the scene, for example, Midori (a well-known Japanese-born SM educator) described some of the ways she disrupts stereotypes about Asian women in the United States as either delicate flowers or dragon ladies. She told us she liked playing with some of these stereotypes and used as an example an East Asian prisoner-of-war scene, in which she was a cruel "dragon lady" imprisoning, torturing, and interrogating a prisoner in a tiger cage. Doing such a scene, she said, can "take away the negative power of stereotypes" through hyperbole. She also pointed to the possibilities of discordant moments, telling us that she enjoyed being particularly sadistic while wearing a traditional kimono, thus mixing the "delicate flower" image with hard-core sadism. She felt that this presentation challenged racial expectations, in much the same way as the gender discordant readings I discussed in the previous chapter.

Similarly, during a conversation about Nazi uniforms in the scene, Bonnie, an Asian American masochist, told me that she had a friend who planned to get a latex burka made: "Not a traditional burka because she wanted it in clear latex, so it would be—it's like satire." For Bonnie, satire means that "we bring things that make us uncomfortable into our everyday lives" in order to "poke fun" at them. Lady Hilary, a white mistress, told me that she thinks latex Nazi regalia is hot because "we're taking it and cartooning it." In these readings, satire, parody, or hyperbole can displace norms, exposing the non-naturalness, noninevitableness, or indeterminacy of social power. So, in a series of similar moves, I read the slave auction as performative resignification.

Yet even when I wrote that conference paper, the Asian man and the black slave refused this pat analysis, remaining stranded, as Roger Lancaster puts it, between "parody or praise, subversion or intensification, deviation or norm, resistant or enabling" (1992, 568). In part, this is because theories of performativity—especially as they are used by most cultural critics—do not easily lend themselves to a more materialist analysis of social structures or embodiment. In part, this is because anthropological, performance studies, and queer and feminist analysts want to validate the subcultural performances of our informants as countercultural. But these frameworks also mean that, as Saba Mahmood's critique of Butler makes clear, when these binary choices are our only critical options, we cannot see the more everyday ways in which norms are embodied, lived, and cultivated, as well as contested (2004).

This point is made by Deborah Elliston, who argues that " 'sex' is not a free-floating signifier available for any social project that comes along. It is structured, embedded, and motivated" (2002, 306; see also Allison 2000). Elliston points out that anthropologists are "ideally positioned" to analyze the specific social relations, cultural contexts, and symbolic logics through which sex is produced. This is where an embedded, ethnographic reading is critical. For it is impossible to talk about the politics of this slave auction—to make claims about what these performances actually did—without understanding the social relations, tensions, and divergent positionalities of the various players, people I did not know that first day at the auction but later met, socialized with, and could locate within a social space. Thus, departing from the more discursive reading that I first attempted, this chapter reads the auction—and other racialized performances—as a cultural performance based on and productive of material relations.

The first significant condition of this performance is audience: the auction was performed in front of an audience that was overwhelmingly white. In the classes, munches, and other events I attended, unless the event was specifically focused on people of color or taught by a person of color, there were generally no more than one or two people of color in a room full of whites. Yet white people rarely noticed how white their scene was—or, if asked to notice, did not feel that this was a community problem. In each of my interviews, I asked practitioners about the racial diversity of the scene, generally by asking: "Why do you think the scene is so white?" Most of my white interviewees gave a version of one of the following answers: people of color aren't into BDSM because they are repressed (by their culture) or can't afford it; there are lots of people of color in the scene (followed by the naming of two or three of the five or so highly visible people of color: "Midori, Mollena, and . . . you know . . .

Cathy, that black woman John was dating?"); or people of color have their own scenes, so they don't need to be in ours. Very few white interviewees felt that racism within the scene, or the construction of the scene as white, might be the reason that there were so few nonwhite practitioners.

These analyses were not, of course, expressed by any people of color with whom I spoke. Much more often I heard that racism made participating uncomfortable, or that people of color were treated like tokens or exotic play partners. Some found the politics of cross-racial playing too difficult to negotiate. Others, including many of the panelists at the people of color panel discussion I describe below, felt trapped between a racist white BDSM community and a kink-phobic racial or ethnic community. Instead, some play only with other people of color in the mostly white scene, or find scenes for people of color only. Yet these scenes are quite limited in size and scope. The Mahogany Munch, a munch "for people of color and the people who like them," was the one pansexual people of color munch in the Bay Area while I was doing fieldwork. It was usually held at a Mexican restaurant in Oakland; fewer than twenty people typically attended. The day I went, I was one of four white people, out of a total of ten attendees. The founder, Darrell, told me he started the munch because, when he entered the scene in the early 1990s, there were only one or two other people of color. He wanted to bring more people out and provide a safe space for them within the larger scene. Darrell does not exclude white people from the munch, but it is tricky for him to balance being inclusive and responsive (to, for example, mixed-race couples) and creating a safe space (for example, he explained that some white men attend the munch to prey on black women). With few exceptions, then, practitioners of color must negotiate the white scene: the organizations, classes, munches, parties, and other community structures that produce and simultaneously justify white, but unmarked, participation and belonging.

Here, whiteness is not merely a demographic issue; whiteness is a nonracial, universal subject position in relation to the visibility of raced —nonwhite—practitioners. For example, the standardization of SM bodily techniques presumes that the body is white: in classes on branding, differences in skin scarring and pigmentation are rarely discussed. This impacts the legibility of what counts as race play, or even play that references race. I was continuously surprised during my fieldwork to find that participants did not connect the slave auction to race. Ouchy—a white, bi top/sadist in his early forties—and I were discussing why, as he put it, the scene was "superwhite," and why there were not more people of color involved in SM. I asked him whether he thought that things like slave auctions, or Master/slave play, might be related to the whiteness of the scene. He replied: "To be honest with you, I've never even thought about it in that way. I've never thought about it being racial. Master/slave seems to be kind of transcending—racism in America is bad, but . . . that doesn't seem particularly race-oriented to me." Ouchy is not ignorant of racism; indeed, he works at an organization founded by radical black activists. Instead, he is voicing a common white perception: slave auctions and SM in general are about abstract or neutral, not racialized, power.

This is in part due to the ubiquity of the slave auction, which is a common fundraising and party event in pansexual communities across the United States. The Society of Janus holds one every year: it is one of the three major yearly parties (the other two are for Valentine's Day and Halloween). At many of the national SM conferences, auctions are a special event; major teachers and well-known players are auctioned off for either the host organization or for charity. During the eighteen months of my fieldwork, I attended six or seven auctions, including a Santa's Slave Auction hosted by a leather bar in the East Bay, and I missed perhaps the same number. Because of this ubiquity, and because the events are simultaneously fun (most are held right before a large play party) and philanthropic, many white people attending such events do not view them as race play, or even referencing race.

Annalee, a white, genderqueer pervert, said to me as we discussed a couple in a 24/7 Master/slave relationship: "I mean, they're both white so there's no racial aspect to it." Talking about Master/slave terminology, Stephanie, a white dominant, explained: "So much of the scene is based on Master/slave with men and men, with women and women, with white people and not white people, and nobody really thinks about it until it's a people of color panel." She was not alone in crediting the Janus-sponsored People of Color Panel Discussion, held in March 2002, with bringing racial issues into view. It appeared to me that, before the panel, most of the white practitioners I interviewed had never really considered the racial overtones of toys, relationships, and scenes that obviously (to me) mimed racialized slavery. At the same time, however, it is the presence of visible, marked nonwhite bodies that makes this connection: a Master/slave scene between whites is "not racial."

This, oddly, makes almost all interracial play scenes race play by default. Mollena, an African American bottom who is very interested in race play, explained that her first public play, with a white top, was perceived as race play, even though "it was a straightforward fuckin' rope scene with whips and shit." Because Mollena often plays with white men, "I do race play by default in the eyes of most people."[3] Estrella explained, as a white top who has had several black partners, even without "overt name calling or plantation scenarios, just the whole idea that me, a white person, was beating a black person—that's race play right there with our history." In this construction, *race play* does not refer only to scenes, roles, or dynamics that reference racialized history, such as slave auctions or Master/slave terminology. Because BDSM is fundamentally about power, and because the vast majority of SM practitioners in the semipublic scene are white, SM sex play reanimates racialized social structures of dominance and submission that themselves forge racial and gendered subjectivities.

This creates divergent racialized social positionalities, with white practitioners seen as simply SM practitioners (and their scenes as "just" about power exchange), and nonwhite practitioners excluded from the scene in both mundane and more fundamental ways. Nonwhite practitioners, in other words, cannot participate in a (or, indeed, the) "neutral" scene, nor are they the normalized subjects of such a scene. This exclusion means that people of color rarely experience their SM practice —or politics—as disconnected from embodied racialization. Tijanna— an African American, lesbian bottom in her late thirties—tells me that she "won't even go" to a slave auction because, in her words, "it's just too": "Oh yeah, I'd be a great notch on somebody's belt, but I'm not going up there for that. A slave auction! Can't they think of another word? You know, a 'sub auction'? Slave auction! Come on! Shit." Tijanna emphasizes the ways in which race bears on her SM practices:

MARGOT: So is it difficult to play with white women?

TIJANNA: Yeah, for me. I'm mostly a bottom, and I just don't want to bottom in public to white women . . . There's certain things I won't do, any of that Master/slave stuff, I don't think so. I don't want to be flogged on the back. It's just too much like slavery.

MARGOT: . . . When you play, do you avoid things that have that [racialized] meaning?

TIJANNA: . . . As far as the Master/slave stuff goes, yes, definitely yes . . . I suppose I'm always conscious of race and my position when I'm playing—when I'm bottoming, I guess I am very conscious of that . . .

MARGOT: Would you top a white woman? I mean, would that be easier?

TIJANNA: Sure that'd be easier, oh yeah. I could do that in a minute, yeah, that's no problem . . . I wouldn't top her like maliciously or meanly or in retaliation, but yeah, I'd be much more open to that, much more open to that.

Tijanna's unwillingness to be flogged on the back, do Master/slave play, or bottom to a white woman in public illustrates that SM play and power in the scene is based on larger, national meanings and histories of race. Her concern is both over her own positionality and, crucially, how she would be read publicly: she needs to be conscious of the racial ramifications of bottoming to a white woman in the context of this history. And, for Tijanna, this kind of dilemma cannot be overcome by distancing the scene (where all power is in flux and negotiable) from the real of social inequality (a space of hierarchical social and institutional racism) but must instead be worked out in practice, based on audience, context, and positionality (public or private scene, white or nonwhite partner, kinds of scenes and toys used).

In contrast, many of my white interviewees felt that the safe, sane, and consensual scene worked precisely to disconnect the social real (of racism) from power exchange. Atheris, a white dominant, explained: "I personally don't think there's anything wrong with emotionally charged or racially charged [play], even though I have personal issues in the real world about that [racism]." She continued: "Let's say a black person really wants to be in that scene and be called a nigger—it's not real. I mean, it's just not real. You're taking a part of history that happened that you know is not going to—you're not going to [be] oppressed again. And you can play with it; I think it's safe now. It wasn't safe when it was real." Like Ouchy, these practitioners felt that Master/slave play and slave auctions "transcended" racism in America: they could be seen as a neutral script for SM play—emptied of any specific historical or social meaning, or rendered "not real" by the bracketing function of the safe, sane, and consensual scene.

Other white practitioners could understand that people of color might be sensitive to these racialized connections but felt that the scene, in concert with the United States as a whole, had progressed beyond these meanings. In our interview, Anton and Jezzie, whites in a Master/slave relationship, discussed the implications of their own language. I asked if anyone had ever suggested that the terms might be racially problematic, and Anton told me: "Once or twice I've seen the attitude that using the term *slave* evokes black racial slavery in the United States and hence, it's inappropriate and instead you should use *submissive* or something like that. But . . . this is an educated person's sport, and most people . . . are sophisticated enough to realize that that's a very superficial connection and isn't really terribly relevant." For Anton, the "educated" and "sophisticated" SM practitioner (a universalized white, professionalized practitioner) knows that trans-Atlantic chattel slavery isn't relevant to SM Master/slave play. Although others (especially people of color) might have a problem with the evocation of "black racial slavery," for Anton and other practitioners, the SSC scene works to separate out the fantasy of Master/slave from any real referents. This enables white practitioners to imagine their play divorced from and irrelevant to racial inequality, as play with no politics.

In these understandings, whiteness is not only social context and unmarked universal, but also a social logic that both produces and justifies unequal social relations, a discourse made material through play. This is the logic of race "colorblindness." Most white people in the scene, like many Americans, subscribe to a colorblind attitude toward racial difference, an attitude commonly understood as antiracist. As Lee Baker cogently argues, this logic denies institutionalized racism in favor of American cultural mythologies of meritocracy, autonomy, personal responsibility, and individualism (2001). For example, Vicki, discussing her "initial reaction" to the word *slave* told me: "I was a little bit worried about the word because it would cause people to think of historical evil instead of what is [today]." But then, she thought: "First Amendment, freedom of expression. So [to] the people who find it upsetting—get over it." This argument is, as Howard Winant argues, part of a neoliberal racial project, a white dualism where such "colorblindness" gives white people the fantasy of an escape from racism without giving up the material benefits of whiteness (1997, 45–47). In this racial project, claims that a white social context doesn't matter bolster whiteness as the basis for universal, individual agency, simultaneously justifying racism inside and outside the scene.

Gretchen told me: "I really believe in freedom of exploration . . . I firmly believe that people have the right to play with Nazi interrogation or Master/slave type scenes." The emphasis here on choice, free will, and individual agency simultaneously separates the scene (and the space of individual desires) from social structures and inequalities and gives some (white) people the privilege of being progressive, sophisticated, or at least tolerant and open to difference. This language of "transcendence," as Ouchy put it, splits apart the bad racism in America and the race-neutral—thus race-free—scene. Because of larger mythologies of neoliberal whiteness and American progress, SM practitioners are, like most whites, inclined to endorse this reading: that there is no relationship between Master/slave play and racism or racial history. For these practitioners—most, but not all, white[4]—the politics of this scene is moot: racial roles can be freely chosen and thus are politically neutral.

My interview with Anton was conducted with his wife and slave, Jezzie, who disagreed with him: "I've had more of a problem with the term [*slave*] than he has . . . I'm not crazy about that word at all." She continued: "It does seem in a way to kind of dismiss the trauma of somebody who's taken into slavery against their will, and I wish there were a comfortable way around it . . . I think there's a common thread that makes it legitimate for us to use the term, but it's such a vast difference that it's not comfortable. And I can certainly see how, in this context—with modern America, with racism as it is—a black person would be uncomfortable with the term. I wouldn't begrudge them that. I wouldn't tell them that they shouldn't be uncomfortable with it." For Jezzie, M/s terms within the SM scene raise the specter of appropriation, an appropriation that is not "comfortable" for her. In other words, she partially accepts the argument made by radical feminists and others who suggest that, by co-opting or appropriating the traumatic experiences or histories of people of color in the United States, SM performances trivialize *real* social power.[5]

These kinds of borrowings simultaneously rely on a referent of racial inequality and obscure this referent through a language of choice. Like Eric Lott's reading of blackface minstrelsy, such borrowing simultaneously depends on and obscures "the material relations of slavery" (1993, 3; see also Klesse 2007). In Lott's analysis, this obfuscation worked not only by "pretending that slavery was amusing" (1993, 3), but also through the racial fantasies and emotional connections that motivated working-class whites to appropriate African American cultural forms in the nineteenth century (a dynamic central to race and class boundary making). In contrast, in SM play with race, although such appropriations consolidate whiteness, they are typically either disavowed or refused—a refusal that takes its most banal form in the refusal of many white people to play with people of color for fear of acting the part of a racist. Tina Portillo, an SM dyke of color, writes: "Frankly, it surprised me that some white leatherdykes didn't want to play with me unless they were bottoming for me . . . whenever a white butch is 'worried' about topping me and isn't sure if she can hit me because she doesn't want to 'hurt' me, I hasten to calm her fears and convince her just how badly I would like her to hurt me" (1991, 50; see also Berlinger 2006; V. Johnson 1999). As Portillo notes, many white people are uncomfortable topping, but not bottoming to, people of color; as with gender play, race play that mimics social power is more difficult for practitioners than play that reverses it. Mollena explains that "reverse race play" is empowering "for people of color who are stepping outside of roles. I mean for a black woman to submit to a white man, well that's just the way it's been," whereas a black male top with a white female bottom, that's a "big score, considering that they're doing something that fifty years ago might have gotten them killed." This mapping of scene to social power combines with the desire of most white people to be—and to be seen as—good, antiracist white people, creating the desire to simply avoid such loaded scenes (at least in public).

Refusing to play with nonwhite people and simultaneously denying the racial referents of SM play produces a situation in which well-meaning white people are exempted from the politics of SM racial projects. The concern about the public politics of such scenes is also a desire for unmarked sex—sex outside of politics—that relies on the universalization of whiteness. So, Annalee, like Jezzie, sees many of the "trappings of SM" as "reminiscent of American slavery" and tells me that she thinks it might "feel creepy" for people of color to come into a community "where people are playing with roles that are a little too close to the truth sometimes." That "truth" is a truth of racialized embodiment:

it is people of color who may feel uncomfortable, not the white people planning and performing these scenes. In this fantasy, white people transcend racism in neutral scenes, while people of color—cast, most often, as black[6]—are materially excluded by becoming the bearers of race and racism. And the production of the scene as separate from the social real is another way in which the whiteness of the SM community is performatively produced, and neoliberal whiteness as social privilege maintained.

With this, I will return to the slave auction. The single most disturbing picture I have from that day was the African American female slave, displayed by her white master. His hand, holding her dress to display her shaved genitals, smoothing back her hair, smacking her ass; the audience's discomfort—or was that my fantasy?

Juxtaposed to the banality of software engineers and toy vendors, hot dogs and small talk, I was drawn to the uncomfortable production of racialized, gendered, and sexual difference—my own, just as much as anyone else's. After the auction, I came back again and again to these scenes, scenes that became so critical to my fieldwork and this book. My desire to understand the politics of such spectacular visibility was continuously frustrated, impotent, insufficient. The spectacular tableau, the enactment and dramatization of hierarchies of race, sexuality, and gender alongside the normalness of these white practitioners, challenged me, again and again, to account for—in a richer way than my analytical framework allowed—what was happening in these scenes. These reworkings, however, eventually pushed me past a concern for this woman's well-being to what I came to recognize as my well-meaning whiteness disturbed by the scene. And instead of taking refuge in these dynamics, I looked again at how whiteness is produced as a universal background for the scene: producing privilege along with the transgressive performances and sexual radicalness to which I was already attuned.

In these moments of performative play, the sudden, spectacular hypervisibility of race reveals, as Robert Reid-Pharr (among many others) has argued, whiteness as a racial position (2001, 88–89). In the context of a community so defined by whiteness, it requires a certain spectacular dramatization to unsettle whiteness as the universal basis of community belonging, of normalness. And so, for me, focusing on the social, economic, and political investments in maintaining the invisibility of whiteness—the forms of privilege, power, and knowing and not knowing that enable whiteness (and other forms of social privilege) to function as universal and thus unseen—finally dislodged my concern for the black slave and my discomfort with her white master's commanding grasp on her hair, and instead prompted a closer look at my simultaneous attraction to and revulsion from such loaded scenes.

My responses are not, to be sure, those of everyone who was at the auction that day or who is reading these words now: particular SM scenes produce differential political effects. But the conditions of a performance are more than context; rather, they begin to unfold the complex circuit between an SM scene and a "real life" referent, a circuit that—depending on how public/private, social/fantasy, real/scene are mapped, produced, and received by practitioners and audiences—produces differential social relations. In what follows, I unfold the thickness of such loadedness in terms of personal, community, and, crucially, national imaginaries. I chart the effectiveness of these social tensions—between the banal and spectacular, visible and invisible, public and private, consensual and nonconsensual—when they are preserved, in fetishistic form, in SM scenes, objects, and dynamics.[7] And finally, I show the effect of emotional engagement—disgust, desire, discomfort—in both producing and drawing attention to the typically unmarked, even disguised, production of difference and power.

NAZI AND OTHER PLAY

AFFECTIVE RESPONSES AND NATIONAL IMAGINARIES

On July 24, 2008, the British High Court ruled in favor of Max Mosley, then the president of the International Automobile Federation—the international governing body of motor sports, including Formula One racing. Mosley had sued the *News of the World* for "breach of confidence and/or the unauthorized disclosure of personal information" after the tabloid published an illustrated story about Mosley with the headline "F1 Boss Has Sick Nazi Orgy with Five Hookers" in March 2008. Mosley is the son of Britain's 1930s fascist leader, Sir Oswald Mosley; as most newspaper stories noted, Mosley's parents married in 1936 at the home of the Nazi propaganda chief Joseph Goebbels, and Adolf Hitler was a guest of honor (Burns 2008b). The story included phrases like: "the son of infamous British wartime fascist leader Oswald Mosley is filmed romping with five hookers at a depraved NAZI-STYLE orgy in a torture dungeon . . . barks ORDERS in GERMAN as he lashes girls wearing mock DEATH CAMP uniforms and enjoys being whipped until he BLEEDS."[8]

In the case, Mosley argued that his rights to and expectation of privacy for his consensual, private SM parties were violated by the story and the secret video recording paid for by the newspaper. The paper countered that revealing Mosley's sexual activities was necessary for the public interest because, as the *News of the World*'s editor, Colin Myler, stated, "taking part in depraved and brutal S&M orgies on a regular basis does not, in our opinion, constitute the fit and proper behaviour to be expected of someone in his hugely influential position."[9] Key to this depravity, of course, is the alleged "Nazi role play" in what was variously characterized as an SM scene, a party, and an orgy. In other words, a "Nazi theme" or "quasi-Nazi behaviour," in the paper's argument, rendered this scene both public and political.[10] Thus, part of the case for the judge, Justice David Eady, to decide was whether there was a Nazi or concentration-camp theme to the scene, which could deprive Mosley of his right to privacy.

In the judgment, over twenty pages are devoted to this question. If there was a Nazi theme, Eady reasons, the paper's allegation that Mosley was "parodying Holocaust horrors" and "mocking the humiliating way Jews were treated" could constitute a public interest question—or, at least, it "would be information which people arguably should have the opportunity to know and evaluate" in terms of his public role in the International Automobile Federation.[11] Thus, the judge proceeds methodically through the video, discussing whether, for example, shaving or medical examinations are particularly Nazi or just, as Mosley's attorney James Price argued, "standard" in SM prison scenes. Eady notes that "in the first scenario, when the Claimant was playing a submissive role, he underwent a medical inspection and had his head searched for lice. Again, although the 'medical' had certain unusual features, there is nothing specific to the Nazi period or to the concentration camps about these matters. Moreover, no German was spoken at this stage." Later he writes: "The Claimant was 'shaved.' Concentration camp inmates were also shaved. Yet, as Mr. Price pointed out, they had their *heads* shaved. The Claimant, for reasons best known to himself, enjoyed having his bottom shaved—apparently for its own sake rather than because of any supposed Nazi connotation."[12] The fascinating contortions in the case—is speaking German during a "juridical" scene necessarily Nazi? What constitutes a "routine" SM prison scene?—are intended to separate "regular" SM from SM that mimics, and thus mocks, instances of historical trauma like the Nazi concentration camps. Or, as John Burns, the *New York Times* reporter, puts it, was the scene's theme "a Nazi concentration camp . . . or, as the participants say, an occasion when the use of guttural commands in German, an old Luftwaffe jacket and military-style caps and boots had nothing at all to do with Nazi fantasies?" (2008c).

The judge decided that "there was no such mocking behaviour and not even, on the material I have viewed, any evidence of imitating, adopting or approving Nazi behaviour"; thus the public interest portion of the case was dismissed.[13] However, Burns's question lingers, resisting a resolution into the either/or required by a court ruling and much critical theory, where the question to be settled is whether Mosley is or is not a Nazi (or at least an anti-Semite), or whether this scene is or is not about concentration camps. Indeed, this story is haunted by the disingenuousness of the claim that there might be a "standard" or neutral German prison scene, that the eroticism of such a scene at this particular historical moment is not already dependent on a collective memory of the Third Reich.

In an essay about the relative normalization of the swastika as an icon in gay leather pornography, Arnie Kantrowitz argues that such uses cannot but glorify Nazis. Criticizing his fellow gay leathermen who see and use the symbol as "just part of the look" or "only an image of power," Kantrowitz writes: "The private romanticization and trivialization of Nazism is not merely a sexual matter. It is political" (1991, 206–7). This critique suggests that imagining Nazi symbols as emblems of power—neutral forms—is a denial of the historical meaning of the swastika; such use can never be merely private/sexual but is always public/political. Indeed, such a mechanism works by evacuating historical specificity (the Holocaust) while retaining its sinisterness by way of an alibi. The disavowal of the connections between the emblem and its social meaning is facilitated by a split between desire and politics: imagining that the swastika is an empty signifier of power, imagining that its use in private and sexual scenes has nothing to do with the Holocaust.

We can read Nazi play—in Mosley's case and otherwise—through this lens and argue that the way such scenes work is to draw on racialized history to make hot scenes, while simultaneously emptying the specificity out of them, allowing the charge to be smuggled back into a scene that, on the outside, is only a prison scene. Such scenes affirm a break between the private (a space of sexual desire, to which one has a right) and the public (a place of real social violence, in which political claims might be made). When this circuit—put into place and then denied—is active and effective, it allows people to experiment with more than they own up to: to play with and also disavow the specific histories upon which such scenes rely. This seems to account for the epistemological attachment to not knowing about race voiced by many white people. Here, as in white racial dualism, freedom is also the freedom to transgress oppression, to be beyond racial or ethnic trauma. As Kantrowitz writes, the swastika is erotic in part because it conveys "the stigma of the forbidden," an appeal especially attractive to those "who perceive themselves as sexual outlaws" (1991, 197). For these men, "the powerful oppressor is perceived as hot sex because of his willingness to transcend the limits of morality" (194–95). This kind of transcendence is the ability to use, appropriate, or borrow signs of oppression in order to achieve the status of outlaw: a person who transgresses the bounds of normal/vanilla morality via a depoliticized, privatized sexuality.

My interviewees, however, often voiced much more complex and ambivalent positions on Nazi play than that allowed for by this reading: they simultaneously emptied out and acknowledged the specificity or particularity of these referents. Annalee notes: "I'm Jewish, and even though I know that Nazi fantasies are totally disconnected from real life, when I go to a party and I see someone in a Nazi uniform, I totally would never want to play with them. Even though I have plenty of fantasies about domination and plenty of ways of eroticizing [power]." Annalee cannot quite separate that uniform from its social and historical meaning, even though she knows that SM community rules and rationalities require this bracketing. This shows the more complicated ways in which practitioners understand the relationships between the real and the pretend, the known and not known, the dependent and the disavowed.

These relationships have to do with charting the ambivalence that practitioners feel about their expression of individual rights and social rights—about, in other words, collective responsibility for the community and broader social norms. Take, for example, two fantasies of a realistic slave auction offered by very differently positioned practitioners during my interviews. The first is from Edward, a white top, who explained to me that he'd "always wanted to do a slave-ship scene, but there's not enough African American people in the scene to carry [it] out." I asked him about the politics of such a scene, and he responded:

EDWARD: Inside the community, I don't think it'd be a big problem. If somebody caught wind of it outside the community, it'd probably be a problem . . . They'd see it as promoting, you're disrespecting slavery or the things that happened to the African American people in our country. I'm just doing it for a kink, 'cause it actually happened and I think parts of it may be erotic. Reenacting some of it—but I wouldn't go so far as to tell somebody to clean my yard and "you're going to be my slave for an entire month." I don't do stuff like that. I don't promote racial violence or anything like that; I'm not that kind of person. I don't think I am. But I would definitely want to see a scene of a slave being taken down off a ship and slaves hung up in the market square and people bidding on them. They had slave auctions all the time in San Francisco . . . it may touch a raw nerve with people, but . . . I think people, there'd be a lot of people in the scene that are kinky enough to want to do that.

MARGOT: Do you think it's exciting because it's historical?

EDWARD: Well, it's exciting because you've got bondage and you've got the drama of it. You've got everything all in together and it's just—it's tailor-made for a fantasy. And then the best part of that is: when you're done, you're done. It's not like something [that]'s going to be around for 400 years, like they actually had to go through. At the end of the night . . . when everybody's packed up and done, it's done.

In this scene, the realism of such an auction is a defining characteristic. Unlike the typical charity auction, here the resemblance between, on the one hand, contemporary, in-scene bodily technologies like bondage and D/s dramas and, on the other hand, historical slave ships, auction blocks, and human bondage is center stage.

However, for Edward, when the scene is done, "it's done"; this means that he can play with the erotics of such a scene without "promoting racial violence" or "disrespecting" black people or the history of slavery. He does not see a real-world impact of creating such a scene "inside the community"; as long as everyone has consented, the scene would enact racial history fully within the play frame (the SSC scene), and the effects of such a scene would be limited to the erotic, defined in opposition to and outside the political or the social.

This circuit—drawing on but obscuring the real—is more complex than simple appropriation, in which such bracketing vacates the specificity of the cultural trauma that is set into play. As bell hooks argues, white appropriation of black cultural experience is a way of "getting a bit of the Other," "wherein whatever difference the Other inhabits is eradicated, via exchange, by a consumer cannibalism that not only displaces the Other but denies the significance of that Other's history through a process of decontextualiztion" (1992, 31). Appropriation, in this way, "denies the specificity of" the Other when "it recoups it for its own use." Paralleling Kantrowitz's reading of the swastika, this kind of cultural appropriation not only trivializes slavery; it simultaneously produces and justifies the privilege of appropriating white subjects who might treat systematic, historical trauma as a choice, or as a playful game.

Yet the fantasy that the specificity of the real referent—slavery, the Holocaust—can be stripped away, and the scene might stand only for power qua power, a neutral form of power, is itself riven with contradiction. To unpack this, I'll focus on one part of Edward's statement: "I'm just doing it for a kink, 'cause it actually happened and I think parts of it may be erotic." This complex, ambivalent statement simultaneously avows and disavows Edward's larger point: playacting, or miming slavery for an erotic kink, is not racist (or racial appropriation); at the same time, "it actually happened"—a comment that seems out of place unless we acknowledge that the materiality of slavery is absolutely critical to the production of the kinky slave auction. In this way, the reenactment that Edward wants to stage is uncanny in the Freudian sense: the uncanny as a familiar scene that had been repressed and then returns (Freud [1919] 1955), but also as an epistemological effect of the unstable relationship between fantasy and reality. The circuit at work relies on a known unknowingness that makes enacting such a scene possible: the difference between reenacting the bondage, the drama, and the narratives of slave auctions as a scene or a performance and the real thing—"slavery or the things that happened to the African American people in our country"—is that between copy and original, performance and real. At the same time, the erotics of the scene serve to obscure what are, in fact, the necessary links between both kinds of slave auctions, the past and the present.

This takes us beyond the epistemology of whiteness that many people in the scene voiced about Master/slave play and charity slave auctions, an unknowingness that imagines that power can be neutral and detached from its social meanings. Edward's comments illustrate how this unknowingness encapsulates the known. Yet through these machinations, the alibi remains in place, keeping the politics of such a scene firmly in the private space of "just . . . a kink." At the same time, like the German prison scene, these scenes require enough of the real to work—black bodies or German commands and uniforms. This requirement is obscured, leaving a formal outline with a broken link to its real: a historical moment as the perfect setting, "tailor-made for a fantasy." This dynamic continuously produces and dissolves a split between the fantasy and the real, which maps on to the split between private (neutral) desires and public (particular) politics.

This sort of private—a depoliticized space of personal desires—is also the crucial issue in Nazi play. Unlike Master/slave play or fundraising slave auctions, which facilitate denial or disavowal and are read as racially neutral (and thus politically neutral), both the realistic slave auction and Nazi play are seen as political. However, the politics of such play is centrally about publics and privates: what can be done in private, in semiprivate ("inside the community"), or in public. Larry, the owner of the Scenery, explained to me that although "we [the Scenery] have had people come in and do Nazi uniform takedowns, police uniform takedowns . . . we've never had a KKK cross burning kind of scene."

MARGOT: Right. Would that be okay?

LARRY: I doubt it. I doubt it. It would depend on who it was, how it was set up, and if it was intended to intimidate anyone other than their play partner. If it was strictly between them and their play partner, I would probably not have a problem with it . . . if someone came in to do a "Nazi Germany, we're going to round up the Jews and persecute them" [scene] in the Scenery, I'll probably not have a problem with that if they come in with an entourage of their own to have that

> scene between themselves and the players they brought with them . . . simply because their scene is not my business, even though I might have a personal point of view on that type of activity. I'm [of] American Indian descent so I'm probably more sensitive to racial issues than most people . . . [but] I'm probably not going to interrupt their scene provided they keep it within themselves and [are] not disturbing the other people in the dungeon. As soon as it becomes a disturbance, something is going to be done to ensure that it's no longer a disturbance.

Larry stresses that the critical thing is whether a scene would "disturb" someone else; otherwise, there is nothing inherently problematic about a Nazi scene. The disturbance potentially created has to do with the boundaries between public and private space, which maps onto tensions between social and personal rights and responsibilities.

Community debate over Nazi play or the use of Nazi paraphernalia tends to cluster around two positions: a libertarianism that resents rules against edgier forms of play and a liberalism concerned that Nazi play might violate other people's rights. The former should be familiar by now; it is the rationality of practitioners who, like Vicki, subscribe to a fiercely individualist understanding of rights: "Let's say you want to wear a Nazi uniform. Let's say I'm offended by that. I take offense that you're wearing this uniform. Bummer for me; not your problem, not your fault." The latter position was also couched in the language of rights, but here, practitioners were concerned with an audience's right to consent. Bailey explained that Nazi play is considered "edge play in the community. There are people [who] cannot handle the fact that other people want to play that way. In general, people who want to play that way are aware this can push other people's buttons and tend to do it at invite-only parties or in private." For these practitioners, since SM must be consented to and bystanders cannot consent, it is not safe, sane, and consensual to do public scenes that are likely to upset an audience (this was also the common argument against playing in busy public spaces).

Thus, unlike slave play, Nazi play does not operate on an axis of visibility/invisibility, nor is it disguised as private and sexual. Instead, since such play is already marked as political, the critical distinction is whether such scenes are "private"—in the sense of one's right to one's desires—or "public"—in the sense of violating a larger community's right to consent. Crucial, in other words, is a tension between rules and freedom, a construction, as I explored in chapter 2, that is less about whether practitioners follow or flout the rules, and more about how the rules incite a certain kind of self-subjectification, a way of becoming an SM practitioner. Formulating one's own political position on Nazi-themed scenes is simultaneously a means of self-cultivation and a way of producing a community organized around a particular distribution of individual (private) and social (public) rights.

This distribution of rights, couched as self-work, has to do with the desire to be and to appear to be a particular kind of antiracist, progressive person. Thus the key question for many practitioners is what kinds of scenes they would do "in public" and what kinds of scenes they would do "in private." Public, here, is semipublic; it means in front of other SM practitioners. With the community as audience, practitioners often felt that they had less control over a potential interpretation of themselves as racist, an interesting recoding of the SSC scene as unsafe, risky, or dangerous to self-presentation, as I discuss below. Paul, for example, explained that, although Mollena has asked him to play with her (by "screaming 'nigger' at her in a scene), "one reason why I wouldn't do it with her is because I don't know how people out there are going to [react]. I mean I'd do it private maybe . . . But in public, no fucking way. There's no way." Estrella explained, while discussing race play, that "when I do really edgy stuff, I make sure to inform people around me, or do it in a private room, or in my private home." Although Estrella voiced a concern with "offending" or nonconsensually harming other people, like Paul she also worried that such play might amount to a public acknowledgment of one's racism, or at least one's desire for or eroticization of racialized dynamics. Annalee commented: "I think that there is such a taboo in our public culture against being racist that even if people might be fantasizing in their heads about these things, they wouldn't say out loud, 'I'm imagining that you're my nigger slave' or whatever." Instead, because of white people's desire to be antiracist, postracial, or maybe just PC, these scenes rarely happen in public: although many practitioners discussed the politics of Nazi play, I did not witness a Nazi scene during my fieldwork. But the complex forms of attachment and disavowal at work in such scenes make them ideal fodder for community debates about the relationships between personal/erotic desire and political/social good.

The other realistic slave auction, imagined by Mollena, frames this tension between the political and the erotic, expressed in terms of public social norms and private desires, quite differently. Her scene also draws on the iconography—the real, material history—of the slave trade. She explained: "A lot of [SM] toys have their origins in stuff that was designed to subjugate people, like spreader bars, but they've been modified . . . and I see ['the traditional trappings of slavery'] when I look at them." But she wondered if others do, too; the ubiquity of the charity slave auction made her wonder "if people think about the idea of what a slave auction in the Americas might actually have been like" when they attend a kinky slave auction. She continued: "What would it be like if you walked into a Society of Janus auction and had the usual people chatting and then suddenly someone was dragged in from outside kicking and screaming and crying and pleading for mercy, and then stripped naked and inspected by a crowd of four or five people? And then sold off, while personally begging for this not to happen? And the idea that they don't want to be pulled away from their children—how shocking would that be? . . . I think it would be a profound political and social statement, and it would rock people's worlds. And maybe not in a good way, but I think sometimes a smack upside the head is not a bad thing." Mollena's desire is to make the resemblance between racialized history and SM dramatically visible. For her, the realism of the scene—dragging in unwilling slaves, stripping, and inspecting them while they scream not to be separated from their children—would "rock people's worlds": intervene in the social world by smacking it "upside the head." This sort of performance, a spectacular enactment that neither denies nor occludes racial history, is a way of contesting, through the dramatization of, the preservation of such histories in SM play dynamics.

Calling attention to the real referent of these scenes—the material basis of slavery—Mollena sees her scene as a way of getting people to "think about the idea of what a slave auction in the Americas might actually have been like," to think about historical referents as ambivalent presences that haunt the SM scene today. This visibility, in other words, is epistemological. By dramatizing, often spectacularly, the social meanings of race, the invisibility of whiteness (as race), and the trace of a US history of slavery, this play provides an opportunity to challenge the colorblind white social logics that produce and justify the community. She imagines that such play would not only dramatize but also disrupt the veil of invisibility that enables and produces forms of racial privileging, creating a shocking or jarring reminder of racial history and disturbing the scene's placid whiteness. When this resemblance is neither denied nor effaced, these scenes have the potential to replay power in ways that are neither appropriative (because they are decontextualized or departicularized) nor parodic (because they exaggerate or display forms of inequality). Instead, Mollena hopes that such a scene might transform players and audiences by putting into place a circuit that shocks the "usual people"—the professional, privileged Society of Janus crowd—into a recognition of the connection between the social and the scene.

Moreover, the circuit not only strives to expose the traffic between the charity slave auction and US slavery. It also strives to address the invisibility of people of color and the racism in the SM scene. Disrupting the invisibility of race, Mollena's scene makes sure that racism cannot be denied through neoliberal fantasies of being postracial or colorblind—about being a certain kind of white person (the good, antiracist kind) in relation to a progressive (postracial) America. Instead, this exposure would also intervene into the ways that people in the scene see their own stakes in and production of racialized social belonging, disrupting white American fantasies of universal citizenship. Mollena's play, in other words, relies on making these ongoing racial projects *public* in the sense of collective and political. This entails making public not only racialized history, but also SM's current and disavowed erotic attachment to such dynamics. She plans scenes that will get race, racism, and racialization "out into the open," making them visible to various publics and demanding a reaction to such play. Crucially, Mollena's play asks audiences and players to reflect on the eroticization of racial history, connecting personal desire to social history and thus resisting the privatization of SM that situates the erotic outside collective social dynamics.

During our interview, Mollena told me a story: She was sitting around with some people, and they were talking about their favorite fantasies. Half joking and half serious, she said to them: "Unfortunately I don't think I'll get to have one of my most heavy fantasies acted out, because I don't think they'll let someone into a party wearing [a] Klansman's outfit. Dressed up as the grand dragon, the imperial wizard guy." People were uncomfortable during this exchange, and later Mollena was taken to task on a people of color e-mail list she is on. She was accused, she told me, of "betraying people of color" and "being an Uncle Tom"; "[her] commitment to [her] race" was questioned. I said, in response to this KKK fantasy, "but you know it would be quite shocking at a play party." She answered: "Yeah, no one would like that. No one would like it. It would just be cool, and I can't even say if I would like it. I just wonder what would happen. Part of what's fascinating about it is the fact that it's so huge a thing for everybody. It's not just me, and part of that energy, that revulsion or that horror or that disgust or that shock—that's a big deal. That's the type of energy I'm very serious about." Crucial to such a scene, for Mollena, is the way that it would prompt an affective response. She isn't even sure she would like this scene—that it would be erotic for her—but she knows it would be a "huge thing for everybody." She explained: "I've heard stories of people being asked to remove Nazi emblems and stuff from outfits at parties [because] it's going to upset people . . . so doing that kind of thing privately, sure. But my curiosity is to how everyone else would react around it." Here, it is not a realistic scene that Mollena is after, but a scene with enough charge—that's "so huge a thing for everybody"—to generate a kind of reflective political energy. This type of scene is targeted not at people of color, but at the larger SM community, calibrated to its disavowed—because privatized—erotic attachments to nationalized racial hierarchies. Crucial to these scenes is an audience's affective response, a kind of emotional involvement that prompts some sort of reconfiguration or reaction. Crucial too is some public recognition of the referents of what becomes simultaneously taboo or publicly off limits, and densely erotic.

Mollena classifies race play as part of a larger set of play styles she calls "taboo play." For her, rape play, incest play, religious play, and race play are all forms of taboo play, "play around . . . traditionally abused or victimized groups." In a class called "Playing with Taboos" that she taught at the Black Rose Conference in Washington, D.C., in November 2002, Mollena explained to her audience that with taboo play, you are "taking years of experience and putting it into a scene." What I found interesting about this remark is that, with the word *experience*, Mollena is talking not only of her own personal history but of larger, social relations. In a recent online interview, she explained that, of course, she has "never lived in the South on a plantation and felt the terror of [her] life every moment at the hands and whims of an owner or of another slave with an agenda."[14] However, because she has experienced racism, "in a very real emotional sense, [she has] tasted what that is like."

Mollena's introduction to her 2002 class was followed by one of the strangest demonstrations I saw. Mollena had traveled to Washington with a friend from San Francisco, James. As Mollena talked, James—a Latino man dressed in a hairnet, a blue flannel shirt buttoned only at the top, gold chain, and sunglasses—appeared at the side of the stage, and suddenly, taking Mollena by surprise, rushed onstage. She called him a "wetback," and he began shouting "Yo, bitch, yo nigger!" right in her face. Mollena began to cry: "I'm sorry. What are you doing? Please don't!" James pushed her onto the floor, kicking her side and yelling at her. He called her a "black bitch," a "Jemima," and threatened to cut her with the knife he produced from his pocket if she didn't give him her money. As he leaned over her, she looked terrified; she was crouched down, covering her head and pleading with him: "I don't have any money . . . please don't hurt me." The audience was silent through this mock mugging, watching but unresponsive. There was none of the excited whispering, laughing, or gasping that usually happens during a class demonstration.

I found the demo odd in part because I had witnessed James's transformation in the hotel bar after Mollena left to prepare for her class. James had gone out to a local strip mall in search of his outfit and, as he dressed in the bar while we chatted, I couldn't help but laugh at his transformation from serious San Francisco guy to Latino gang banger. But when he strutted onstage and took Mollena down, I was uncomfortable for several reasons: it wasn't so much that I was watching a mugging filled with racial epithets, but my nagging suspicion that the performance wasn't working. The juxtaposition between Mollena's jovial presentation and this Latino-on-black everyday kind of crime was awkward. I was also intrigued that Mollena had chosen such an everyday taboo to play with and on—intrigued theoretically, but not moved. It was a scene of the urban present, and, although it was about crime, fear, gender, race, and class all at the same time, I suspected that it was too mundane to make good erotic drama.

The Klansman scene, the realistic slave auction, and Nazi play and paraphernalia contrast with this mugging scene in interesting ways.

SM scenes do not just draw on material social relations; they draw selectively, seeking deeply affective, culturally shared scenarios. Indeed, effective scenes find and push hot buttons, buttons that access the power that coheres within national imaginaries that structure citizenship, belonging, and subjectivity through affective relations (on national imaginaries see Appadurai 1996; Bell and Binnie 2000; Berlant 1997; Povinelli 2006).[15] A hot-button issue is one that links individuals, through affective involvement, with cultural and national imaginaries. Not every scene is available for such dramatization; there are many forms of racial and ethnic play—Native American play, for example—that I have never heard described as such. And this, surely, is not because these dynamics are not crucially American, but rather because the selection of racialized inequality for SM scenes relies on broader national constructions of race, most crucially a black/white racial dichotomy. Effective race play, in other words, generates a complex circuit between affective response, erotic attachment, and national imaginaries, tapping into complex veins of shame and desire—the "charge" that animates national belonging.

These racialized belongings, of course, also intersect with other axes of power: sexuality, gender, age, and so forth. In the SM scene, cultural trauma play is tightly focused on black/white race play, Nazi play, rape play, and incest play. Interviewees, when describing one, would slip smoothly into another; they seemed to be structurally related. As Larry explained to me, this kind of play "triggers primal buttons." "They are looking to press someone's trigger to get a specific reaction: 'Okay, you are a (button) slave. You will do as you're told.' 'Yes, Massa!' They are looking to push that button to put them into that head space. You see women do it to men a lot. Maybe not necessarily racially mixed, but you see women tops tell men, 'You're a worthless male worm, and you will worship me as a worm should worship a goddess.' They are pushing that same button, and I don't care if it's male over female, black over white, white over black, Nazi over Jew—to me it's all the same button." These forms of play re-encode particularly loaded, culturally meaningful power inequalities. These cultural performances work when they tap into complex and dynamic circuits of affect and social power. They work particularly well when they reference a real (of racism, if not slavery; of exploitation, if not incest) that is shared and elaborated as trauma safely in the past—a mimetic performance of a durable, if disavowed, structure of inequality.[16]

Such fantasies organize self-cultivation around an affective response to national imaginaries. Sometimes, this affirms a privatized relation to power, as Edward's narrative reveals, in part because facing one's personal issues is a community norm—part of the project of becoming a practitioner. Atheris, a white prodomme, explains to me that she knows a regular client who likes being called "nigger" and being forced to be a slave. Although she isn't willing to play with this client, she explains: "I think exploring things that make you uncomfortable is a good thing . . . I think people that go, 'oh my God, that's horrible,' and walk away are not—don't really know themselves or don't want to know something about themselves. And I'm not afraid to look at myself; if something makes me uncomfortable, I want to know why." Atheris voices the value that the community places on knowing oneself, on exploring one's own desires, boundaries, and rules. Understanding and learning about oneself and one's SM desires, communicating one's individual desires in clear and direct terms, and examining and moderating one's own affective responses—especially shame, disgust, and desire—is a crucial way practitioners become practitioners.

This kind of work on the self lies in the personal labor of figuring out one's individual relationship to SM, structured through affective response and individual self-cultivation. When SM pushes individuals beyond their comfort levels or personal boundaries, it can enable practitioners to reexamine, explore, and create new versions of themselves as practitioners. Stephanie explained: "One of the things that's enthralling to me [about SM] is that it is so real . . . I mean, it's a whole different life afterward . . . as I always say to them [submissives]: 'You will look at yourself differently in the mirror tomorrow morning when you're shaving. You'll remember what happened at our house last night.'" But even as a project of self-cultivation and mastery, the value of personal discomfort as a path to self-knowledge is ambivalently connected to broader social imaginaries. Gretchen, discussing race and other cultural trauma scenes, explained: "I think that they're sort of revolutionary. They're really on the edge of exploring who we are, and the people who are exploring those issues are the ones who are really strong because they're willing to expose themselves to that vulnerability. I admire them." I asked her why such scenes were "revolutionary," and she said: "It gives you the opportunity to say, 'I have a violent response to this, a violent emotional, personal, psychological response.' What's that about? What does that say about us as a culture, then, and who I am as a person, and what power do I have over that versus what power does that have over me?" In these cases, rather than simply reaffirming one's sense of self or one's boundaries, pushing buttons can initiate a more recognizably collective racial project.

During our interview, Anthony, a white dominant, told me that he had been asked to "dress up in a Ku Klux Klan outfit" for a scene. He would not do the scene partly because he would be concerned that people might think he was a real racist. Because he has a Southern accent, grew up in the segregated South, and, as a boy, acted "overtly" racist, this kind of play is, as Stephanie put it, very close to "where we live literally and figuratively." But for Anthony, although such play is "dangerous in terms of my identity" (in the scene), it also has the potential to connect the personal/affective with the social/national. He explained: "Public scenes now for me are less about the scene itself, although I'm totally into my partner when I'm doing it. The scene to me has to include the onlookers, and I have to do something—I'm compelled to do something—that will touch them somewhere . . . with the racial thing, it would be more to touch their buttons in terms of their own racial issues and their racial taboos and make it [public] . . . That would be something I would want to achieve in a race scene." For Anthony, like Mollena, race play can push buttons by tapping into hot-button issues, social issues that interface complexly with the particular positionalities and experiences of individuals. As with Anthony's story of reenactment I discussed in the previous chapter, part of the way this works is by finding someone's button, the trigger that "get[s] her where she lives." Finding someone's trigger means creating an effective circuit between their individual eroticization and the social charge of loaded play.

Race and ethnicity, as well as gender, are hot buttons or triggers because they are central conduits between the affective/subjective and the social/structural/national. These themes in play provoke emotional and affective individual responses to SM scenes. This kind of self-cultivation enables forms of self-mastering (especially for white practitioners to "overcome" race and racism through choice, consent, and so on), but it also creates the possibilities for this play to transform practitioners, giving them new ways to understand themselves and, crucially, the social relations they produce and reproduce. This, then, is another way to read the self-cultivation of SM practice: as generating particular affective responses within players and audiences, responses that might transform what is a fundamentally individual project of self-making into collective, or public, politics.

In her introduction to the demonstration in Washington, Mollena explained that there is always shame involved in taboo play, both for the people involved in the scenes and for the communities and histories that such scenes reference. "I've been accused of setting the race back by doing race play," Mollena told us. This collective shame is one index of the way that sexual desires are produced through discomforting power relations, racist histories, domination, and inequality; it reveals a collective, rather than a personal, responsibility for racialization. In our interview, Mollena told me that she was particularly interested in scenes that "push that envelope with people" and "freak people out." I asked her what she wanted out of such scenes, and she explained: "I know that there are some people who I've talked to personally who said, 'I've never seen that type of play done before. It made me really uncomfortable. I had to kind of examine why.' And so I do and say some things that make people think outside of their lives and that, for me, is again educational and that's the push that I like to get." Educational scenes "challenge people to observe and think about their own history that they bring into the scene, their own prejudices they bring into the scene." In this way, Mollena's SM is less about sex-desire as a personal, private, affective relation and more about sexual performance as a social, cultural, and public dramatization of power, a dramatization that forces SM practitioners to reflect on their eroticization of and reliance on racialized national belonging. Making the referents of a scene public and generating an affective response can, she hopes, be educational; her desire is to create scenes that demand a public recognition of what is normally unspoken or unseen, by making people connect what they do in a scene with their own history, a larger national history.

Crucial to an effective cultural performance is audience involvement: an ambivalent, affective connection. Mollena's scene with James failed as a cultural performance, at least for me, because we did not have to become involved. In contrast, doing a hard resistance scene with a white top with a Southern drawl or enacting a realistic slave auction or a KKK scene stages race in ways that make other people uncomfortable—and here I mean people watching such a scene, but also the people at Mollena's classes, the people she talks to about this, me, and you, the reader. This discomfort can, she hopes, force an audience to become emotionally involved in a social, political, and collective way; can allow the disruptive force of the social to erupt in the privatized scene. As she explained, "making a private act like that that involves sex . . . to have that shared with people . . . to me, that's a pretty profound political statement." The audience, "whatever their reaction is," makes possible the "politicization of gender and race and sex and all those things." This affective involvement is ambivalent; Mollena names many forms of emotional reactions including energy, revulsion, horror, disgust, shock, and becoming upset—and I would add the more typical desire, lust, joy, and pleasure. This circuit means that political SM play involves the audience in a way that can disrupt the obfuscation of race and racism, and open up new ways to think about, and challenge, the links between individual erotic attachment and more-collective racial dynamics.

The forms of disavowal we can see in the Mosley case are ways of bracketing or shielding the "tensive social issues" on which SM depends through a "protective veneer of the performative" (Alexander 2004, 502). As long as this veneer or barrier—what Bryant Alexander calls the "prophylactic" of performance (503)—is in place, racialized spectacle can be emptied of its referent, becoming neutral or just play. This form of denial can also take a more ambivalent turn; when it is confined to the consensual, private, and individual, such play can simultaneously reveal and conceal the real stakes of such performances. Both of these effects can further the disavowals of privilege and power under the guise of neutral subjectivity. However, when SM play touches players and audiences where they live—connects individual (private, sexual, affective) buttons with social (public, political, national) imaginaries—such play exposes practitioners and audiences to the vulnerability of play, to the shared responsibility we have for producing unequal social relationships. When this happens, when SM play creates a way for practitioners to reimagine the responsibility they have for social relations, the play breaks down the split between personal desire and public politics that obscures, via neoliberal rationalities, a collective sense of responsibility for the ways that race structures and restructures subjectivity, community, and belonging.

At these points, BDSM scenes are troubling or discomforting because they disrupt certain ideological constructs—what I have been calling alibis—that separate the social and the sexual. They suggest that, contrary to community ideology, SM isn't equally available to everyone, an unmarked, universalized practice; rather, racial, gendered, and classed difference is at the center of SM practice. They disrupt the idea that sexuality springs from a private, innate, sexual essence deep inside the body, and instead insist that desire is forged in the crucible of history, community, and nation. And they challenge a narrative of historical progress, where we (urban, progressive, alternative white people) are beyond race, along with America itself—instead showing that we remain affectively and erotically bound to precisely the forms of difference that we might desire to overcome. This discomfort is the effect of seeing, and of being jarred by one's complicity in, the violence of whiteness. BDSM play produces political possibilities when it encourages—even forces—practitioners to take responsibility for erotic practice as part of a larger community. This responsibility is what is effaced in neoliberal denials of the circuit between the scene and the social. And so this form of discomfort can be transformational when it capitalizes on the density of affective responses to bring into relief a wider social world, when it connects an individual's self-making project with the social responsibility we all share. When this happens, SM play puts into place a circuit that can challenge a neoliberal prioritization of personal responsibility in favor of one much more resonant with a social responsibility to others.

THE SCENE THAT WORKED ALL TOO WELL

THE MATERIALITY OF DISCOURSE

> Lynndie England . . . [is] not just the face of Torturegate; she's the dominatrix of the American dream.
>
> —RICHARD GOLDSTEIN, "Bitch Bites Man!"

My final scene—the Abu Ghraib torture photographs—shifts from racialized politics in the SM scene to the "sadomasochistic" imaginary of a larger US nationalism. But, like the slave auction or the Nazi scene, this scene must also be read in terms of the fetishistic tensions embedded within mimetic performance, the relations between public/private and social/individual that guide a political reading of performance. And here, too, audience, positionality, and discursive productions set up the complicated circuits of affect and effect upon which power—not only of the safe, sane, and consensual variety—relies.

In spring 2004, I read a scene report—a written description of a consensual BDSM play scene—in the Janus newsletter. The scene took place at a San Francisco dungeon in late March 2004. It was an interrogation scene, involving a colonel, a captain, a general, and a spy. The spy was hooded, duct-taped to a chair, and slapped in the face. As she resisted, the spy was threatened with physical and sexual violence, stripped naked, cut with glass shards, vaginally penetrated with a condom-sheathed hammer handle, force-fed water, shocked with a cattle prod, and anally penetrated with a flashlight. The scene ended when the spy screamed out her safeword: "Fucking Rumsfeld!"

Ending a neutral interrogation scene—with its stock characters of colonel and spy—with this particular safeword illuminates the complex politics of SM scenes. I read the "joke" of Rumsfeld-as-safeword as both a gesture to the real of imperialist power from which SM draws much of its symbolism and a mockery of that power. Like the interrogation scene I described in the introduction, many SM play scenes rely on the iconography of torture and military or imperial dynamics. Indeed, practices focused on the breasts and genitals are called both play and torture: tit torture, nipple play, genitorture, CBT (cock and ball torture), genital play. Play themes like interrogation, military, torture, terror or fear, and abduction are common topics for SM classes and workshops. These scenes work through mimetic resignification; they draw on forms of state power available as historical or cultural signage, staging military, imperial, or colonial relations of power in performative ways. In this scene, co-opting the extraordinary power of the name while subverting its claims to rule (*Rumsfeld* can be exchanged with other safewords, like *red* and *pineapple*), Rumsfeld-as-safeword is a form of political critique in which one can get off on and enact power at the same time.

BDSM scenes work, as I have argued, by tapping into something powerful or realistic enough to be effective; to touch people where they live. These scenes—along with many other scenes in this book—worked for me and for practitioners because they effectively produced emotional responses, forcing players and audiences to get involved with the play. By restaging military techniques, or performing violent intimacies between guard and prisoner, or cop and victim, interrogation scenes might be parodic: they might undermine the remote power of authority through creative reenactment. They might be a redeployment, allowing us to reimagine on our own terms our lack of power over the war, over state power, and over intimate violence like rape, incest, or racism. They might make a mockery of imperial power, recostuming or camping it up; they might give the lie to such power (in the humor-as-politics of a scene in which *Rumsfeld* means stop). They might reproduce a structure of feeling, an attachment to authority, that can be harnessed by the state to ensure our compliance. I do not want to close down the complexity of such scenes; SM play with imperialism is not always, or necessarily, politically interventionist. However, by dramatizing power in often spectacular ways, satisfying SM play effectively creates a circuit between the individual, private, or erotic and the social, national, or public routed through affective response.

If this, as I have been arguing, is how we might begin to read the political effects of SM play scenes with cultural or national trauma, what about actual torture practices? This question was prompted by a flurry of e-mail messages on SM mailing lists in late May and early June 2004, two months after I read about that Rumsfeld scene. BDSM practitioners were both offended by and anxious about the way the media continuously linked SM to the torture practices and photos from the Abu Ghraib prison after Seymour Hersh broke the story in the *New Yorker* (2004). For example, the *San Francisco Bay View* billed Lynndie England the "cigarette smoking, dominatrix prison guard" (Damu 2004). After members of Congress viewed an additional 1,800 photographs that were not released to the public, the *Los Angeles Times* reported Representative Barney Frank's comment: "It had nothing to do with trying to break them . . . It was sadomasochistic sexual degradation" (quoted in Serrano and McDonnell 2004). Joanna Bourke wrote in the *Guardian* that "the pictures of American soldiers humiliating Iraqi detainees are reminiscent of sadomasochistic porn" (2004).

In this context, practitioners were eager to claim that consensual BDSM had nothing at all to do with nonconsensual torture, that BDSM was not sadism. And, of course, BDSM is not the same thing as torture. Still, what do we make of the uncomfortable similarities between BDSM play and prison torture? Of the easy slippage from guard to dominatrix, from torture and interrogation to sadomasochistic sex play? These crossings point to an uncanny resemblance between the photographs and SM scenes: similar body technologies (hooding, bondage, sexual humiliation, emotional manipulation) and similarly careful staging (the arranged bodies, the props, the audience). It is politically appealing, although ultimately dishonest, to argue that these scenes are unrelated, that they exist outside of or can be fully bracketed from real torture, military interrogation, or imperialism. SM, as I have argued, depends for its erotic power on precisely these real-world relations, within which it is given form and content.[17]

Such scenes, then, are neither precisely the same nor completely unrelated, but instead might be productively juxtaposed in order to reveal not only their contrasting contexts, but also their different discursive and material effects. Both the SM interrogation scene and the Abu Ghraib photographs create circuits or exchanges between the real (the social, public, political) and the scene (the performance, private, erotic). And both BDSM play and the photographs of torture at Abu Ghraib spectacularize power inequality; they both render relations of domination in dramatic, staged, and framed ways. Yet politicized SM practice strives to be more than just play; politically effective SM sutures performance to the social, creating social and relational exchanges between players, and between players and audiences, that force recognition of and reflection on the social basis of subjectification. The photographic representation in Abu Ghraib, on the other hand, destroys relational exchange, transforming a political and national real—torture—into an individuated, sexual fantasy.[18] In this way, the relationship between these two performative events is more properly chiasmic: SM scenes can enable an intervention into the social world through affective involvement, while the Abu Ghraib photographs close off a social response to torture through affective disengagement.

Take, for example, the notorious photograph of Lynndie England holding a leash attached to a naked Iraqi detainee, a photograph that reminded many of a dominatrix pose. In the *Telegram and Gazette*, Dianne Williamson called England a "deranged dominatrix" (2004); the *Toronto Star* used "diminutive dominatrix" ("Sex, Sexism Drive Prison Coverage" 2004). Susan Sontag wrote in the *New York Times Magazine* that "the pictures seem part of a larger confluence of torture and pornography: a young woman leading a naked man around on a leash is classic dominatrix imagery" (2004, 27). Though diminutive, England is no dominatrix; describing her in this way facilitates a disavowal of institutionalized torture by framing the abuse as her personal psychosexual predilection, even as she (and thus this slippery mechanism) became the circulated and recirculated image of the scandal at Abu Ghraib. This commentary borrows from the icon of the dominatrix (a figure usually encased in skintight black leather or latex, not military fatigues) to pathologize England, offering us the story of a woman with individuated deviancy.[19]

This discourse of sadomasochistic pathology is also at work in the final independent panel report on the scandal, the Schlesinger report. The opening sentences of the report read: "The events of October through December 2003 on the night shift of Tier 1 at Abu Ghraib prison were acts of brutality and purposeless sadism . . . The pictured abuses . . . represent deviant behavior and a failure of military leadership and discipline" (Schlesinger et al. 2004, 5; see also 43). Even as the report places responsibility on the chain of command, the environment, and the reclassification of interrogation techniques, it also states: "The aberrant behavior on the nightshift in Cell Block 1 at Abu Ghraib . . . [has] a unique nature fostered by the predilections of the noncommissioned officers in charge. Had these noncommissioned officers behaved more like those on the day shift, these acts . . . would not have taken place" (13; see also 29). "Deviant" "predilections" and "*purposeless* sadism"—these repetitions throughout the document refigure torture as sadistic, personal pathology, decontextualized and atomized: "Some individuals seized the opportunity provided by this environment to give vent to latent sadistic urges" (29).

The slippage between dominatrix and military guard, between "deviant" behavior and military plans, shows us the effectiveness of naming this violence "sadomasochism." This discursive production has two important political effects: it pathologizes BDSM practitioners, and it works to shield US military operations. Calling the practices depicted in these photographs sadism instead of torture draws attention to the sex in these pictures, and then frames this sex as the depraved practices of individuals, rather than institutionalized military practice. This mechanism is made possible through the discourse of sadomasochism as individual perversion: a discursive production with terrifying material effects.

"It's not a pretty picture," then–Defense Secretary Donald Rumsfeld commented shortly after the photographs were released ("Rumsfeld

Testifies Before Senate Armed Services Committee" 2004). The acts depicted, Rumsfeld goes on to say, are "acts that can only be described as blatantly sadistic, cruel and inhuman"; they are "fundamentally un-American." Contesting these statements to document the Americanness and unexceptional nature of sexualized forms of torture, as well as the context of a much larger US war strategy, is not enough. Rather, we should recall that the problem is the efficacy of the framing and staging of these photographs as sadomasochism: the materiality of sadomasochism as a discursive production.

In a context where viewers have very little information about Iraq, the war there, or international politics, the reception of these photographs as sadomasochistic perversion simultaneously produced patriotic Americans and screened off torture as a technique of imperial power. Mark Danner writes that the "aberrant, outlandish character of what the photographs show—the nudity, the sadism, the pornographic imagery—seems to support" President Bush's statement that the behaviors do not represent America (2004). On May 24, 2004, on a visit to the Army War College, Bush dismissed the prison scandal as "disgraceful conduct by a few American troops who dishonored our country and disregarded our values" (Bush 2004). The argument that the photographs are the rogue, late-night actions of a few bad apples is more than disavowal; it is also a way of pressing the pathologization of sadomasochism into imperial service, and using this taint to shield the workings of power. Danner argues: "Behind the exotic brutality so painstakingly recorded in Abu Ghraib . . . lies a simple truth, well known but not yet publicly admitted in Washington: that since the attacks of September 11, 2001, officials of the United States, at various locations around the world . . . have been torturing prisoners . . . [T]he bizarre epics of abuse coming out of Abu Ghraib begin to come into focus, slowly resolving from what seems a senseless litany of sadism and brutality to a series of actions that, however abhorrent, conceal within them a certain recognizable logic" (2004). Rather than the sadistic actions of a few bad apples, the torture was part of a much larger course of action carried out around the world as part of US military and political strategy.[20] Yet focusing attention on the particular bodies of the perverse guards instead of on the larger US military and political strategy was effective on multiple levels. Indeed, in the aftermath of the scandal, although nine of the reservists who served at Abu Ghraib were convicted at a court-martial or pled guilty to charges of abuse (eight were sentenced to jail time), the only officer charged, Lieutenant Colonel Steven Jordan, was cleared of all criminal responsibility in 2008 (White 2008). No senior US civilian or military officer—Secretary of Defense Donald Rumsfeld, CIA Director George Tenet, Lieutenant General Ricardo Sanchez (the top US commander in Iraq), and Major General Geoffrey Miller (commander at Guantánamo Bay)—was investigated.

The effectiveness of the images from Abu Ghraib relies on a spectacularization that pins an audience's attention to the surface of a photograph, obscuring the geopolitical reality of US military imperialism. This is not because the photographs did not incite affective response; even as the viscerality of the images fades, the photographs' circulation and reproduction elicited shock and outrage. For some, this galvanized demand for intervention in the war because a "line was crossed," an argument that had political effects. Yet perversely, the "line crossed," as Jasbir Puar notes, is one of sexuality, not death or violence—or, more important for my purposes, torture (2005, 13). As others have shown, the production and refiguring of a split between what Brian Keith Axel terms "national-normative" and "antinational" sexuality (2002, 420) yokes together gender and sexuality to secure empire on the backs of racialized Others. But what these critical commentaries miss is the discursive use of sadomasochism to transfer our feelings of discomfort or disgust with torture onto the perverse practices of individual US soldiers.[21]

Mobilizing this sadomasochism performatively produces an American public that is unified and good and decent, as Alphonso Lingis puts it, in contrast to the "visual fascination" or "voluptuous anxiety" aroused by the photographs (2006, 85). This is fascination in Baudrillard's sense: a state of "narcoticized" spectatorship, in which being mesmerized by the visible surface dissolves meaning into sheer spectacle (1994; see also Debord [1967] 1995). Through this mechanism, torture, dehumanization, and imperialism are transmuted into the "sadomasochistic" practices of US soldiers, closing down a social or political response. This mechanism allows the spectator to remain insulated from these photographs—safely distant through our disembodied viewing, denied an access point or a means of intervention. And, although this is the risk of all photographic representations, the photographs from Abu Ghraib make a performance phantastical, moving torture from a space of the real (the prison) to the space of fantasy (sadism). The US audience for these photographs from Abu Ghraib is enabled, through these circuits, to think about the scandal (and its larger geopolitical context) in terms of a particular, pathological relationship between sex and violence called "sadomasochism," rather than torture. The sex—blurred out anuses, naked bodies, thumbs-up signs—an overwhelming, sensationalistic, and outrageous surface—leaves only the echo or shadow of what it displaces.

At the press conference for the release of the report, Schlesinger said: "It was kind of *Animal House* on the night shift" (Graham and White 2004). This reference parallels some of the comments in the media that the torture had been for the "amusement," "entertainment," or "fun" of the guards (Higham and Stephens 2004; Scelfo and Nordland 2004, 41).[22] Yet describing torture as "fun" requires the trivialization of sex rendered as merely individual: an inability to see the relations produced or destroyed by sexuality as both deadly serious and deeply embedded in national modalities of power—as social and political problems, rather than pathological, private desires.

How, then, do we make sense of the relationship between consensual SM and photographic representations of torture?[23] Effective SM can put into place circuits that force audience involvement, that can serve as performative interventions into and productions of social relations. Yet it can also put into place circuits that facilitate disavowal, that enable practitioners to imagine themselves as outside—exempt from—the social relations on which they depend (and that they create), especially when such circuits reproduce material and social relations of whiteness, individualism, and personal rights and responsibility. Similarly, the photographs from Abu Ghraib show us that these other circuits depend not only on a disavowal, facilitated through alibis and fantasized separations, but also on the materiality of discourse: sadomasochism as individual—and not social, military, or structural—perversion. This relies, in turn, on the figuration of sexuality as personal, private, and trivial, as opposed to the real of political, economic, and international relations.

It is for these reasons that we should read SM scenes and their referents as neither parallel nor oppositional—not a case of original and copy—but rather in terms of their specific performative effects. And here, with the case of the interrogation scene and the photographs of torture, we see a chiasmic relationship between socialized power in SM and sexualized power in imperialism. In her reading of the torture in Abu Ghraib, Rosalind Morris (2007) argues that the sexualization of torture techniques produces dehumanization—a nonrelation, a social unmaking—that is grounded in the racialization of religious otherness. This opens up one way to differentiate torture from SM: effective SM produces social relations through affective involvement; effective torture destroys them. SM can be transformational when it connects the scene to the social real—when, even in the safe space of a classroom demo, and even for me, the anthropologist in the room, the "just for play" becomes real, and the audience must risk identification with the bodies and social imaginaries at play. In contrast, the Abu Ghraib photographs work when they disconnect the scene from the political real. Reading Lynndie England as a sadistic dominatrix forecloses identification and relationality: she becomes sick, and we (the audience) are shocked by what human beings—other human beings—can do. This distancing from England's particular body is, crucially, a distancing from the United States as body politic, and an effective veiling of the military and imperial scene in Iraq.

These insights allow us to refigure the relationship between SM and torture, moving beyond the liberal distinction: that of consent. In late 2002, several newspapers breathlessly revealed that Jack McGeorge, a munitions analyst deployed to Iraq to find weapons of mass destruction, is also a leader in the BDSM scene (McGeorge is a founder of Black Rose and an officer in the NCSF and the national Leather Leadership Conference). McGeorge became the butt of jokes on late-night talk shows, in cartoons featuring him in a leather harness, and in news articles with clever pun-titles like "The UN's Foray into Saddamasochism" (Steyn 2002)—each analogizing BDSM practices and Saddam Hussein's torture techniques. In an essay supporting McGeorge, David Steinberg argues that "enjoying pain is not the same as getting beaten up on the street" and that "consensuality is the defining difference between empowerment and abuse" (2003). My interviewees agreed. Jezzie explained that her discomfort with Master/slave terminology has to do with the "fundamental differences" between nonconsensual and consensual slavery: "Nonconsensual is so fundamentally destructive and horrifying, and consensual in my life is so fundamentally constructive and wonderful that it's not a comfortable connection to draw." Yet this dichotomy, as I have shown throughout, is inherently unstable. The Abu Ghraib photographs, as Morris argues, produce "consent" retrocitationally: "The detainee's submission to the torturer's very command is made to appear as the source of the detainee's own enjoyment" (2007, 112; see also Mirzoeff 2006, 26). The fantasized sexual and racialized deviancy of the detainees transformed torture into consensual sex, a performative abjection that produces deviant, masochistic objects. In contrast, SM's claim to consent relies on, and simultaneously disrupts, the liberal, autonomous subject. Requiring *nonconsensual* social inequality and power differentials for erotic charge, but also the fantasy of a subject free to choose and perform in such scenes without social consequence, SM's unstable and ambivalent relations between consent and nonconsent highlight social tensions between agency and coercion. In the BDSM community and in particular scenes, this relies on the construction and validation of a kind of neoliberal subject—a race-, gender-, and class-neutral rational agent enacting its own private, empowered desires in the sexual marketplace—whose very production belies its dependence on social hierarchy.

Thus, although we can contrast these two scenes in terms of their modes of operation, as well as their social, performative, and ideological contexts, the interrogation scene, with *Rumsfeld* as the safeword, reminds us that the efficacy of SM scenes is dependent on violent referents, unstable relations, and social audiences—just as the spectacular performance of the photographs as and of torture shows us new, disturbing forms of organizational efficiency and representational efficacy. We should not valorize minoritarian performances in terms of transgression, imagining a split between those performances that enforce social power and those that uproot it. Rather, both scenes, through repetition, encode or coalesce bodies both individual and social; both are performances that produce and respond to power organized around effective performance. We must, then, trace the complex circuits that sexuality travels as it connects private selves and social power—revealing, distorting, connecting, involving.

READING SM PERFORMATIVE MATERIALISM

The stories with which I opened this book—the charity slave auction, Mark's bondage party, Estrella's incest play scene, and the juxtaposition of the Abu Ghraib photographs and consensual interrogation scenes—

reveal the dense connections between materiality and performance that are crucial to SM sexuality, subjectivity, community, and belonging. To read these scenes, I have moved beyond typical analyses of performative politics, resisting the question, "Which SM performances subvert social power?" to ask instead, "What political effects are produced in the complicated circuits between bodies, players, audiences, and readers created by SM?" Performance and materiality must be read together through a performative materialism that neither ignores the materiality of discourse nor effaces the performativity of material inequality.

SM is a social practice that links bodies and subjects, selves and communities, private desires and public politics. When we parse the circuits that sexuality creates between individuals and social relations—in the history and economy of the Bay Area, in commodity and energy exchanges between SM bodies, and in gendered and racialized power exchanges dependent on larger systems of inequality—we see the dynamic relationship between subjects and social hierarchies. Such circuits are productive: they draw on and reproduce the social horizon against which subjects, communities, and political imaginations gain force and legibility. The complicated circuits put into place through SM sex connect the embodied subject and the social body through commodity exchanges, through creative embodiments, through the ambivalences of gender and sex, and through the hierarchies of racial visibility. Not always subversive nor always capitulative, these exchanges *are* always productive; performances both depend on and produce material relations.

Communities like BDSM are dependent on capitalism; changing forms of community, identity, and commodity exchange produce BDSM and its pleasures. The economic underpinnings of BDSM are both consolidated —legitimized—and disavowed by neoliberalism as a cultural formation, a political rationality that champions market logics of personal responsibility, free choice, privacy, and individual agency. Imagining the scene as a *private* public, play as privatized desire, risk or safety as personal responsibility, and SM roles as freely chosen and personal proclivities both produces this new SM community and justifies a neutral or universalized social belonging within it. In other words, replaying social norms in the privacy of our home dungeon might obscure the institutionalized systems of domination in and through which such scenes arise.

At the same time, such scenes are mobile, multiple, and ambivalent.

As I have argued, effective performances work when they connect individual with social and national imaginaries, when they touch you "where you live." What happens next, however, depends. Sometimes, as I have shown, making sex public can disrupt fantasies of autonomous individualism, personal pathology, individuated responsibility, the privateness of desire, or sex removed from the social. Sometimes, too, circuits can reproduce, reinforce, even establish forms of disavowal and unknowing that enable social privilege and help to justify it. There is no single reading of the SM scene, because scenes depend on the active production of the materiality of social differentiation by players, audiences, and readers.

In this way, I have sought to reframe the analysis of SM away from a binary—transgressive, queer, counterpublic practice versus hegemonic, heteronormative lifestyle—and toward, instead, the "contingent yet foundational ways in which practices of everyday life rework, within a range of limitations" larger economic, political, and institutional forces (Boellstorff 2007, 15). To read the political effects of performances that produce social relations requires a lens trained on ambivalence, on what is uneven, contradictory, and multiple in both SM performances and the material social relations that form and are formed through such scenes. Following Bhabha, Lott shows that the cultural performance of blackface is "less a repetition of power relations than a signifier of them—a distorted mirror, reflecting displacements and condensations and discontinuities between which and the social field there exist lags, unevenness, multiple determinations" (1993, 8). Similarly, SM performance is not a repetition of social power; it carries and produces the complexities of social relationships, relationships shot through with contradictions unresolved—indeed, erotically and politically powerful precisely because they remain in tension.

And here, although sexuality is imagined as a break from material social relations, sexuality is, instead, the raw material of these circuits, the route through which these bodies—individual, social, national—link and join; where ideologies of public and private, of rights and responsibilities, are produced and contested. Reid-Pharr argues: "What we think when we fuck is not so much dictated by race, gender, and class but instead acts itself as an articulation of the structures of dominance —and resistance—that create race, gender, and class" (2001, 92). Indeed, the "fantasy of escape is precisely that which marks the sexual act as deeply imbricated in the ideological process by which difference is constructed and maintained . . . the task that awaits all of us, then, is to speak desire plainly, to pay attention to what we think when we fuck . . . the work before us is precisely to put our own bodies on the line" (98). The task for audiences, readers, and critics is to attend to our involvement, our affective responses, our investments in the study—and the politicization—of sexuality. If we can do this, we can understand sexuality as a social relation—interarticulated with hierarchies, institutions, national imaginaries, and local spaces of practice—rather than an escape. And we might also begin to see how our own commitments, subjectivities, and communities—sexual or otherwise—are constituted through social relations of power.

APPENDIX 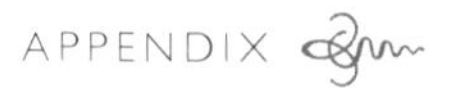

INTERVIEWEE VIGNETTES

Each person chose a name and provided the following biographical information. All ages and dates are at the time of the interview.

ANNALEE is a thirty-two-year-old white woman. She is bisexual, partnered, and poly, and she identifies as a genderqueer/pervert/voyeur. She works as a newspaper columnist and freelance writer and lives in San Francisco. She moved to the Bay Area fourteen years ago, from Southern California. She has been in the SM scene for three years. Interviewed 2002.

ANTHONY is a fifty-six-year-old white man. He is bisexual, married, and poly, and he identifies as a dominant. Retired from the military, he lives in Solano County with his wife, STEPHANIE. He moved to the Bay Area fourteen years ago, from Florida, and has been in the semipublic scene for four years. Interviewed 2002.

ANTON is a twenty-five-year-old white man. He is heterosexual and married, and he identifies as a master. He works in the IT industry and lives in San Francisco with his wife and slave, JEZZIE. He moved to the Bay Area three years ago, from Pennsylvania, and has been in the semipublic scene for three years. Interviewed 2002.

ATHERIS is a thirty-five-year-old white woman. Partnered and monogamous, she identifies as a dominant. She works as a professional dominant and lives in Alameda County. She moved to the Bay Area four years ago, from Florida, and has been in the semipublic scene for six years. Interviewed 2002.

BAILEY is a forty-three-year-old white woman. She is heterosexual and single, and she identifies as a bottom. A technology consultant, she lives in San Mateo County. She moved to the Bay Area eight years ago, from North Carolina. She has been in the semipublic scene for about six years. Interviewed 2002.

BONNIE is a twenty-six-year-old Asian American woman. She is heterosexual, partnered, and monogamous, and she identifies as a masochist. An office manager, she lives in Alameda County. She moved to the Bay Area four years ago, from Southern California. She has been in the semipublic scene for three years. Interviewed 2002.

CARRIE is a forty-four-year-old white woman. She is bisexual, married, and poly; she identifies as a bottom/submissive. A massage therapist and mother, she lives in Santa Clara County. She is from the Bay Area and has been in the semipublic scene for seven years. Interviewed 2002.

CATHY is a thirty-nine-year-old white woman. Pansexual and partnered, she identifies as a dominant/switch. She works in retail and lives in San Mateo County. She moved to the Bay Area three years ago, from Washington, D.C. She has been in the semipublic scene for two years. Interviewed 2002.

CHRIS is a thirty-five-year-old white man. He is heterosexual, married, poly, and he identifies as a dom. He works as a market researcher and lives in Santa Clara County. He has been in the semipublic scene for about eight years. Interviewed 2002.

COVENANT is a forty-five-year-old white man. Heterosexual and partnered, he identifies as a top. He works in software development and lives in Santa Cruz County. He moved to the Bay Area from Massachusetts. Interviewed 2002.

DOMINA is a forty-nine-year-old white woman. She is bisexual, married, and also partnered with her submissive, HAYDEN; she identifies as a dominant/sadist. She is a professional dominant and lives in Stanislaus County. She has been in the semipublic scene for eight years. Interviewed 2000.

DON is a forty-year-old white man. He is straightish and poly and identifies as a service top. A computer consultant, he lives in San Mateo County. He moved to the Bay Area thirty-nine years ago, from Colorado. He has been in the scene for eleven years. Interviewed 2002.

DYLAN is a thirty-five-year-old white woman. She is bisexual/lesbian and single and identifies as a submissive. A web designer and student, she lives in Alameda County. She moved to the Bay Area thirteen years ago, from Southern California. She has been in the semipublic scene for seven years. Interviewed 2002.

EDWARD is a thirty-three-year-old white man. Heterosexual and single, he identifies as a dominant. He is a warehouse manager and lives in Alameda

County. He moved to the Bay Area five years ago, from the East Coast. He has been in the semipublic scene for six years. Interviewed 2002.

ESTRELLA is a thirty-nine-year-old white woman. She is lesbian, married, mostly monogamous, and identifies as a femme top. She works as a prodomme and lives in Alameda County. She moved to the Bay Area four years ago, from New Mexico. She has been in the semipublic scene for fourteen years. Interviewed 2003.

FRANCESCA is a forty-eight-year-old white woman. She is bisexual and single, and identifies as a pain slut bottom. She works as a consultant and lives in San Mateo County. Born in the Bay Area, she has been in the semipublic scene for eleven years. Interviewed 2002.

GRETCHEN is a forty-one-year-old white woman. She is bisexual, partnered, monogamous, and identifies as a bottom/submissive. She is a civil engineer and lives in San Mateo County. She moved to the Bay Area twenty years ago, from Southern California. She has been in the semipublic scene for six years. Interviewed 2003.

HAILSTORM is a fifty-three-year-old white man. He is heterosexual and single, and identifies as a top. A network administrator, he lives in Napa County. He grew up in the Bay Area. He has been in the semipublic scene for seven years. Interviewed 2002.

HAYDEN is a twenty-eight-year-old white woman. She is lesbian, collared to DOMINA, and she identifies as a masochist/slave. She works in the computer industry and lives in Alameda County. She moved to the Bay Area four years ago, from Texas. She has been in the semipublic scene for four years. Interviewed 2000.

IKANDI is a thirty-five-year-old white woman. Married and monogamous, she identifies as a voyeur. She works in public relations and lives with her husband, OUCHY, in Alameda County. She moved to the Bay Area six years ago, from North Carolina. She does not consider herself a part of the SM community. Interviewed 2002.

J. is a forty-two-year-old white man. He is heterosexual, partnered (with S.), and monogamous, and he identifies as a top. He works in the mental health field, is a student, and lives in Santa Cruz County. He moved to the Bay Area four years ago, from Hawaii. He has been in the scene for two years. Interviewed 2002.

JAY is a fifty-three-year-old white man. He is heterosexual, single, and identifies as a switch with top leanings. A student, he lives in San Francisco. He moved to the Bay Area thirty-five years ago, from Indiana. He has been in the semipublic scene for twenty-eight years. Interviewed 2003.

JEFF is a thirty-eight-year-old white man. He is heterosexual, married, poly, and identifies as a dominant top. A student, he lives in San Francisco with his wife and their 24/7 submissive, RACHEL. He moved to the Bay Area four years ago, from Texas, and has been in the semipublic scene for six years. Interviewed 2000.

JEZZIE is a twenty-four-year-old white woman. She is bisexual, married, and poly; she identifies as a slave. She is in graduate school and lives in San Francisco with her husband and master, ANTON. She moved to the Bay Area three years ago, from Pennsylvania, and has been in the semipublic scene for three years. Interviewed 2002.

KB is a fifty-seven-year-old white woman. She is het/bi and partnered. She is a professional dominant and lives in San Francisco. From the Bay Area, she has been in the scene for twenty-five years. Interviewed 2002.

KC is a fifty-eight-year-old white woman. She is married (with two primary partners and one M/s relationship) and poly; she identifies as a submissive/slave. She is the housemother of a domination house and lives in Contra Costa County. She moved to the Bay Area thirty-seven years ago, from Southern California. She has been in the semipublic scene for twenty-five years. Interviewed 2002.

LADY HILARY is a thirty-three-year-old white woman. A lesbian in a 24/7 Master/slave relationship, she is poly and identifies as a femme top. She works as a nurse, attends school, and lives in Santa Clara County. She was born in the Bay Area and has been in the scene for thirteen years. Interviewed 2002.

LADY THENDARA is a forty-one-year-old white woman. Bisexual and married, she identifies as a top. She is an insurance adjuster and lives with her husband, LATEX MUSTANG, in San Mateo County. She moved to the Bay Area twenty years ago, from New York, and has been in the semipublic scene for seventeen years. Interviewed 2000.

LARRY is a forty-seven-year-old American Indian man. He is bi, life-partnered, poly, and identifies as a dominant/master. He owns the Scenery dungeon, and lives in Santa Cruz County. He is from the Bay Area and has been in the scene for thirty years. Interviewed 2002.

LATEX MUSTANG is a forty-year-old white man. He is heterosexual, married, and identifies as a bottom/pony. He is a manager in the computer industry and lives with his wife, LADY THENDARA, in San Mateo County. He moved to the Bay Area about ten years ago, from New York. He has been in the semipublic scene for three years. Interviewed 2002.

LENORA is a twenty-year-old white woman. She is bisexual, partnered in an M/s relationship, monogamous, and identifies as a switch/slave. She is a college student and lives in Santa Clara County. She is from the Bay Area and has been in the semipublic scene for two years. Interviewed 2002.

LILY is a twenty-nine-year-old white woman. Heteroflexible and partnered, she identifies as a bottom/sub. She is an editor at a technology magazine and lives in San Mateo County. She moved to the Bay Area six years ago, from Southern California. She has been in the semipublic scene for three years. Interviewed 2000.

MALC is a thirty-eight-year-old white man. He is heterosexual, single, and identifies as a dominant, mostly. He works in intelligence/computing and lives in San Francisco. He moved to the Bay Area six years ago, from England. He has been in the semipublic scene for six years. Interviewed 2002.

MARCIE is a white transwoman in her forties. She is lesbian, partnered, and poly, and she identifies as a switch. She works in the computer industry and moved to the Bay Area eight years ago, from Nevada. She has been in the semipublic scene for ten years. Interviewed 2000.

MARK is a forty-six-year-old white man. He is heterosexual, single, and identifies as a switch. He works as a marketer in the computer industry and lives in San Francisco. He grew up in the Bay Area. He has been in the SM scene for fourteen years. Interviewed 2002.

MARK F. is a forty-eight-year-old white man. He is gay, multiply partnered, and poly, and he identifies as a top. The manager of a sex club, he lives in San Francisco. He moved to the Bay Area seventeen years ago, from New York. He has been in the leather and motorcycle scene for thirty years. Interviewed 2003.

MAXX is a twenty-four-year-old white man. Bisexual and single, he identifies as a switch/bottom. He goes to college and lives in Alameda County. He is from the Bay Area and has been in the semipublic scene for three years. Interviewed 2000.

MEG'GAN is a twenty-nine-year-old white woman. She is lesbian and single and identifies as a butch bottom/sometimes switch. She is in college and works as a housecleaner. She lives in Alameda County. She was born in the Bay Area and has been in the scene for three to four years. Interviewed 2002.

MIGUEL is a Latino man in his fifties. Gay and partnered, he identifies as versatile. He is an artist, theater designer, consultant, and landlord and lives in San Francisco. He moved to the Bay Area twenty-two years ago, from Florida. He has been involved in the men's leather and motorcycle scenes for twenty-two years. Interviewed 2002.

MOLLENA is a thirty-three-year-old African American woman. She is bi, single, poly, and identifies as a submissive bottom. She is an administrative assistant and an actress, and lives in San Francisco. She moved to the Bay Area six years ago, from Southern California. She has been in the semipublic scene for five years. Interviewed 2002.

MONIQUE ALEXANDRA is a thirty-three-year-old Latina woman. She is bisexual, partnered, and monogamous, and identifies as a bottom/submissive/masochist. A student, she lives in Santa Clara County. She moved to the Bay Area eight years ago, from Maryland. She has been in the semipublic scene for one year. Interviewed 2002.

NONI is a fifty-two-year-old white woman. She is bisexual, single, dominant, and polymorphously perverse. She is a poet. She moved to the Bay Area twenty-eight years ago and lives in San Mateo County. She has been in the semipublic scene for twenty-four years. Interviewed 2002.

OUCHY is a forty-year-old white man. Bi, married, and poly, he identifies as a top/sadist. He is a professional dominant/clown, an asset manager, a meeting facilitator, and a DJ/performance artist, and he lives in Alameda County with his wife, IKANDI. He moved to the Bay Area from Texas. He has been in the scene for five years. Interviewed 2002.

PAM is a white woman in her fifties. She is bisexual, in a Master/slave relationship with her master, VINCE, and identifies as a slave. She is from the Bay Area and has been in the scene since her twenties. Interviewed 2000.

PANTHER is a forty-four-year-old Asian American man. He is heterosexual and single, and he identifies as a dominant top. He works in healthcare and lives in Alameda County. He moved to the Bay Area fifteen years ago, from Washington State. He has been in the semipublic scene for six years. Interviewed 2003.

PAUL is a forty-year-old white man. He is heterosexual, single, monogamous, and identifies as a dominant top. He is currently unemployed, on disability; he lives in San Francisco. He moved to the Bay Area twenty-one years ago, from Southern California. He has been in the semipublic scene for fifteen years. Interviewed 2003.

PHIL is a fifty-five-year-old white man. He is heterosexual, married, monogamous, and identifies as a switch/bottom/slave. He is unemployed, on disability, and lives in Alameda County. He moved to the Bay Area thirty-six years ago, from Utah. He has been in the semipublic scene for twelve years. Interviewed 2003.

RACHEL is a twenty-one-year-old white woman. She is bisexual, bipartnered, and bi-amorous; she identifies as a pain fetishist/submissive. A teacher, she lives in San Francisco with JEFF. She moved to the Bay Area from Southern California. She has been in the semipublic scene for three years. Interviewed 2002.

ROBERT is a white man in his early forties. He is heterosexual, single, and identifies as a top. A financial planner, he lives in Alameda County. He moved to the Bay Area five years ago, from Southern California. Interviewed 2000.

ROBERT D. is a forty-four-year-old white man. He is gay, partnered, and identifies as a leatherman. He is a writer and publisher, and lives in San Francisco. He moved to the Bay Area six years ago, from Wisconsin. He has been in the men's leather scene for twenty years. Interviewed 2002.

S. is a white woman. Heterosexual and partnered (with J.), she identifies as a bottom. She is an administrative assistant in healthcare and is also in graduate school. She lives in Alameda County and is from the Bay Area. She is not in the public scene. Interviewed 2002.

STEPHANIE is a fifty-four-year-old white woman. She is bisexual, married, and poly, and she identifies as a dominant/sadist. A consultant, she lives in Solano County with her husband, ANTHONY. She moved to the Bay Area twenty-six years ago, from New York, and has been in the semipublic scene for close to thirty years. Interviewed 2002.

SYBIL is a fifty-three-year-old white woman. She is bisexual and single, and she identifies as a dominant/mistress. A prodomme and therapist, she lives in San Francisco. She moved to the Bay Area thirty-three years ago, from Massachusetts. She has been in the scene for thirty-three years. Interviewed 2002.

TERAMIS is a forty-six-year-old Arab American woman. She is lesbian and single, and she identifies as a slave. She is a student and lives in San Francisco. She moved to the Bay Area seven years ago, from Southern California. She has been in the semipublic scene for eighteen years. Interviewed 2002.

TIJANNA is a thirty-seven-year-old African American woman. She is lesbian and single and identifies as a bottom. She works in the biotech field and lives in San Francisco. She moved to the Bay Area seventeen years ago, from Oregon. She has been in the semipublic scene for six years. Interviewed 2002.

TOM is a white man in his fifties. Bisexual, partnered, and mostly monogamous, he identifies as a switch. He is semiretired from computer work and lives in Napa County. He moved to the Bay Area twenty-one years ago, from New York. He has been in the semipublic scene for about twenty years. Interviewed 2000.

UNCLE ABDUL is a white man in his sixties. He identifies as a bi technosadist. An electrical engineer, he lives in San Francisco. He has been in the semipublic scene for about twenty years. Interviewed 2002.

VICK is a forty-five-year-old white woman. She is lesbian and single, and she identifies as a daddy/top. An environmental consultant, she lives in San Francisco. She moved to the Bay Area thirty-nine years ago, from Iowa. She has been in the semipublic scene for eight years. Interviewed 2002.

VICKI is a fifty-two-year-old white transwoman. Lesbian and single, she identifies as a dominant (who occasionally bottoms). She works as a software engineer and lives in Santa Clara County. She moved to the Bay Area when she was a teenager, from New Mexico, and has been in the semipublic scene for ten years. Interviewed 2002.

VINCE is a white man in his mid-forties. He is gay and in a Master/slave relationship, with PAM. Originally from Texas, he is unemployed and lives in San Francisco. He has been in the scene for about thirteen years. Interviewed 2000.

WALDEMAR is a thirty-two-year-old white man. He is bisexual and single, and he identifies mostly as a top. He works for a computer company and lives in Santa Clara County. He moved to the Bay Area eight years ago, from Massachusetts. He has been in the semipublic scene for five years. Interviewed 2002.

NOTES

TERMINOLOGY

1 The current *Diagnostic and Statistical Manual of Mental Disorders: DSM-IV-TR* (American Psychiatric Association 2000) defines "sexual masochism" as:

A Over a period of at least 6 months, recurrent, intense sexually arousing fantasies, sexual urges, or behaviors involving the act (real, not simulated) of being humiliated, beaten, bound, or otherwise made to suffer.

B The fantasies, sexual urges, or behaviors cause clinically significant distress or impairment in social, occupational, or other important areas of functioning.

"Sexual sadism" is:

A Over a period of at least 6 months, recurrent, intense sexually arousing fantasies, sexual urges, or behaviors involving acts (real, not simulated) in which the psychological or physical suffering (including humiliation) of the victim is sexually exciting to the person.

B The person has acted on these sexual urges with a nonconsenting person, or the sexual urges or fantasies cause marked distress or interpersonal difficulty.

An updated version, *DSM-V*, is due in 2013. According to the American Psychiatric Association, the proposed revisions for "sexual sadism" and "sexual masochism" involve striking the phrase "real, not simulated" and adding a threshold number ("two or more nonconsenting persons on separate occasions") to criteria "B" for sexual sadism. The Paraphilias Subworkgroup spearheading the revisions has also proposed a diagnostic change that would distinguish between a paraphilia (just the "A" criteria) and a paraphilic psychiatric disorder (both "A" and "B"), where only the latter would necessitate psychiatric intervention. As the working group specifies, "this approach leaves intact the distinction between normative and non-normative sexual behavior, which could be important to researchers, but without automatically labeling non-normative sexual behavior as psychopathological" (American Psychiatric Association, "*DSM*-5 Proposed Draft Revisions to *DSM* Disorders and Criteria," "Proposed Revision to Sexual Sadism," http://www.dsm5.org/; see also Krueger 2010a and 2010b). This is a mixed blessing, in my view: in the new edition, sexual sadism could be either a paraphilia ("sexual sadism") or a paraphilic disorder ("sexual sadism disorder"), but in either case, it would be classified as deviant sexuality under the broad diagnostic heading "Sexual and Gender Identity Disorders." BDSM practitioners are divided on the inclusion of sadism and masochism in the *DSM*: some feel it is helpful to differentiate nonconsensual, violent sadists from the SSC community, while others feel that it can only entrench the pathologization of any form of sadomasochism, consensual or otherwise (see also Moser and Kleinplatz 2005).

2 National Coalition for Sexual Freedom, "Sound Bites for the SM-Leather-Fetish Community," June 17, 2007, http://ncsfreedom.org/.

3 For example, Freud ([1924] 1961) argues that sadism/masochism is a dual drive, while Deleuze ([1967] 1991) argues that, based on their literary, psychic, and cultural differences, Sacher-Masoch's masochistic "universe has nothing to do with that of Sade" (13).

4 Readers with a particular interest in this lexicon and its variations can refer to one of the very informative SM guidebooks, such as *Bound to Be Free* (Moser and Madeson 1996), *Consensual Sadomasochism* (Henkin and Holiday 1996), *Different Loving* (Brame and Brame 1996), *SM 101* (Wiseman 1998), *The Bottoming Book* (Easton and Liszt 1998a), or *The Topping Book* (Easton and Liszt 1998b), as well as the countless online dictionaries of BDSM terms.

INTRODUCTION

1 I want to clarify that I am not claiming that the number of people who engage in BDSM sex practices has changed. Statistics on sexual practices are at best uncertain, but the latest Kinsey Institute estimate of the number of people practicing some form of BDSM in the United States is between 5 percent and 10 percent (Reinisch 1990). Charles Moser, a sexologist and physician specializing in BDSM, estimates that "about ten percent of the general population are actively involved in SM with some recognition that their interests are specifically sadomasochistic; another twenty to forty percent may engage in SM behaviors without knowing their activities could be so defined" (Moser and Madeson 1996, 44). Although this estimate may seem high, SM behaviors span

quite a range. Some practices are about erotic pain; others, like bondage or dominance, are about erotic power; and still others are about a fetish (like feet or leather) or invoke a role (like headmistress or pony). Pinning one's partner to the bed, sexual taunting, wrestling, wearing blindfolds, spanking, pinching, and biting are all forms of SM play, as are the more iconographic practices like flogging, chaining, whipping, bondage, and caning.

2 Another way to frame this conjoining is by bringing together what Nancy Fraser terms a politics of "redistribution"—class and economic justice—and "recognition"—status and visibility/identity politics (1997a). Judith Butler's contestation, along with Fraser's reply (1997b), guide my analysis here.

3 My analysis is indebted to Joseph's understanding of the Derridean supplement: the structure "constitutively depends on something outside itself, a surplus that completes it, providing the coherence, the continuity, the stability that it cannot provide for itself, although it is already complete. But at the same time, this supplement to the structure supplants that structure; insofar as the structure depends on this constitutive supplement, the supplement becomes the primary structure itself" (2002, 2).

4 There is a long tradition of theorizing the relationship between sexual norms, intelligibility, and subjectivity. In Lacanian work, for example, the subject comes into being through a regulatory ideal of binarily sexed materiality: the sexed body (Butler 1997b; Grosz 1990; Lacan 1977; Lacan, Mitchell, and Rose 1985). In the Foucauldian tradition, modern Western subjectivity itself depends on the regulation of sex and sexuality; the subject emerges through a disciplinary mode of identifiable and thus regulatory fixed sexual identity. Foucault argues that "it is through sex—in fact, an imaginary point determined by the deployment of sexuality—that each individual has to pass in order to have access to his own intelligibility . . . to the whole of his body . . . to his identity" ([1976] 1990, 155–56). Butler emphasizes the role of cultural intelligibility within social norms: "'Sex' is, thus, not simply what one has, or a static description of what one is: it will be one of the norms by which the 'one' becomes viable at all, that which qualifies a body for life within the domain of cultural intelligibility" (1993, 2). In this way, sexuality (as a discourse) simultaneously enables and restricts the possibilities for subjectivity; it is, in Foucault's terms, a necessary "stumbling-block" ([1976] 1990, 101; see also Butler 1991). Foucault writes: "There are two meanings of the word subject, subject to someone else by control and dependence, and tied to his own identity by a conscience or self-knowledge" (1983, 212).

5 At the first mention, I identify my interviewees with the name and BDSM terms they use to describe themselves, along with their general age, sexual orientation, and race or ethnicity. More biographical details, including relationship status, type of employment, county of residence, and how long they had been in the scene when I interviewed them, can be found in the appendix. I give pseudonyms to practitioners I did not formally interview, unless they are public figures.

6 In this way, BDSM challenges sexual identity understood as a stable taxonomy based on dimorphously sexed bodies, complementary gender, and binary sexual orientation. Scholars from Freud and Foucault to Eve Kosofsky Sedgwick have highlighted the centrality of identity—a binary identity as man or woman, heterosexual or homosexual—in Western conceptions of sexuality and, even more critically, subjectivity. At the same time, these scholars also point out that identity, as a stable, fixed, and essentialized form of being, is not a particularly accurate description of sexuality as it is lived across time and place (see, for example, Sedgwick 1990; Weeks 1977 and 1995). I think here of Sedgwick's classic list of the various elements "that 'sexual identity' is supposed to organize into a seamless and univocal whole," a list that includes biological sex, gender assignment, personality, appearance, procreative choice, preferred sexual acts, sexual organs, fantasies, emotional bonds, and cultural and political identification (1993b, 7–8).

Anthropologists have made strong contributions to this project by documenting the tremendous range of sexual practices, roles, and identities across cultures; the diverse connections made—and not made—between sexual acts and sexual identities; and the ways that sexuality responds to and shapes local and global conditions of change (Allison 1994 and 2000; Altman 2001; Blackwood and Wieringa 1999; Boellstorff 2005, 2007; Cruz and Manalansan 2002; Elliston 1995; Herdt 1984; Kulick 1998; Kulick and Willson 1995; Lancaster 1992; Lewin and Leap 1996; Padilla 2007a, 2007b; Patton and Sánchez-Eppler 2000; Rofel 2007; Wekker 2006). This work has produced an exciting new perspective on the cultural, economic, and historical linkages between sexual subjectivity and desire. Yet these rich problematics are rarely applied to sexualities in the United States (notable exceptions include Frank 2002; Gray 2009; Lapovsky-Kennedy and Davis 1993; Lewin 1993; Manalansan 2003; Newton 1979, 1993; Valentine 2007; Weston 1991). And, as David Valentine argues, ethnographies on sexuality in the United States *not* organized by identity—gay and lesbian identity, in particular—are even scarcer (2003, 124).

7 Some notable academic exceptions include essays in three collections (Langdridge and Barker 2007; Moser and Kleinplatz 2006; Weinberg 1995a) and several essays (in particular, Bauer 2008; Duncan 1996; Hale 1997; Langdridge and Butt 2005; Taylor and Ussher 2001; M. Weinberg, Williams, and Moser 1984; Woltersdorff 2011). Staci Newmahr's (2011) sociological study of pansexual BDSM communities, *Playing on the Edge: Sadomasochism, Risk, and Intimacy*, was published too late for me to incorporate here. There is also a large body of journalistic, essayist, and practitioner-oriented texts; those that focus on SM community and politics include Mains (1991), Samois ([1981] 1987), Scott (1993), and Thompson (1991).

8 For example, philosophers have linked sadism and masochism to Western rationality and explored SM in terms of the transgression of, and resistance to, unified subjectivity and identity (see, for example, Deleuze [1967] 1991; Foucault [1975–76] 1996 and [1984] 1996; MacKendrick 1999). Cultural theorists

and literary critics have examined SM as a narrative convention in fiction (see, for example, Barthes 1989; Sawhney 1999). These studies are valuable, yet the meaning of SM in these fields is wildly discordant, standing at once for problems of Oedipality and object relations, modern relations between writer and readers, and celebrations of bodily excess. In feminist theory, sadomasochism has been a generative object of political and ethical debate (as I explore in chapter 4). See, for example, Chancer's (1992) and Bartky's (1990) work on power relations of dominance and submission applied to American culture and gender oppression, respectively, as well as the deep archive of writing on SM in the context of the feminist "sex wars" (Califia 1987; Hart 1998; Linden et al. 1982; Reti 1993b; Rubin 1987; Samois [1981] 1987).

9 Work in social psychology and psychoanalysis—the largest body of work on SM—tends to focus on individual etiology and SM as a pathological perversion. From Freud onward, psychoanalysts have explored SM in terms of pathology, deviance, and the inherently paradoxical nature of pleasure (see, for example, J. Benjamin 1988; Ellis [1905] 1942; Freud [1924] 1961; Stoller 1991). More-recent work on SM from this post-Freudian perspective has focused on sadomasochism as a pathological, destructive, or dangerous drive or perversion (see, for example, Grossman 1986; Hanly 1995; Person 1997), not as a consensual, community-based practice. In part, this is because it is unlikely that a client who engages in consensual SM as part of her sexuality (and has no desire to rid herself of this activity) will generate a clinical paper on sadomasochism. But it is also because these psychoanalytic analyses of masochism and sadism tend to pathologize SM practitioners, reifying a normative, heterosexist conception of sexuality and sexual practice.

The sexological literature tends to emphasize easily quantifiable data, like the percentages of practitioners with particular sexual and SM orientations, or the average age of "coming out" or first awareness of SM interests. See, for example, work on the differences in sexual arousal between male and female college students (Donnelly 1998); demographic and psychosocial characteristics of SM practitioners (Breslow, Evans, and Langley 1985; Levitt, Moser, and Jamison 1994; Moser and Levitt 1987; Richters et al. 2008); and differences in preferred SM activities between women and men, and between gay and heterosexual men (Alison et al. 2001). These researchers tend to generalize from very small samples and across subject populations, comparing, for example, results from a study conducted in Finland to a study based on questionnaires handed out at SM organizations in the United States, without emphasizing the likely differences between these findings.

10 I do not mean to collapse all of these theories into one, as there are critical differences that these terms encode. David Harvey (1997), for example, draws attention to new systems of flexible accumulation (the creation of new systems of production and marketing, based on flexible labor processes and markets, geographic mobility, and rapid shifts in consumption) and space-time compression (the acceleration in exchange and consumption, as well as the horizontal

speeding up of time bound to capitalist accumulation). Fredric Jameson (1992), drawing on Ernest Mandel, understands late capitalism as the third industrial revolution, a shift to electronic technology, media and spectacle, and multinational capitalism (from earlier market and monopoly capitalisms). Although these are important differences, I am less interested in debates around periodization and terminology and more interested in the transformation of the relationships between commoditization, consumerism, technology, sociality, and the body—a transformation that many theorists of contemporary US capitalism have noted (see also Castells 2000; Fischer 1998; Fraser 2003; Rose 2007).

11 Deleuze argues that contemporary societies operate under "control" (1995b), not Foucauldian "discipline" (Foucault [1975] 1995; see also Deleuze 1995a; and Foucault 2003, for his later analysis of biopolitics). Discipline, Deleuze explains, is about discrete sites of confinement—a prison, hospital, school, or family—each with their own laws; a modern set of techniques, methodically calculated, for administering, controlling, and training people and bodies to make them useful, productive, and docile. Instead, he argues, we live in a control society in which, rather than fixed sites, we have networked, diffused, flexible, digital modes of control that operate in dispersed, open circuits with continuous control and instant communication (1995a, 174; see also Hardt and Negri 2001). Discipline is about limiting and regulating bodies; control is flexible and modulated, generative. This shift corresponds to changes not just in networks of power, but also in capitalism and social organization. One can map a "discipline society" onto modernist or Fordist production, and a "control society" onto late capitalism. Fraser begins this work in "From Discipline to Flexibilization? Rereading Foucault in the Shadow of Globalization," arguing that just as Foucault was theorizing a "disciplinary normalization," a new regime of what she terms "flexibilization" was taking shape. She argues that discipline is a Fordist mode of social regulation: "totalizing, socially concentrated within a national frame, and oriented to self-regulation" (2003, 164). "Flexibilization," on the other hand—the regime of a neoliberal, globalized, post-Fordist economy—is "multi-layered as opposed to nationally bounded, dispersed and marketized as opposed to socially concentrated" (166). Taking inspiration from Jon McKenzie (2001), I explore this shift to flexibility in terms of performative efficacy.

12 The phrase *cultural performance* was used by the anthropologist Milton Singer in the 1950s to describe a performance (a drama, ritual, or dance) that is marked off from the social field and that communicates and builds social meanings with the audience (cited in Turner 1986, 22–23). As Victor Turner and others have expanded the concept, cultural performance now includes a broad range of events, ranging from more formal dramas to everyday gestures that are set apart in imaginative and spatial—not only, or even primarily—temporal terms. The cultural performance is critical to Turner's exploration of the social drama (see also Schechner 1985; Turner 1980).

13 Neoliberalism is not only an economic theory that, as Harvey writes, "proposes that human well-being can best be advanced by liberating individual entrepreneurial freedoms and skills within an institutional framework characterized by strong private property rights, free markets, and free trade" (2005, 2). It is also, as scholars like Lisa Duggan and Wendy Brown, following Foucault (2008), have argued, a form of governmentality aimed at "extending and disseminating market values to all institutions and social action" (Brown 2005: 39–40; see also Duggan 2003). As Catherine Kingfisher and Jeff Maskovsky argue, neoliberalism "desires" to "remake the subject, reassert and/or consolidate class relations, realign the public and the private, and reconfigure relations of governance—all with direct implications for the production of wealth and poverty, and for raced, gendered and sexualized relations of inequality" (2008, 118). There has been much debate among scholars on the likely demise of neoliberalism, given the recent economic collapse. I steer clear of these predictions not only because neoliberalism, as anthropologists have shown, is a culturally variable formation with durable social effects (Ong 2006; Rofel 2007), but also because the formation is crucial to understanding the particularities of the SM scene in San Francisco in the late 1990s and early 2000s.

14 I am drawing on Omi and Winant's concept of "racial formation," the "sociohistorical process by which racial categories are created, inhabited, transformed and destroyed" (1994, 55) through "racial projects," an approach that brings together representation (ideology) with structure (the organization and distribution of resources). They write: "A racial project is simultaneously an interpretation, representation or explanation of racial dynamics, and an effort to reorganize and redistribute resources along particular racial lines" (56).

15 See chapter 4 for a discussion of the relationship between mimesis (the imitation of an original by a copy) and resignification (repetition with a difference), drawing on queer, critical race, and feminist theories of performativity (Butler 1990, 1991, 1993, and 2004; Jackson 2001 and 2005; E. Johnson 2003; Muñoz 1999; Reid-Pharr 2001) and cultural and social theories of mimesis (W. Benjamin [1966] 1986; Bhabha 1984 and 1985; Taussig 1993).

16 For further discussion of the parallels and disjunctures between the SM interrogation scene and the "sadomasochistic" torture at Abu Ghraib, see chapter 5 and Weiss 2009.

17 McKenzie argues that, since the close of the Second World War, we have entered what he calls an "Age of Performance": "Performance will be to the twentieth and twenty-first centuries what discipline was to the eighteenth and nineteenth, that is, an onto-historical formation of power and knowledge" (2001, 18). In McKenzie's account, performance has become increasingly important across a range of fields, from academic theories of performativity (and performance studies) to employee performance reports, on-the-job performance, high-performance computing, and technological performance. These various iterations of *performance* are bound by linked conceptualizations of efficacy, efficiency, and effectiveness: performance studies, the academic field,

investigates the *efficacy* of cultural performances in relation to social norms; organizational performance, a field of management, is concerned with corporate *efficiency* managed by maximizing employees' satisfaction, creativity, and innovations; and technological performance, a military and industrial field, seeks to build more *effective* products and technologies for both the United States as a nation-state and for consumers.

18 As part of a shorter project on mainstream understandings of BDSM, I also conducted twelve interviews with nonpractitioners, which are discussed more fully in Weiss 2006a.

19 For every possible scenario, play scene, behavior, or role there are a wide variety of interpretative frameworks and motivations. For some practitioners, the idea of being in tight, restrictive bondage is arousing because of the loss of control; for others, it is about the feel of latex or leather against bare skin; for some, it is about imagining how one's body looks encased in tight material; for others, it is about doing something difficult as a test for oneself or because it gives someone else pleasure. Female-on-male fellatio can be an expression of submission and service, but it can also—as a class called "Tooth and Nail: A Femdom [female dominant] Perspective on Fellatio" promises—be an expression of control, power, and dominance (see also Hale 1996; Langdridge and Barker 2007; Taylor and Ussher 2001). Similarly, just as there is no single interpretation of BDSM roles or behavior, neither is there a single motivation. People who get off on incest play, for example, may have been abused as children, or they may simply enjoy the frisson of socially unacceptable play. They may be parents or childless; they may view such play as healing, therapeutic, shocking, performative, exciting, disorienting, or just fun. During my fieldwork, practitioners provided a wide range of personal reasons for doing SM. Some people I talked to said that they "always knew" that they were into BDSM: they liked to tie their childhood friends to trees, or lock themselves in their bedrooms, devising self-bondage techniques. Others said that they felt like something was missing for them, sexually, but they didn't know what it was until they found BDSM. Still others were introduced to BDSM through a partner or friend, or just by living in the Bay Area. They found the social and sexual scene exciting and appealing, so they stayed.

ONE SETTING THE SCENE

1 There was also a dispersed heterosexual fetish and SM network (or imagined community) formed through professional dominants and the circulation of pornographic films and fetish booklets. This network dates from the 1930s, but it was not localized in a community until recently (see Bienvenu II 1998).

2 As much work on the development of gay and lesbian communities shows, small community businesses (like bars) have helped solidify alternative, sexuality-based enclaves or counterpublics (see, for example, Berlant and Warner 1998; Bell and Valentine 1995; Dangerous Bedfellows 1996; D'Emilio 1983; Herdt

1992; Ingram, Bouthillette, and Retter 1997; Lapovsky-Kennedy and Davis 1993; Leap 1999; Newton 1993; Warner 2002; Weston 1998).

3 "The Great Exception: San Francisco's SoMa Neighborhood," NewGeography .com, August 8, 2008.

4 The Folsom Street Fair originated with Kathleen Connell and Michael Valerio, two gay/lesbian activists who met while advocating for affordable housing, community-centered development, local school renovation, small business assistance, and social services in the SOMA area. In 1983, Connell and Valerio began to plan a SOMA street fair modeled on the Castro Street Fair, which Harvey Milk had successfully transformed into a political mobilization tool for the gay community. The new fair, initially called "Megahood," was intended to support local businesses, as well as to bring the diverse SOMA populations into contact with each other and to give the public a sense of the local residents as something other than disposable slum dwellers. The first fair was held in 1984; 30,000 people attended. Through the 1980s, the fair became increasingly leather focused with the increased involvement of gay community activists and businesses, as well as AIDS organizations (see Connell and Gabriel 2001 for a more detailed history of the fair).

The Up Your Alley Fair began in 1985 and moved to Dore Alley in 1987; it now draws about 10,000 to 12,000 people to SOMA for an early summer leather street fair. In 1990, the Folsom Fair and the Up Your Alley Fair merged into SMMILE (South of Market Merchants' and Individuals' Lifestyle Events), the precursor to Folsom Street Events. SMMILE continued to emphasize community issues and local quality of life. The funds raised by the fairs go to charity and community organizations; in 2000 the fairs raised $250,000 for AIDS agencies, clinics, homeless shelters, and the local elementary school, in addition to the charities designated by the San Francisco Police and Fire Departments (Connell and Gabriel 2001).

5 Barbary Coast ran along Pacific Avenue from Kearny Street to the Embarcadero. The area's establishments provided residences, entertainment, and labor contractors for the ship workers and dockworkers of the time. By the beginning of the twentieth century, Barbary Coast was packed with bars and clubs, including several gay and drag bars, clubs, baths, and hotels. Boyd notes that there was one saloon for every ninety-six residents, twice the ratio for either New York or Chicago (2003, 26). Barbary Coast was the home of many single immigrant men who worked as seasonal laborers; the boarding rooms, bars, and brothels provided work, a place to live, and a social environment. Burlesque shows, strip shows, and brothels; gambling houses; and bars and dance halls lined the streets until 1917, when several years of antivice legislation pushed the sex workers west into the Tenderloin and closed the brothels.

6 This is not to downplay the role of immigration in San Francisco's history. In 1880, for example, more than 60 percent of the population was foreign born or first-generation American; 10 percent were Chinese (see Wollenberg 1985, 142). Migrants from East and Southeast Asia and from Latin America have

settled in the Bay Area in successive waves; the 2000 US Census estimated that 37 percent of the city's population was foreign born. Yet, as the history of Chinese exclusion shows most strikingly, immigrants to San Francisco were not celebrated as ideal citizens of the city (see, for example, Shah 2001). In contrast, progressive intellectuals and writers—from the bohemian writers and artists of the 1860s through the early 1900s (including Ambrose Bierce, Jack London, Frieda Kahlo, Diego Rivera, and Upton Sinclair) to the Beats of the 1940s and 1950s (such as Neal Cassady, Jack Kerouac, Lawrence Ferlinghetti, and Allen Ginsberg)—are central to the city's national reputation as eclectic, radical, and tolerant (see Peters 1998).

7 *Queerness*, here, refers not only to gay and lesbian communities and cultures but to a more general sense of sexual license aligned against a straight or mainstream norm.

8 All population figures are from the 2000 US Census unless otherwise indicated. The era also saw the first large migration of African Americans to the Bay Area from the South to work in the shipyards and other industries. In addition, Chinese, Central Americans, and Mexicans were recruited to work alongside women in jobs related to the war, or formerly held by white men who had been deployed.

9 As D'Emilio argues, a combination of enlisting young, unmarried men with no children; asking questions about homosexuality; and providing crowded same-sex housing, sleeping, and living situations made the military both a feasible escape from small towns into same-sex companionship for men who identified as homosexual, and a breeding ground for same-sex emotional, physical, and sexual exchanges for men who did not. The same was true for women, although to a lesser extent, as fewer than 150,000 women served in the Second World War (D'Emilio 1983, 27). More salient, for women, was the possibility of independent wage labor during the war, which often meant moving away from family and hometowns to live in boarding houses with other women.

10 In 1953 the Mattachine Society, begun in Los Angeles, spread to the Bay Area, with branches in Berkeley, Oakland, and San Francisco. Del Martin and Phyllis Lyon formed Daughters of Bilitis in San Francisco in 1955 as a social club for lesbians. Martin and Lyon were issued the first same-sex marriage license in San Francisco in February 2004.

11 "Now That's a San Francisco Treat," NBCBayArea.com, October 21, 2008.

12 In 1776 local Coast Miwoks and Ohlones together numbered about 10,000, but there were fewer than 2,000 of them by the 1830s, due largely to crowded living conditions, disease, dramatic diet change, and regimented labor. Throughout the gold rush (1848 through the mid-1850s), Native Californians were openly exterminated: public hatred, the rapid influx of miners, and local, state, and federal bounties on Native scalps—as well as paid expenses for the posses that hunted Native Californians—decimated Native populations in the area.

13 The Bay Area also has a long history of radical antiracist activism. It is a central node in radical black activism (the Black Panther party was formed in Oakland

in 1966), Asian activism (for example, the yellow power movement in Berkeley), Latino activism (such as the farm-labor organizing of Cesar Chavez), and Native American red power activism (including the Indian take-over of Alcatraz in 1969).

14 Population figures from 2000 put San Jose at 894,943 residents, San Francisco at 776,733, and Oakland at 399,484.

15 The development of new access roads and bridges encouraged the suburban development of the Bay Area. In 1940, Santa Clara County, for example—formerly wheat, fruit, and vegetable farmland—had a population of 50,000 who lived primarily in Palo Alto (around Stanford University, founded in 1891) and San Jose (the old pueblo, now the commercial center of the region). The area between these towns was largely rural until the late 1940s and 1950s, when a combination of industrialization related to the Second World War, Stanford University land grants, and the mass suburbanization taking place across the country transformed the area into what is now the Bay Area's most populous county.

16 For purposes of comparison, the census estimates that the Bay Area population is 7.5 percent African American, 58.1 percent white, 19 percent Asian, and 19.4 percent Hispanic/Latino (of any race).

17 Others lived in outlying counties—Solano, Contra Costa, and Napa—and Santa Cruz and Stanislaus, neighboring counties not officially part of the Bay Area.

18 By 1999, the Bay Area accounted for 8.9 percent of all Internet hard links in the United States (Townsend 2001, 49). In addition, the Bay Area is home to the first nodes connected by ARPANET, which began in 1969 as a project of the Department of Defense (in 1995 it was decommissioned and privatized, becoming the backbone of today's Internet).

19 Academics and SM practitioners alike find the word *community* vexing. Some practitioners reject the word because the gay men's and pansexual scenes are rarely in the same place, others because they see gaps between what they want from "the community" and what they get (see also Rubin 1995). Indeed, except during the Folsom Street Fair, the "leather community" is in many places at once, or no place at all. But at the same time—through national, regional, and online networks of teachers, conferences, contests, and activists—there is also a sense of shared belonging, commonly referred to as *community*. I retain the word in the spirit of Joseph's critique of the "romance" of community belonging.

20 In an influential and problematic book, Putnam (2000) bemoans the decrease of voluntary organizations like the Kiwanis or bowling leagues in the United States. Although the number of US voluntary organizations has grown steadily since the 1960s, the time and energy people devote to these groups is declining. Putnam links this to a decline in civic or community engagement. Like many, I contest this reading of community throughout.

21 The Scenery closed at the end of 2003 and a new dungeon in San Francisco—the SF Citadel—opened. It moved to its current SOMA location in 2005.

22 This produced the ambivalent position of being "out" but "not out." Panther

says: "I'm not going to call [my family] and say, 'Hey, Dad, guess what? I'm kinky!'" Others explained that "there's no need to advertise" (Chris), or "a lot of my friends would not care for that at all so I don't see why I should irritate them" (Waldemar), or "I don't think it's appropriate to talk about sex at work . . . it's not professional . . . and so it makes no sense for me to be out at work because I'd never get into that discussion" (Latex Mustang). Some practitioners told me that they were "selectively out," or that their SM involvement was an "open secret," and many used "don't ask, don't tell" as a metaphor. For example, Bailey told me: "I don't hide what I am, and if somehow [my parents] caught wind of it, I would be happy to discuss it with them. But it also feels like it's not right for me to rub" their noses in it.

TWO BECOMING A PRACTITIONER

1 The first answer (a) is correct.

2 The Journeyman II Academy was a two-year training program held in San Francisco. Old—or at least older—guard SM practitioners, well known in the San Francisco scene, taught classes to trainees, called cadets. The classes were held over two full days, one or two weekends a month, and designed to give students some training in SM, old guard style. Gayle Rubin's speech is titled "Old Guard, New Guard." The speech was reprinted in *Cuir Underground* issue 4 (2) (Summer 1998); an excerpt of the speech is archived at the Black Rose website: http://www.black-rose.com/cuiru/archive/4-2/oldguard.html.

3 E-mail confidentiality requires that this comment remain unattributed.

4 For example, many practitioners believe that the new guard is much less rule oriented, with a loose, anarchistic, hippie style, while the old guard was quite rigid about roles (top or bottom, not both), apprenticing, leathers (and when one earned the right to wear them), and other markers of community. Yet, as I will show, what characterizes the new guard—at least in its most recent iteration—is a commitment to a certain kind of formal and rigid training method. The new guard is not less rule oriented; rather, what have changed are the kinds of rules, who issues them, and their social effect. The shift is from a strict hierarchy and apprentice system located within a small community to a formalized, professionalized organizational structure located within a larger, diffuse community.

5 Opened for Saturday night fisting parties in 1975, the Catacombs was a private house converted to a sex club in San Francisco's Mission district. Cynthia Slater (a Janus founder) was one of the first women involved in this space primarily devoted to men; she brought in several other prominent lesbian and bisexual women (including Rubin, Pat Califia, and Cleo du Bois) who were later involved in the founding of Cardea and Samois (see the next note) and critical to the development of the San Francisco scene. As Rubin put it, the Catacombs was "home and clubhouse for the nascent San Francisco lesbian S/M community" (1991, 131). The Catacombs was known for its massive quantities of Crisco,

excellent fisting and flogging music, cleanliness, diversity, and warmth (see also Mains 1991, 125–41).

6 The original Janus meetings drew heterosexual couples and professional dominants (cofounder Cynthia Slater was a prodomme). In its first year, however, Janus restructured itself and became a primarily gay male organization. Jay told me that back then, Janus "was mostly gay. I went to my first Janus presentation sometime in 1977, and it was like 85 percent gay men, in the classic black leather biker thing, and about 13 percent leatherdykes, and literally a sprinkling of heterosexuals and bisexuals—we sort of stood out." In the early to mid-1980s the population of Janus shifted from mostly gay male to mostly heterosexual: more and more heterosexual men started attending Janus meetings, while HIV/AIDS and the formation of the 15 Association in 1980 (a gay men's SM group) decreased potential gay male members. In a parallel development, when Cardea—the women's SM group formed in 1975 to bring more women into Janus—folded, several other groups rose in its place: first Samois (formed by Califia and Rubin in 1978), then the Outcasts (formed by Rubin in 1984), and now the Exiles (formed in 1996; for women's SM history, see Califia 1987; Rubin 1996). These groups were more attractive than Janus to many lesbian and queer-identified bisexual women. Thus, although Janus still claims to be a pansexual group, much of the true pansexuality—the mix of lesbian, gay, bi, and straight—of the early Janus has been lost.

7 In 2008, NCSF received 489 requests for assistance: 27 percent had to do with criminal charges based on SM practice, 4 percent with employment discrimination, 31.5 percent for child custody or divorce issues, and 15.5 percent were related to SM, leather, or fetish group issues, such as police busts.

8 NCSF, "Violence and Discrimination Survey," 1999, https://ncsfreedom.org/. NCSF conducted a follow-up survey in 2008: out of 3,058 respondents, 37.5 percent had experienced discrimination, harassment, or violence based on BDSM; and 11.3 percent had been discriminated against by service providers (doctors, for example). The 2008 survey is available at https://ncsfreedom.org/resources/bdsm-survey/.

9 Some argue that the Backdrop Club is actually the first SM organization in the Bay Area. Many people who played active roles in the founding and development of Janus and the pansexual San Francisco scene began their SM "careers" at Backdrop. Backdrop was almost exclusively heterosexual; it emphasized male-dominant/female-submissive fantasy play. This is part of the reason why many people left Backdrop, and possibly the reason Slater started Janus. Fantasy Makers is the current incarnation of the "sessions" part of Backdrop.

10 From Janus's bylaws, excerpted in the group's bimonthly newsletter, *Growing Pains*.

11 In fact, I heard about only one instance during my fieldwork, which involved a man who said at his orientation that he was interested in beating up women. This seemed to be a nonconsensual desire, and thus, given Janus's policy of "safe, consensual and non-exploitive" SM, this man was denied membership.

12 Michelle Zornes, "Interview with the Society of Janus." The interview was posted at http://www.lashtales.org/LinkSpotlight/Janus.htm but is no longer available.

13 As the organization's archivist, I arranged for Janus to donate its archival material (a full run of *Growing Pains*, organizational materials, ephemera such as flyers and photos, taped interviews, and other material) to San Francisco's Gay and Lesbian Historical Society so that it might be cared for and preserved.

14 *Mr. Benson* was first published serially in *Drummer* in 1979 and later released as a novel by San Francisco's Alternate Publishing in 1983.

15 Guy Baldwin, "The Leather Restoration or Sacred Cows Make the Best Hamburger," speech at the Sixth Leather Leadership Conference, Los Angeles, April 14, 2002. The speech is available at Madoc's Place website, http://www.madoc.us/sacredcows.shtml.

16 Jay Wiseman's two essays, written in the late 1990s, "I Want My 'Precaution B'!" and "The Medical Realities of Breath Control Play," are available in updated and edited form on his website: http://www.jaywiseman.com/.

17 Here, SM both is and is not an institution: its more nebulous spatial characteristics, for example, and its alternative ethos, locate it outside the bounds of a normative social institution. At the same time, the development of the new SM scene is not, as Foucault argues, "fluid." He writes: "What strikes me with regard to S/M is how it differs from social power," because social power "has been stabilized through institutions," and thus social relations of power are limited, fixed, or rigid ([1984] 1996, 387). SM, on the other hand, is a "strategic game" of power (388). I take up this purported fluidity below and in chapter 4.

18 David stein's essay "Safe, Sane, Consensual" was presented in a workshop at the Leather Leadership Conference in Washington, D.C., in April 2000 and is archived at the Leather Leadership Conference website: http://www.leatherleadership.org. An updated version was published in 2002 as "Safe, Sane, Consensual: The Making of a Shibboleth" in *VASM Scene* 20 (September/October).

19 This is not to say that all people negotiate; for example, most people in 24/7 (full-time) or M/s relationships do not use safewords or negotiate with each other, although they may use safewords, limits, and negotiation when they play with others. Many people also cease using safewords and negotiation when they know their partner well. For example, Bailey, who is usually a bottom, told me that she decided to top her partner: "It was awesome because I knew him long enough that I knew he didn't want to negotiate. He just wanted it to happen. I wouldn't normally do that with people if I didn't know them really well, but that's the cool part about really knowing your partner. You can make judgment calls like that."

20 The Antioch rules were created in 1992 in response to the crisis of consent in legal and social definitions of rape, especially date rape (see Soble 1997). Anton reminded me of this link when he said he thought that SSC "has sort of infected the community with . . . this sort of safety-first mentality that I don't agree with at all . . . There are some people who I think take [it] too far. You have to go

through a rigorous checklist before you do anything—you know, this sort of . . . what is that college, the university that put those rules for dating in place where you had to ask people before you could—'May I touch your breast?' " "Antioch?" I asked, and he replied "Antioch, yeah, these sort of Antioch rules for BDSM."

21 "Two squeezes" is a way for a top to check in on a bottom. The top squeezes the bottom's arm or leg twice; if all is well, the bottom gives two squeezes in return. A "safe signal" or "drop safe" is a non-verbal safeword, such as an object that the bottom can drop on the floor.

22 For example, Lady Thendara told me: "It's [SM] different than anything else. Relationships and discussions that we have, you never have—can you imagine on a vanilla date saying to someone 'Now, if you want to kiss me, you can kiss me. But if you want to touch me under my shirt, you can't do that.' Nobody would ever do that, but you really do [in SM] . . . You might say 'I'm going to tell you at the outset, tonight I just want to get to know you. I don't want there to be any sex or sexual overtures or anything.' . . . I mean very explicit discussions go on and they're the norm, and I think that's really neat. . . . It's really important to talk about and I love that. The men in the scene really understand if you say 'You can do this but you can't do that.' "

23 Mustang is referring to an online community service managed by Race Bannon called "Kink Aware Professionals," a list of kink-friendly doctors, therapists, and lawyers across the United States.

24 Gary Switch's essay, "Origin of RACK; RACK vs. SSC," was originally posted on the Eulenspiegel Society's (TES) e-mail list in the late 1990s. An archived version of the post can be found at http://www.leathernroses.com/generalbdsm/garyswitchrack.htm.

25 Alison Moore's speech, "Out of the Safety Zone: Codes of Conduct and Identity in SM Communities," was presented at the Bob Buckley memorial discussion for Sydney Leather Pride Week, April 25, 2002. It is currently archived at: http://tngc.org/tngc/NC_safetyzone.html.

26 This is similar to what Califia advises in his section on breath play: "Avoid any activity that may injure or kill someone . . . on the other hand, it's very common for a top to briefly cut off the bottom's air with the palm of their hand. I think this can intensify excitement in a low-risk fashion. So please don't call the S/M police if you see this being done" (2002, 203).

27 The wording is based on Miller v. California, 413 U.S. 15 (1973). Challenges to the Communications Decency Act (CDA), which regulates pornography on the Internet have recently tested US obscenity law (see Nitke v. Gonzales, 547 U.S. 1015 [2006]), and a federal case brought against the distribution of "extreme pornography" (Extreme Assoc. v. United States, 547 U.S. 1143 [2006]).

28 In one case in New York, the Columbia University graduate student Oliver Jovanovic was charged with kidnapping, assaulting, and sexually abusing a Barnard undergraduate on a date the two had arranged after exchanging SM interests via e-mail. His defense was that she had consented; the judge, invoking the Rape Shield Law (which prevents a consideration of the victim's prior

sexual conduct), barred the consideration of e-mail evidence and instructed the jury that consent is not an available defense on a charge of assault (People v. Jovanovic, 176 Misc. 2d 729 [N.Y. Supp. 1997]; see also "Memorandum of Law of Amicus Curiae" filed by the National Coalition for Sexual Freedom and available on their website: https://ncsfreedom.org/). Jovanovic was convicted and sentenced to fifteen years. In 1999, the Appellate Division reversed his conviction, finding that this was an erroneous invocation of the Rape Shield Law, and in 2001, just before his retrial, the New York District Attorney moved to dismiss the charges (People v. Jovanovic, 263 A.D.2d 182 [N.Y. App. 1999]; Fritsch and Finkelstein 2001; see also Hanna 2001 for a legal discussion of consent, including the Jovanovic case).

29 In October 1999 the San Diego vice squad raided a pansexual play party held by Club X and issued misdemeanor citations for lewd behavior and/or nudity in a public space to six attendees. The first of the six to be tried was unanimously found not guilty in February 2000, and charges against the remaining five were then dropped (see Ridinger 2006; "Club X Legal Defense Fund and Information" from October 1999, archived at http://www.madoc.us/sd6.shtml). In July 2000, Attleboro, Massachusetts, police raided a private play party and arrested the host, Benjamin Davis, and one guest, Stefany Reed. Davis was arraigned on thirteen counts (ranging from keeping a house of ill fame to possession of a dangerous weapon), while Reed was charged with assault and battery with a dangerous weapon: a wooden kitchen spoon (hence the incident's nickname, "Paddleboro"). The prosecution dropped all but two charges a year later (see Lawrence 2000; Parker 2001).

30 This is linked to, although differentiated from, Roy Baumeister's (1988) explanation of masochistic SM practice as a cathartic escape from the pressures of modern identity. MacKendrick eschews this kind of systematic analysis, instead arguing that SM practice is itself a form of rupture. See Hart (1998) and Barker, Gupta, and Iantaffi (2007) for a critique of the healing or therapeutic narrative of BDSM.

31 Guy Baldwin, "The Leather Restoration or Sacred Cows Make the Best Hamburger," speech at the Sixth Leather Leadership Conference, Los Angeles, April 14, 2002. The speech is available at Madoc's Place website, http://www.madoc.us/sacredcows.shtml.

THREE THE TOY BAG

1 I am wearing one of my two standard pansexual play party outfits: black jeans and a dark maroon T-shirt that has a vaguely Indian squiggly circle design on the chest (the other outfit is jeans with a dark red, long-sleeved velvet shirt); both are Renaissance Faire–lite. I also have a leatherdyke-lite look (classic Levis, a fitted black T-shirt, and black boots) and two fetish-lite looks (latex pants, a black shirt, and a latex jacket, and a black, lace-up dress and biker boots).

2 CyberNet Entertainment (Kink.com) runs several specialty websites, including fuckingmachines.com, whippedass.com, and hogtied.com. Kink.com's studios are headquartered in San Francisco's former National Guard Armory and Arsenal, which the company purchased in 2006 amid city-wide controversy (Freedenberg 2008; Rubenstein 2007).

3 Whip makers in the 1980s, especially Jay Marston and Fred Norman, introduced many of the artisanal techniques common today, such as quality leather, finishing knots, and balanced handles (Rubin 1994).

4 For a critique of the emphasis on consumption rather than production in queer studies, see Jeff Maskovsky (2002). He argues that an emphasis on identity based on consumerism—the urban gay men who, as Michael Warner puts it, "reek of the commodity" (1993, xxxi)—erases class.

5 These variations determine the price. The least expensive flogger—a short (fifteen-and-one-half inch), lightweight (deerskin), standard (with 24 tails)—is $135; the most expensive—a two-foot mop (with 150 tails)—is $300. Heartwood's customized floggers cost even more.

6 And price range: Mr. S's paddles range from $27 to $198 and have names like "The Belter," "Thumper," "Thwacker," and "Abrasive Slapper." These descriptions evoke both the sensations and the intended uses of the paddles.

7 There is concern in the scene that beating a woman's breasts increases her risk of developing lumps, tumors, or cysts.

8 Although not usually the primary focus of classes, top injuries are important. The top risks carpel tunnel and other repetitive injuries, as well as muscle straining and pulling and fatigue, which can be minimized with certain techniques.

9 From a speech Gayle Rubin gave at the graduation ceremony for the Journeyman II Academy on October 4, 1997. Rubin's speech is titled "Old Guard, New Guard." The speech was reprinted in *Cuir Underground* issue 4.2 (Summer); an excerpt of the speech is archived at http://www.black-rose.com/cuiru/archive/4-2/oldguard.html.

10 From a two-part dialogue edited by Christine titled "Talking Class: Working Class SM Dykes Shoot the Shit." The dialogue was printed in issues 3 (1992) and 4 (1993) of the zine *Brat Attack: The Zine for Leatherdykes and Other Bad Girls*. Parts of the zine are archived at http://classic-web.archive.org/web/20030202100658re_/home.earthlink.net/~devilfishtattoo/brat/.

11 Paddles sold for table tennis or other games, purchased at a game or toy store, were frequently mentioned as good pervertables, whereas floggers and whips are harder to find in vanilla form. Many people told me that Home Depot (jokingly called "Home Dungeon") was a great resource, not only for DIY dungeon furniture, eye bolts, and rope, but also for various kinds of sensation toys. Hayden says: "Those little wooden paint stirrers? Great, stingy paddles!" Latex Mustang and Lady Thendara are fans of the portable clothing bars sold at Target: "If you attach ankle restraints," she tells me gleefully, "they make great spreader bars!"

12 A "cat-o'-nine" or just "cat" is a whip with nine rounded, braided tails.

13 Some practitioners thought that since women, in general, have less money to spend on toys than men, the leatherdyke community was not as toy-centered as the pansexual scene. Teramis argues that "men have more economic power and they like toys: boys and their toys . . . when you go to pansexual parties . . . you are going to see more widgets." Although this comment points to differential gendered access to toys, I found that the saturation of and desire for toys (and the concomitant anxiety about connection) was common across these linked, albeit distinct, communities.

14 In an essay on adultery, Laura Kipnis (2000) argues that modern marriage is about extracting labor, and that marriage-type relationships are about work. Her essay makes explicit the sense that there is something bad about working so hard at sex. For Kipnis, following Marcuse, sexuality should be free from labor, work, and capitalist regimentation. In contrast, BDSM practitioners are concerned that toys eliminate the labor or work necessary to SM.

15 The sexual fetish is an object or a part of the body that has been objectified; detached, it stands in for sexual relations between people. For Freud, "a certain degree of fetishism is . . . habitually present in normal love," but it becomes pathological when "the longing for the fetish passes beyond the point of being merely a necessary condition attached to the sexual object and actually *takes the place* of the normal aim, and, further, when the fetish becomes detached from a particular individual and becomes the *sole* sexual object" (Freud [1905] 2000, 20; italics in original). Freud theorized that the fetish stands for the lost penis of the mother; the boy, upon seeing the missing penis, is threatened with castration, and so the fetish stands in for, while disavowing, the lack. In its most mechanistic form, the fetish (fur or feet) is the part of the mother's body seen just before the fearsome gap (see also Freud [1927] 1961).

16 For Marx, a commodity is an object that masks the realities of its own production. The "mysterious" and "mystical" character of the commodity is fetishistic because the object "reflects the social characteristics of men's own labour as objective characteristics of the products of labour themselves, as the socio-natural properties of these things. Hence, it also reflects the social relation between objects, a relation which exists apart from and outside the producers" (Marx [1867] 1990, 164–65). In commodity fetishism, social relationships appear to form between commodities, not between people: "The definite social relation between men . . . assumes . . . the fantastic form of a relation between things" (165).

17 Appadurai argues that the substitution of things for social relations is subject to a second substitution: a situation, as with advertising, in which "the images of sociality (belonging, sex appeal, power, distinction, health, togetherness, camaraderie)" are focused on the "transformation of the consumer to the point where the particular commodity being sold is almost an afterthought." This "double inversion of the relationship between people and things," he continues, "might be regarded as the critical cultural move of advanced capitalism" (1988, 56).

18 Haraway defines the cyborg as a "hybrid creature, composed of organism and machine" (1990, 1). The cyborg marks the blurring of boundaries between human and animal, organism and machine, and physical and nonphysical.

19 Thinking about SM as a form of connection or spiritual exchange resonates with the BDSM literature on euphoria, transcendence, and spirituality. Patrick Califia, among others, has described SM as transcendent: "There's the opportunity to worship, in the person of the beloved, a representation of the divine. One can see sexuality as a form of ministry which generates joy [and] . . . that joy is often a conduit into a transcendental state which can lead one to experience a sense of unity with the divine" (Sensuous Sadie, "Interview with Patrick Califia, Author and Activist," SCENEprofiles, 2003. The interview is archived at http://www.sensuoussadie.com/interviews/patrickcalifiainterview.htm. See also Califia and Campbell 1998; Mains 1991; Thompson 1991). Mira Zussman writes that SM play "results in feelings of transcendence, absolute faith, trust, safety, protection, and euphoria . . . Play gives practitioners a feeling of union with the divine, or even a sense of having achieved divinity oneself, and it is, for the most part, ineffable" (1998, 35). Zussman argues that this spirituality is more articulated in lesbian and gay SM than in heterosexual communities. I did not find such a division; people of all sexualities with whom I spoke described SM as spiritual in some way. In San Francisco, the "modern primitives" community explicitly spiritualizes forms of SM; Fakir Musafar, "father" of the modern primitives movement, demonstrates his practice in many pansexual spaces. For example, I saw a ball dance ritual at Black Rose, the large, pansexual Washington, D.C., SM conference. Seventeen dancers were hooked through the chest with large piercing hooks attached to ropes. Partners held the ropes, and—to the accompaniment of drumming, rattle shaking, invocations to various goddesses, and burning incense—the dancers were pulled through the room. Fakir replays these rituals, drawn from Native American and Asian religious rites, in SM and other spaces (see Klesse 2007 for a critique of such appropriations).

20 Similarly Patrick Califia, not a romantic when it comes to SM, opens his book *Sensuous Magic: A Guide to S/M for Adventurous Couples* with the line: "This is a book for people who love each other" (2002, 1).

21 Nelson argues that the prosthetic device fills a gap or lack. Her master metaphor of amputees and artificial limbs positions the prosthesis as a substitution, something grafted to the body or body politic to fill an absence. In contrast, the prosthesis in SM does not require a lack; instead, it is about creating new possibilities for, and extending, connection.

22 For example, some practitioners argued that there is more fat acceptance in the SM scene than in the vanilla world. The value of being fat in the scene has to do with the usefulness of flesh: fat bodies have better padding, are more protected, and can do more than thin bodies. This is because the fat body is not evaluated only on the basis of technique (how much or how well it can take or give), but also as a larger, better canvas or object (for a bottom) or as a heavier, more powerful top.

23 There is a semiserious opinion in the scene that computer programmers make the best bondage tops because they have the (human) engineering knowledge necessary for the mastery of bondage, especially technically difficult suspension bondage.

FOUR BEYOND VANILLA

1 I define *radical feminism* as the theory that the oppression of women, as a sex-class, is the fundamental form of oppression. In this way I am marking the continuity between antipornography feminism and earlier radical feminism, which flourished from the late 1960s to the mid-1970s; both were centrally concerned with individuals' sex practices, nonegalitarian fantasies, and desires in the context of the oppressive structure of heterosexual patriarchy. For more on the history of radical feminism, see Alice Echols, who argues that early radical feminism saw sexuality as a source of both pleasure and danger, while later antipornography feminists saw only the danger. Both, however, argued that compulsory heterosexuality or heterosexual patriarchy conditions sexuality and desire (Echols 1989, 290).

The "sex wars" centered on the politics of sadomasochism, pornography, and lesbian butch-femme dynamics. In 1980 the National Organization for Women (NOW) passed a "Delineation of Lesbian Rights" that declared that both sadomasochism and pornography were issues of "exploitation" and "violence, not affectional/sexual preference" (this resolution was not amended until 1999, after years of pressure from the NOW S/M Policy reform project. See Lynda Hart [1998] for the text of NOW's resolutions). Between 1980 and 1981, several key antipornography texts were published, including Andrea Dworkin's *Pornography* (1981). In 1982 the infamous Barnard conference "Towards a Politics of Sexuality" was picketed by antipornography feminists; radical feminist papers covered the conference, including an unrelated women's SM play party (for the papers from this conference, see Vance 1984; see also Duggan and Hunter 1995; Love 2011; Rubin 2011).

In 1993 an updated radical feminist critique of sadomasochism appeared, titled *Unleashing Feminism: Critiquing Lesbian Sadomasochism in the Gay Nineties* and promising to address the ways that "virulent racial and sexual violence . . . [has] permeated the lesbian community" and to question "to what extent . . . sadomasochism itself power[s] this racism" (Reti 1993a, 2). Echoing the earlier critique, SM is seen to "replicate" existing racist and heterosexist structures of domination; this replication strengthens these structures of domination because the sexual is also the social. The volume is also, as Irene Reti writes, "an earnest plea for a revitalized, powerful feminism—in an era where earnestness is caricatured more and more as old-fashioned and silly, uncool, uptight" (1993a, 2). This echoes many contemporary debates about queer theory and feminism, which are often cast, as Biddy Martin puts it, as a battle between "dull, literal-minded, uptight" feminism and the "sexually-ambiguous, fun, performative" queer theory (1994b, 104; see also Butler 1997a; Wiegman 2002). There are, of course, many other anti-SM perspectives, some feminist and some not (for example, psychoanalytic and psychiatric, philosophical, and ethical). See Hart's excellent analysis of anti-SM feminist critiques (1998, especially chapter 2).

2 This Butlerian language is intentional. Writing as Judy Butler, Judith Butler was one of the contributors to *Against Sadomasochism*; she argued that SM lesbians fail to problematize and historicize consent and desire (1982).

3 Hart's use of "real" is the Lacanian Real; she argues that sexuality is a striving for this real-impossible—not realism, classical mimesis, reality, or truth.

4 For Geertz, the cockfight, because it is "only a game," allows the activation of kin and village rivalries and status tensions in play form (1973, 440). "Deep play," for Geertz, drawing on Bentham, is play with dangerously high stakes, capable of dislocating actors from the social field. Yet expressing status tensions (which could not be directly expressed) in game or play form also has an impact on "real" social structures: "It is this kind of bringing of assorted experiences of everyday life to focus that the cockfight, set aside from life as 'only a game' and reconnected to it as 'more than a game,' accomplishes" (450; see also Weiss 2006b).

5 For Butler, drag is able to expose the nonunity of sex and gender because of a disconnection or rupture between the sexed body and gendered presentation. Similarly, for Judith Halberstam, female masculinities (drag kings, butches, or FTMs) reveal the multiple forms of masculinity that are "actively denied to people with female bodies" (1998, 269). She argues that masculinity becomes visible as a social and cultural construction when its naturalized, hegemonic status is disturbed; female masculinity is one site of such disturbance. In these theorizations, analysis is focused on the potential for a discord between sex and gender to expose or disrupt a naturalized sex-gender linkage. For critiques of these relations of (crossing, gendered) figure to (embodied, sexed, and raced) ground, see B. Martin (1994b), Namaste (1996), Samuels (2003), and Walters (1996).

6 The e-mail description of the event taunted: "Do you have what it takes to be an Iron Dom? If you were stranded on a desert island, with only those things that washed ashore with you, would you still be able to do a scene, or would you sit on the shore and mourn your lost toys? . . . Can you do it? Are you DOM enough?" This is another demonstration of real SM: not about toys, but rather about technique, skill, and creativity.

7 Nancy Fraser defines "subaltern counterpublics" as "parallel discursive areas where members of subordinated social groups invent and circulate counter-discourses, which in turn permit them to formulate oppositional interpretations of their identities, interests, and needs" (1990, 67). Key to this definition and its use today is what Fraser terms "conflict" or oppositionality: counterpublics "contested the exclusionary norms of the bourgeois public" by creating alternative social and political arenas (61).

8 See also work on queer space and queer publics, especially Bell and Valentine (1995); Dangerous Bedfellows (1996); and Ingram, Bouthillette, and Retter (1997).

9 See Caserio et al. (2006) for a debate, and Halberstam (2008) and Muñoz (2007, 2009) for elaboration and critique of the antisocial thesis in queer studies.

10 Among my interviewees, 71 percent of the heterosexual women identified as bottom/submissive (14 percent identified as top/dominant) and 75 percent of the heterosexual men identified as top/dominant (6 percent identified as bottom/submissive).

11 This could be because my research centered on Janus, the primary pansexual organization in the Bay Area. Some feel that Janus is currently, as Cathy, a white pansexual dominant/switch in her late thirties, puts it, "a het dom group. Every single presentation I've ever been to, every class I've ever taken . . . across the board—het dom male." I am uncertain as to the orientation of Janus's membership, but it is true that most presentations are offered by male and female dominants because of the emphasis on technique.

This may also reflect a historical change. Almost all my interviewees who had participated in the scene before the early to mid 1990s commented that there were many more men than women then, and that the few women who showed up at a party or event would be overwhelmed with requests to top these men (see also Weymouth and Society of Janus 1999). It is SM common sense that the majority of practitioners are submissive or bottoms, regardless of gender. In 1987, Rubin argued that most heterosexual sadomasochists are male bottom/female top. However, this claim was based in part on the understanding that heterosexual practitioners are primarily involved with professional domination—most of the female professionals are tops, and most of the male clients are bottoms. However, within the professional community, many female dominants are not heterosexual.

Since Rubin published this analysis, the pansexual, nonprofessional SM scene in the Bay Area has grown tremendously, but there is next to no work on this community. One key text, Gini Graham Scott's *Erotic Power: An Exploration of Dominance and Submission* (1993), is based on her research in the (now mostly defunct) Bay Area female dominant organization SM Church of Mankind and so, obviously, reflects this orientation. A quantitative study from 1978 found that 11.7 percent of women and 43.6 percent of men were tops; 47 percent of women and 42.5 percent of men were bottoms (Levitt, Moser, and Jamison 1994; Moser and Levitt 1987). A 1982 study found that 27.5 percent of women and 33 percent of men were tops, while 40 percent of women and 41 percent of men were bottoms (Breslow, Evans, and Langley 1985). I am unaware of any more-recent quantitative studies in the United States (see Richters et al. 2008 for data from Australia, and Alison et al. 2001 for data from Finland).

12 An emphasis on transgressive potential holds true across performance studies more generally. Richard Schechner argues that performance studies scholarship

emphasizes how "performances mark identities, bend and remake time, adorn and reshape the body, tell stories, and provide people with the means to play with the worlds they not only inhabit but to a large degree construct" (2001, 162). "Play with the worlds" draws attention to performance as actively producing social relations. Yet work in performance studies is most often concerned with the transgression, rather than the affirmation, of social norms. Even for Victor Turner, whose work on performance and ritual set the terms of the anthropological engagement with performance studies, the ways cultural performances might "re-establish" power receives less emphasis than the ways performances might, instead, "radically critique" it (1986, 81). For example, he argues that it is not the case that performance "merely 'reflects' or 'expresses' the social system or the cultural configuration" but rather performances are "reciprocal and reflexive—in the sense that the performance is often a critique, direct or veiled, of the social life it grows out of, an evaluation (with lively possibilities of rejection) of the way society handles history" (22).

13 See David Savran for a thoughtful analysis of how anti-SM feminism relies on a contradiction between, on the one hand, a social system so strong as to be able to thoroughly colonize individuals (internalized oppression) and, on the other hand, individuals with enough free will or autonomy ("bourgeois individualism") to resist this oppression and forge new, nonpatriarchal relations (1998, 217; see also Hart 1998).

14 This iteration of libertarianism emphasizes individualism and personal responsibility, free-market freedom, and the right to privacy and personal property. For the white, heterosexual computer professionals in the South Bay, libertarianism matches some of their concerns: it is seen to protect intellectual property and copyright, support rights to sexual privacy and the decriminalization of sex work, and stress noninterference with pornography and other forms of sexual expression. Not all practitioners are libertarian, of course; I discuss libertarianism here because it is in ideological opposition to radical feminism, and because these belief systems are aligned with neoliberal rationalities. But justifying the freedom to do SM (or to own guns, for that matter) on libertarian grounds depends on the ability to separate the desires of an isolated individual from any larger social context or consequence, and on the production of subjects who act according to free will and free choice, who make decisions as fully autonomous rational agents.

Libertarians in the scene tend to follow mainstream libertarian politics, with a bit more emphasis on sexual freedom. For example, during my fieldwork, Theresa A. Reed (Darklady), an SM practitioner and erotic writer, ran for the Oregon House of Representatives as a Libertarian. She ran for the Oregon Senate in 2004, the same year she won the title of Ms. Oregon Leather, and she currently runs several BDSM parties, including an annual Portland Masturbate-a-thon for charity. This suggests that a "free-sex" libertarian may rely on a different nexus of privacy/propriety/the public than a "free-market" libertarian. Some of the people I interviewed described their politics as libertarian, and modified the term with "anti-authoritarian," "iconoclastic," "open-minded," or "broad-minded."

15 There is overlap here between sexism and what Gretchen called "domism," the sense that "dominants are somehow more valid people than submissives." Teramis agreed, noting that it was sometimes unclear if someone was being sexist or "D/s presumptive": do "you think you can order me to get you a drink" because I am submissive "or is it 'cause you're a sexist pig anyway, and you would do it to any woman who was standing there"? There are similar tensions in the leatherdyke scene around butch and femme, expressed as sexism (although with a different valence): butch tops who don't take femme tops seriously, women who look down on switches, butches who try to "roll" (flip) femme tops.

16 I am using the common definition of *liberal feminism* here: an equality feminism that aims at reform (not revolution); accepts a private/public, sexual/social dichotomy, rather than undermining such binaries; and, like libertarianism, emphasizes the right to noninterference in sexual matters. As Lisa Duggan (2003) argues, new social movements—including feminist, antiracist, and queer activism—have taken increasingly liberal forms since the 1980s, moving away from the Left, radical, and liberationist paradigms that were more common in the 1960s and 1970s.

17 These issues revolve around both sexism and heterosexism. Several interviewees explained that some heterosexual men were also homophobic (about men, *not* women); for example, Carrie told me that her husband (and other men) enjoyed being in a group of all male dominants and female submissives because "they feel uncomfortable" and "would rather not be around" different kinds of couples: "he would not want to be next to a woman topping a guy or a gay male couple." Both of these dyads challenge the parallel construction of gender/sexuality. The homophobia of some heterosexual men in the pansexual scene reflects the way that heterosexual masculinity is founded on the simultaneous disavowal of femininity and homosexuality; it is the community expression of what many have theorized about masculinity. If proper masculinity fundamentally requires the disavowal of both homosexuality and femininity, then gay male sexuality and heterosexual female dominant sexuality are two related scenes of horror.

18 As Annette Schlichter (2004) argues in an analysis of "queer straightness," heterosexual writers who take on a queer identity have a sort of aspirational queerness, linked to a desire to be a "potentially transgressive, queer subject" (544; see also Thomas, Aimone, and MacGillivray 2000). This, Schlichter argues, is based on a problematic "identification with an oppressed or minority position" (2004, 545). In her analysis, the need for recognition and the "self-legitimizing" these authors do can undermine queer critique by instead fostering "an individualist and volunteerist endeavor" of dissociation with the privi-

lege of heterosexuality (555). Like Robyn Wiegman's critique of whites in whiteness studies, this move "renders the formative and regulatory effects of power invisible" (Schlichter 2004, 555; Wiegman 1999). See also Christian Klesse, who argues that "dominant (white) subjects may construe themselves as 'transgressive' through racialized forms of embodiment," especially the cross-racial queer identification of practitioners of "neo-primitive" body modification (2007, 276). I discuss racial appropriation in chapter 5.

19 John Hartigan argues that "seeing emphatic links between whiteness and dominance has generated analyses that powerfully delineate the vast, diffuse scope of white privilege while unproblematically presenting white people as a collective order with a common cultural identity" (1997, 498). However, it is not necessary to see whiteness as a monolithic category in order to see that it is fundamentally constituted by racial domination (see, for example, Frankenberg 1997).

20 Taussig notes that mimesis does not require a good or realist copy; here he draws on Freud, who argues that an effigy does not have to resemble its subject (Taussig 1993, 52). From this, Taussig suggests that, especially in a colonial space, it is nearly impossible to distinguish the copy from the original, the imitator from the imitated (78).

FIVE SEX PLAY AND SOCIAL POWER

1 Some of the play scenes I explore exist only in fantasy, some were told to me during one-on-one interviews, and some are circulated stories. In reading SM play as cultural performance, I am extending the concept to include event scenes, fantasy scenes, and performative scenes in language (and not only ritual events), in line with theorizing about subjectivity itself as a performative (productive) endeavor.

2 I use the problematic term *people of color* throughout this chapter in part because this is the term used in the scene. But I also use it because, although the phrase has been critiqued for collapsing all difference into one difference from white, this dynamic is critical to the ways practitioners understand, talk about, and enact race in race play. Thus, I am retaining this phrasing in part because of its problematic reference to a white/nonwhite racial duality.

3 Andrea Plaid, "Race Play Interview—Part IV (Conclusion)," interview with Mollena Williams, April 9, 2009. The interview is available on Mollena's website, the Perverted Negress: http://www.mollena.com/2009/04/race-play-interview-part-iv/. It is also available on the blog Racialicious: http://www.racialicious.com.

4 Because this is a larger social logic, some nonwhite people share this analysis. Bonnie, for example, explained that in a gay male couple she knows, the master "happens to be white and the submissive happens to be black." "They get a lot of people shaking fingers at them because he is black and the top is white and

people are like 'that's just not right' . . . But that's their thing, that's their kink . . . I mean when I see two people, I don't see their color, I just see their kinks or what they like or what they don't like."

5 For example, many of the contributors to *Against Sadomasochism: A Radical Feminist Analysis* critiqued a scene featuring a lesbian, interracial Mistress/slave couple in a documentary on SM ("One Foot out of the Closet") that aired on KQED in 1980. Alice Walker argues that the scene between the white woman and her "smiling and silent" black slave "trivialized" "the actual enslaved condition of literally millions of our mothers . . . because two ignorant women insisted on their right to act out publicly a 'fantasy' that still strikes terror in black women's hearts" (1982, 207). Hilde Hein argues that "to treat with levity a self-chosen condition of humiliation which is a hated oppression to multitudes of other people is to reduce their suffering to a mockery" (1982, 87). See also Reti (1993b).

6 This underscores a national imaginary of race and visibility. In San Francisco, even though the city is 8 percent African American and 30 percent Asian or Asian American, race means black, and Asian Americans are invisible as people of color. In our group interview, Rachel, Paul, Malc, and Jeff were trying to remember all of the people of color they knew in the scene. After dialogue back and forth ("Wasn't Jared's last bottom Asian?" "Oh—remember that black guy who used to come to the munch?"), Rachel said, "I don't notice the Asians, only the blacks." This remark struck me as typical—race means black and white, a reflection of a larger American construction of race, rather than the demographics of the Bay Area.

7 As Anne McClintock notes, the fetish is "haunted by historical memory . . . [it] embodied the traumatic coincidence of historical memories held in contradiction" (1992, 72). I use this expanded definition of the fetish to track the ways in which unresolved social contradictions and tensions are grafted onto objects and dynamics that, in turn, come to stand in for this displaced ambivalence.

8 Max Mosley v. News Group Newspapers Ltd. EWHC 1777 (QB); [2008] WLR (D); [2008] WLR (D) 259, 8. See also Burns (2008a) and two articles posted on the *BBC News* website: "Mosley Wins Court Case Over Orgy," July 24, 2008, http://news.bbc.co.uk/2/hi/7523034.stm, and "Tabloid Editor Reacts to Libel Defeat," July 24, 2008, http://news.bbc.co.uk/2/hi/uk_news/7523313.stm.

9 *BBC News*, "Tabloid Editor Reacts to Libel Defeat," 2008.

10 Max Mosley v. News Group Newspapers Ltd. 2008, 12.

11 Ibid., 30.

12 Ibid., 12, 13.

13 Ibid., 30.

14 Andrea Plaid, "Race Play Interview—Part II," interview with Mollena Williams, April 7, 2009. The interview is available on Mollena's website, the Perverted Negress: http://www.mollena.com/2009/04/race-play-interview-part-ii/. It is also available on the blog Racialicious: http://www.racialicious.com.

15 Elizabeth Povinelli explores social imaginaries within what she terms "liberal

settler colonies"—Australia and the United States (2006, 3). This is an important link to the forms of liberalism and whiteness at work in settler colonies, where a national origin story and subsequent national belonging require the disavowal of an originary imperialist domination, instead, as she shows, producing discourses of "individual freedom." See also Goldstein (2008) for an analysis of the often obscured relationships between settler colonialism, white colorblindness, and American Indian rights claims.

16 Some practitioners explained that a good scene will draw on events that are both culturally meaningful and safely in the past. For example, after the 2002 interrogation scene class (which I described in the introduction), I asked Domina if she thought there have been September 11 scenes. She said she didn't think so, because it's "too soon." Using Nazi uniforms as an example, she explained that for her, the uniforms are too far in the past for her to feel personally connected to them. Outside of her personal history, they stand as historical signifiers of power and fear, able to be reappropriated within the scene. Her counterexample was Klan uniforms, which—because her father was a Klansman—are too bound up in her own personal history to be available for resignification. This is a reminder of the importance of both personal and national histories, shedding light on the temporality of eroticism and its links to cultural trauma.

17 Similarly, in her analysis of the relationship between Hannah Cullwick and Arthur Munby in Victorian London, McClintock argues that their SM dynamics were grounded in "the central transformations of industrial imperialism": "It is no accident that the historical subculture of S/M emerged in Europe toward the end of the eighteenth century with the emergence of imperialism in its modern, industrial form" (1995, 142).

18 This contrast between SM and torture relies on Elaine Scarry's definition of torture (1985, 51). Scarry differentiates torture from other forms of pain, such as therapeutic pain, based on duration, control, and purpose (34–35). Unlike torture, BDSM is of limited duration, bracketed, controlled, chosen, and consensual. Furthermore, in torture, pain is radically antisocial, while pain in the context of the BDSM scene is relational: pain marks a social exchange between practitioners. This contrast is further explored in Weiss (2009).

19 England's gender, race, and class are also crucial to the story. See Kumar (2004) for a comparison of "masculine" England and the fragile, feminine Jessica Lynch; Sjoberg (2007) for an analysis of Lynch's white hypervisibility in relation to the invisibility of military women of color; and Giroux (2004) for an analysis of the links between the guards' working-class ruralness and sexual deviancy.

20 The torture techniques depicted in the photographs ("water boarding," "stress positions," sensory and sleep deprivation, and even sexual humiliation) have been part of the repertoire of torture and terror for a very long time (see Scarry 1985), and in use by the United States for at least the last fifty years—in Vietnam and in homeland prisons, taught by the School of the Americas, and in

CIA training manuals like KUBARK (see Cohn, Thompson, and Matthews 1997; Pincus 2004; the 1963 KUBARK manual is available on the National Security Archive website: http://www.gwu.edu/~nsarchiv/). As Scarry points out, torture has long had a sexual component; the goal is to turn the prisoner's body against itself, transforming basic bodily needs (food or sleep) and "special wants like sexuality" into "ongoing sources of outrage and repulsion" (1985, 48). This general objective was combined with the no-touch shaming, humiliation, shock, fear, and dehumanizing tactics advocated in the KUBARK manual. The "script" at Abu Ghraib brought together widely used stressful conditions (noise, food and sleep deprivation, and stress positions) with sexual humiliation, rape, and violation (forced masturbation, nakedness, homosexual acts, human pyramids). In this sense, the scenes from Abu Ghraib are part of a long history of sexualizing imperialism (Enloe 2007; McClintock 1995; Stoler 1995, 2002).

21 For an analysis of what is, in some ways, the other side of this scandal, see Jasbir Puar and Amit Rai's reading of the construction of the "Monster-Terrorist" figure as a damaged, deviant, and pathological personality (2002, 123; see also Puar 2005, 27).

22 Rosalind Morris argues that it was the satisfaction and enjoyment we could read in the photographs (the thumbs up, the smiles), rather than the torture itself, that made the photographs disturbing (2007, 103). For Morris, the torturer's enjoyment is based on a reconfiguration of the tortured as satisfied and consenting (123–30). I take up this formulation of consent below.

23 Another way to read the distinction is through Deleuze's differentiation of masochism and sadism. Deleuze argues that Sacher-Masoch's masochism and Sade's sadism are entirely different mechanisms: sadism is institutional, quantitatively repetitive, demonstrative, and hostile to aestheticism, whereas masochism is contractual, qualitatively suspended, imaginative, and aesthetic ([1967] 1991, 134). In this analysis, contemporary, consensual BDSM would be a form of masochism, while the detainee torture would be sadism. Although I find this line of argument interesting, I am not convinced that breaking these forms apart in this way is a particularly useful path out of the discursive problems generated by "sadomasochism," for reasons I show.

REFERENCES

Alexander, Bryant K. 2004. "Bu(o)ying Condoms: A Prophylactic Performance of Sexuality (or Performance as Cultural Prophylactic Agency)." *Cultural Studies/Critical Methodologies* 4 (4): 501–25.

Alison, Laurence, Pekka Santtilla, N. Kenneth Sandnabba, and Niklas Nordling. 2001. "Sadomasochistically Oriented Behavior: Diversity in Practice and Meaning." *Archives of Sexual Behavior* 30 (1): 1–12.

Allison, Anne. 1994. *Nightwork: Sexuality, Pleasure, and Corporate Masculinity in a Tokyo Hostess Club*. Chicago: University of Chicago Press.

———. 2000. *Permitted and Prohibited Desires: Mothers, Comics, and Censorship in Japan*. Berkeley: University of California Press.

Altine, Kenn. 1998. "Folsom Street Fair." *International Leatherman*, no. 20 (September–October): 4–10.

Altman, Dennis. 2001. *Global Sex*. Chicago: University of Chicago Press.

American Psychiatric Association. 2000. *Diagnostic and Statistical Manual of Mental Disorders: DSM-IV-TR*. 4th ed., text revision. Washington: American Psychiatric Association.

Appadurai, Arjun. 1988. "Introduction: Commodities and the Politics of Value." In *The Social Life of Things: Commodities in Cultural Perspective*, edited by Arjun Appadurai, 3–63. Cambridge: Cambridge University Press.

——. 1996. *Modernity at Large: Cultural Dimensions of Globalization*. Minneapolis: University of Minnesota Press.

Apter, Emily S., and William Pietz, eds. 1993. *Fetishism as Cultural Discourse*. Ithaca: Cornell University Press.

Armas, Genaro C. 2003. "S.F. Losing Population Fastest of U.S. Cities: Census Shows Drop of 1.5% to 764,049." *San Francisco Chronicle*, July 10.

Axel, Brian Keith. 2002. "The Diasporic Imaginary." *Public Culture* 14 (2): 411–28.

Baker, Lee D. 2001. "The Colorblind Bind." In *Cultural Diversity in the United States: A Critical Reader*, edited by Ida Susser and Thomas C. Patterson, 103–19. Malden, Mass.: Blackwell.

Baker, Tom, and Jonathan Simon, eds. 2002. *Embracing Risk: The Changing Culture of Insurance and Responsibility*. Chicago: University of Chicago Press.

Baldwin, Guy. 1998. "The Old Guard: Classical Leather Culture Revisited." *International Leatherman*, no. 20 (September–October): 26–31.

——. 1999. "'Old Guard': Its Origins, Traditions, Mystique, and Rules." In *SM Classics*, edited by Susan Wright, 71–79. New York: Masquerade.

Bar On, Bat-Ami. 1982. "Feminism and Sadomasochism: Self-Critical Notes." In *Against Sadomasochism: A Radical Feminist Analysis*, edited by Robin R. Linden et al., 72–82. East Palo Alto, Calif.: Frog in the Well.

Barker, Meg, Camelia Gupta, and Alessandra Iantaffi. 2007. "The Power of Play: The Potentials and Pitfalls in Healing Narratives of BDSM." In *Safe, Sane and Consensual: Contemporary Perspectives on Sadomasochism*, edited by Darren Langdridge and Meg Barker, 197–216. New York: Palgrave Macmillan.

Barthes, Roland. 1989. *Sade, Fourier, Loyola*. Translated by Richard Miller. Berkeley: University of California Press.

Bartky, Sandra Lee. 1990. *Femininity and Domination: Studies in the Phenomenology of Oppression*. New York: Routledge.

Bateson, Gregory. 1955. "A Theory of Play and Fantasy." *Psychiatric Research Reports* 2:39–51.

Baudrillard, Jean. 1994. *Simulacra and Simulation*. Translated by Sheila Faria Glaser. Ann Arbor: University of Michigan Press.

Bauer, Robin. 2007. "Playgrounds and New Territories—The Potential of BDSM Practices to Queer Genders." In *Safe, Sane and Consensual: Contemporary Perspectives on Sadomasochism*, edited by Darren Langdridge and Meg Barker, 177–94. New York: Palgrave Macmillan.

——. 2008. "Transgressive and Transformative Gendered Sexual Practices and White Privileges: The Case of the Dyke/Trans BDSM Communities." *Women's Studies Quarterly* 36 (3–4): 233–53.

Baumeister, Roy F. 1988. "Masochism as Escape from Self." *Journal of Sex Research* 25 (1): 28–59.

Bell, David, and Jon Binnie. 2000. *The Sexual Citizen: Queer Politics and Beyond*. Malden, Mass.: Blackwell.

Bell, David, and Gil Valentine, eds. 1995. *Mapping Desire: Geographies of Sexuality*. New York: Routledge.

Benjamin, Jessica. 1988. *The Bonds of Love: Psychoanalysis, Feminism, and the Problem of Domination*. New York: Pantheon.

Benjamin, Walter. (1966) 1986. "On the Mimetic Faculty." In Walter Benjamin, *Reflections: Essays, Aphorisms, Autobiographical Writing*, translated by Edmund Jephcott, edited by Peter Demetz, 333–36. New York: Schocken.

Berger, Maurice, Brian Wallis, and Simon Watson. 1995. Introduction to *Constructing Masculinity*, edited by Maurice Berger, Brian Wallis, and Simon Watson, 1–7. New York: Routledge.

Berlant, Lauren. 1997. *The Queen of America Goes to Washington City*. Durham: Duke University Press.

Berlant, Lauren, and Michael Warner. 1998. "Sex in Public." *Critical Inquiry* 24 (2): 547–66.

Berlinger, Cain. 2006. *Black Men in Leather*. Tempe, Ariz.: Third Millennium.

Bersani, Leo. 1987. "Is the Rectum a Grave?" *October* 43 (Winter): 197–222.

——. 1995. *Homos*. Cambridge: Harvard University Press.

Bérubé, Allan. 1996. "The History of Gay Bathhouses." In *Policing Public Sex: Queer Politics and the Future of AIDS Activism*, edited by Dangerous Bedfellows, 187–220. Boston: South End.

Bhabha, Homi K. 1984. "Of Mimicry and Man: The Ambivalence of Colonial Discourse." *October* 28 (Spring): 125–33.

——. 1985. "Signs Taken for Wonders: Questions of Ambivalence and Authority under a Tree Outside Delhi, May 1817." *Critical Inquiry* 12 (1): 144–65.

——. 1995. "Are You a Man or a Mouse?" In *Constructing Masculinity*, edited by Maurice Berger, Brian Wallis, and Simon Watson, 57–65. New York: Routledge.

Bienvenu II, Robert V. 1998. "The Development of Sadomasochism as a Cultural Style in the Twentieth-Century United States." PhD diss., Indiana University.

Blackwood, Evelyn, and Saskia Wieringa, eds. 1999. *Female Desires: Same-Sex Relations and Transgender Practices across Cultures*. New York: Columbia University Press.

Boellstorff, Tom. 2005. *The Gay Archipelago: Sexuality and Nation in Indonesia*. Princeton: Princeton University Press.

——. 2007. *A Coincidence of Desire: Anthropology, Queer Studies, Indonesia*. Durham: Duke University Press.

Borden, Mark. 2000. "The Best Cities for Business." *Fortune*, November 27, 218–32.

Bourke, Joanna. 2004. "Torture as Pornography." *Guardian*, May 7.

Boyd, Nan Alamilla. 2003. *Wide-Open Town: A History of Queer San Francisco to 1965*. Berkeley: University of California Press.

Brame, William, and Gloria Brame. 1996. *Different Loving: A Complete Exploration of the World of Sexual Dominance and Submission*. New York: Villard.

Braun, Bruce. 2003. "'On the Raggedy Edge of Risk': Articulations of Race and Nature after Biology." In *Race, Nature, and the Politics of Difference*, edited by Donald S. Moore, Anand Pandian, and Jake Kosek, 175–203. Durham: Duke University Press.

Brent, Bill. 1997. "Queer American Pie." *Black Sheets*, no. 12, 20–36.

Breslow, Norman, Linda Evans, and Jill Langley. 1985. "On the Prevalence and Roles of Females in the Sadomasochistic Subculture: Report of an Empirical Study." *Archives of Sexual Behavior* 14 (4): 303–17.

Brodkin, Karen. 1998. *How Jews Became White Folks and What That Says about Race in America*. New Brunswick, N.J.: Rutgers University Press.

Brodsky, Joel. 1995. "The Mineshaft: A Retrospective Ethnography." In *S&M: Studies in Dominance and Submission*, rev. ed., edited by Thomas S. Weinberg, 195–218. Amherst, N.Y.: Prometheus.

Brooks, David. 2000. *Bobos in Paradise: The New Upper Class and How They Got There*. New York: Simon and Schuster.

Brown, Wendy. 2005. "Neoliberalism and the End of Liberal Democracy." In Wendy Brown, *Edgework: Critical Essays on Knowledge and Politics*, 37–59. Princeton: Princeton University Press.

Buchanan, Wyatt. 2005. "Skeleton in Gays' Closets: Racism." *San Francisco Chronicle*, June 26.

Burns, John F. 2008a. "British Judge Rules Tabloid Report Tying Grand Prix Boss to 'Orgy' Violated Privacy." *New York Times*, July 25.

——. 2008b. "Possible Nazi Theme of Grand Prix Boss's Orgy Draws Calls to Quit." *New York Times*, April 7.

——. 2008c. "Trial about Privacy in Which None Remains." *New York Times*, July 9.

Bush, George W. 2004. "President Outlines Steps to Help Iraq Achieve Democracy and Freedom: Remarks by the President on Iraq and the War on Terror." Office of the Press Secretary. May 30. http://georgewbush-whitehouse.archives.gov/.

Butler, Judith. 1982. "Lesbian S&M: The Politics of Dis-Illusion." In *Against Sadomasochism: A Radical Feminist Analysis*, edited by Robin R. Linden et al., 168–75. East Palo Alto, Calif.: Frog in the Well.

——. 1990. *Gender Trouble: Feminism and the Subversion of Identity*. New York: Routledge.

——. 1991. "Imitation and Gender Insubordination." In *Inside/Out: Lesbian Theories, Gay Theories*, edited by Diana Fuss, 13–31. New York: Routledge.

——. 1993. *Bodies That Matter: On the Discursive Limits of "Sex."* New York: Routledge.

——. 1997a. "Against Proper Objects." In *Feminism Meets Queer Theory*, edited by Elizabeth Weed and Naomi Schor, 1–30. Bloomington: Indiana University Press.

——. 1997b. *The Psychic Life of Power: Theories in Subjection*. Stanford: Stanford University Press.

——. 1998. "Merely Cultural," *New Left Review* 1 (227): 33–44.

——. 2004. *Undoing Gender*. New York: Routledge.

——. 2005. *Giving an Account of Oneself*. New York: Fordham University Press.

Califia, Pat[rick]. 1987. "A Personal View of the History of the Lesbian S/M Community and Movement in San Francisco." In *Coming to Power: Writings and Graphics on Lesbian S/M*, 3rd ed., edited by Samois, 245–83. Boston: Alyson.

——. 1988. *Macho Sluts*. Boston: Alyson.

——. 1994. *Public Sex: The Culture of Radical Sex*. Pittsburgh: Cleis.

——. 2002. *Sensuous Magic: A Guide to S/M for Adventurous Couples*. Pittsburgh: Cleis.

Califia, Patrick, and Drew Kelly Campbell. 1998. *Bitch Goddess: The Spiritual Path of the Dominant Woman*. Emeryville, Calif.: Greenery.

Card, Claudia. 1995. *Lesbian Choices*. New York: Columbia University Press.

Carrette, Jeremy R. 2005. "Intense Exchange: Sadomasochism, Theology and the Politics of Late Capitalism." *Theology and Sexuality* 11 (2): 11–30.

Caserio, Robert L., Lee Edelman, Judith Halberstam, José Esteban Muñoz, and Tim Dean. 2006. "The Antisocial Thesis in Queer Theory." *PMLA* 121 (3): 819–28.

Castells, Manuel. 2000. *The Rise of the Network Society*. 2nd ed. Oxford: Blackwell.

Celsi, Richard L., Randall L. Rose, Thomas W. Leigh. 1993. "An Exploration of High-Risk Leisure Consumption through Skydiving." *Journal of Consumer Research* 20 (1): 1–23.

Chancer, Lynn S. 1992. *Sadomasochism in Everyday Life: The Dynamics of Power and Powerlessness*. New Brunswick, N.J.: Rutgers University Press.

Chapple, Karen, John Thomas, Dena Belzer, and Gerald Autler. 2004. "Fueling the Fire: Information Technology and Housing Price Appreciation in the San Francisco Bay Area and the Twin Cities." *Housing Policy Debate* 15 (2): 347–89.

Cohen, Cathy J. 1997. "Punks, Bulldaggers, and Welfare Queens: The Radical Potential of Queer Politics?" *GLQ* 3 (4): 437–65.

Cohn, Gary, Ginger Thompson, and Mark Matthews. 1997. "Torture Was Taught by CIA." *Baltimore Sun*, January 27.

Comaroff, Jean, and John L. Comaroff. 2000. "Millennial Capitalism: First Thoughts on a Second Coming." *Public Culture* 12 (2): 291–343.

Comaroff, John L., and Jean Comaroff. 2004. "Criminal Justice, Cultural Justice: The Limits of Liberalism and the Pragmatics of Difference in the New South Africa." *American Ethnologist* 31 (2): 188–204.

Connell, Kathleen, and Paul Gabriel. 2001. "The Power of Broken Hearts: The Origin and Evolution of the Folsom Street Fair." In *Folsom Street Fair 2001 Program: Leather Comes of Age*, 12–27, 84–89. San Francisco: HBK Media.

Cruz, Arnaldo, and Martin F. Manalansan, eds. 2002. *Queer Globalizations: Citizenship and the Afterlife of Colonialism*. New York: New York University Press.

Curtis, Debra. 2004. "Commodities and Sexual Subjectivities: A Look at Capitalism and Its Desires." *Cultural Anthropology* 19 (1): 95–121.

Damu, J. 2004. "The Culture of Torture." *San Francisco Bay View*, May 12.

Dangerous Bedfellows, ed. 1996. *Policing Public Sex: Queer Politics and the Future of AIDS Activism*. Boston: South End.

Danner, Mark. 2004. "Abu Ghraib: The Hidden Story." *New York Review of Books*, October 7.

Davis, Katherine. 1987. "Introduction: What We Fear We Try to Keep Contained." In *Coming to Power: Writings and Graphics on Lesbian S/M*, 3rd ed., edited by Samois, 7–13. Boston: Alyson.

Day, Liz. 1994. "'Transgression': The 'Safe Word' in S/M Discourses." *Mattoid* 48:241–53.

"Dear Aunt Sadie." 1987. In *Coming to Power: Writings and Graphics on Lesbian S/M*, 3rd ed., edited by Samois, 148–52. Boston: Alyson.

Debord, Guy. (1967) 1995. *The Society of the Spectacle*. Translated by Donald Nicholson-Smith. New York: Zone.

Delany, Samuel R. 1999. *Times Square Red, Times Square Blue*. New York: New York University Press.

DeLeon, Richard. 1992. *Left Coast City: Progressive Politics in San Francisco, 1975–1991*. Lawrence: University of Kansas Press.

Deleuze, Gilles. (1967) 1991. *Masochism: Coldness and Cruelty*. Translated by Jean McNeil. New York: Zone.

——. 1995a. "Control and Becoming." In *Negotiations, 1972–1990*, translated by Martin Joughin, 169–76. New York: Columbia University Press.

——. 1995b. "Postscript on Control Societies." In *Negotiations, 1972–1990*, translated by Martin Joughin, 177–82. New York: Columbia University Press.

D'Emilio, John. 1983. *Sexual Politics, Sexual Communities: The Making of a Homosexual Minority in the United States, 1940–1970*. Chicago: University of Chicago Press.

Donnelly, Denise. 1998. "Gender Differences in Sadomasochistic Arousal among College Students." *Sex Roles* 39 (5–6): 391–407.

Downing, Lisa. 2007. "Beyond Safety: Erotic Asphyxiation and the Limits of SM Discourse." In *Safe, Sane and Consensual: Contemporary Perspectives on Sadomasochism*, edited by Darren Langdridge and Meg Barker, 119–32. New York: Palgrave Macmillan.

Duggan, Lisa. 2003. *The Twilight of Equality: Neoliberalism, Cultural Politics, and the Attack on Democracy*. Boston: Beacon.

Duggan, Lisa, and Nan D. Hunter. 1995. *Sex Wars: Sexual Dissent and Political Culture*. New York: Routledge.

Duncan, Patricia. 1996. "Identity, Power and Difference: Negotiating Conflict in an S/M Dyke Community." In *Queer Studies: A Lesbian, Gay, Bisexual, and Transgender Anthology*, edited by Brett Beemyn and Mickey Eliason, 87–114. New York: New York University Press.

Dworkin, Andrea. 1981. *Pornography: Men Possessing Women*. New York: Putnam.

Easton, Dossie, and Janet W. Hardy. 2004. *Radical Ecstasy: SM Journeys to Transcendence*. Oakland, Calif.: Greenery.

Easton, Dossie, and Catherine A. Liszt. 1998a. *The Bottoming Book: How to Get Terrible Things Done to You by Wonderful People*. San Francisco: Greenery.

——. 1998b. *The Topping Book: Or, Getting Good at Being Bad*. San Francisco: Greenery.

Echols, Alice. 1989. *Daring to Be Bad: Radical Feminism in America, 1967–1975*. Minneapolis: University of Minnesota Press.

Edelman, Lee. 2004. *No Future: Queer Theory and the Death Drive*. Durham: Duke University Press.

Ehrenreich, Barbara. 1986. *Remaking Love: The Feminization of Sex*. Garden City, N.Y.: Anchor Doubleday.

Ekberg, Merryn. 2007. "The Parameters of the Risk Society: A Review and Exploration." *Current Sociology* 55 (3): 343–66.
Ellis, Havelock. (1905) 1942. "Love and Pain." In Havelock Ellis, *Studies in the Psychology of Sex*, vol. I: part 2, 66–188. New York: Random House.
Elliston, Deborah. 1995. "Erotic Anthropology: 'Ritualized Homosexuality' in Melanesia and Beyond." *American Ethnologist* 22 (4): 848–67.
——. 2002. "Anthropology's Queer Future: Feminist Lessons from Tahiti and Its Islands." In *Out in Theory: The Emergence of Lesbian and Gay Anthropology*, edited by Ellen Lewin and William L. Leap, 287–315. Urbana: University of Illinois Press.
English-Lueck, J. A. 2002. *Cultures@Silicon Valley*. Stanford: Stanford University Press.
Enloe, Cynthia. 2007. "Feminist Readings on Abu Ghraib: Introduction." *International Feminist Journal of Politics* 9 (1): 35–37.
Ferguson, Ann. 1984. "Sex War: The Debate between Radical and Libertarian Feminists." *Signs* 10 (1): 106–12.
Ferguson, James G. 2002. "Of Mimicry and Membership: Africans and the 'New World Society.'" *Cultural Anthropology* 17 (4): 551–69.
Ferguson, Roderick A. 2004. *Aberrations in Black: Toward a Queer of Color Critique*. Minneapolis: University of Minnesota Press.
Fischer, Michael. 1998. "Emergent Forms of Life." *Annual Review of Anthropology* 28: 455–78.
Foucault, Michel. (1975) 1995. *Discipline and Punish: The Birth of the Prison*. Translated by Alan Sheridan. New York: Vintage.
——. (1975–76) 1996. "Sade: Sergeant of Sex." In *Foucault Live: Interviews, 1961–84*, translated by Lysa Hochroth and John Johnston, edited by Sylvère Lotringer, 186–89. New York: Semiotext(e).
——. (1976) 1990. *The History of Sexuality*. Vol. 1, *An Introduction*. Translated by Robert Hurley. New York: Vintage.
——. (1982) 1996. "Sexual Choice, Sexual Act." In *Foucault Live: Interviews, 1961–1984*, translated by Lysa Hochroth and John Johnston, edited by Sylvère Lotringer, 322–34. New York: Semiotext(e).
——. 1983. "The Subject and Power." In *Michel Foucault: Beyond Structuralism and Hermeneutics*, 2nd ed., edited by Hubert L. Dreyfus and Paul Rabinow, 208–26. Chicago: University of Chicago Press.
——. (1983) 1996. "An Ethics of Pleasure." In *Foucault Live: Interviews, 1961–84*, translated by Lysa Hochroth and John Johnston, edited by Sylvère Lotringer, 371–81. New York: Semiotext(e).
——. (1984) 1988. *The Care of the Self*. Vol. 3, *The History of Sexuality*. Translated by Robert Hurley. New York: Vintage.
——. (1984) 1990. *The Use of Pleasure*. Vol. 2, *The History of Sexuality*. Translated by Robert Hurley. New York: Vintage.
——. (1984) 1996. "Sex, Power, and the Politics of Identity." In *Foucault Live: Interviews, 1961–84*, translated by Lysa Hochroth and John Johnston, edited by Sylvère Lotringer, 382–90. New York: Semiotext(e).

——. 1988. "Technologies of the Self." In *Technologies of the Self: A Seminar with Michel Foucault*, edited by Luther H. Martin, Huck Gutman, and Patrick H. Hutton, 16–49. Amherst: University of Massachusetts Press.

——. 2003. *Society Must Be Defended: Lectures at the Collège de France, 1975–76*. Edited by Mauro Bertani and Alessandro Fontana and translated by David Macey. New York: Picador.

——. 2008. *The Birth of Biopolitics: Lectures at the Collège de France, 1978–79*. Edited by Michel Senellart and translated by Graham Burchell. New York: Palgrave Macmillan.

Frank, Katherine. 2002. *G-Strings and Sympathy: Strip Club Regulars and Male Desire*. Durham: Duke University Press.

Frankenberg, Ruth. 1997. "Introduction: Local Whitenesses, Localizing Whiteness." In *Displacing Whiteness: Essays in Social and Cultural Criticism*, edited by Ruth Frankenberg, 1–34. Durham: Duke University Press.

Fraser, Nancy. 1990. "Rethinking the Public Sphere: A Contribution to the Critique of Actually Existing Democracy." *Social Text* 25/26: 56–80.

——. 1997a. "From Redistribution to Recognition? Dilemmas of Justice in a 'Post-socialist' Age." In Nancy Fraser, *Justice Interruptus: Critical Reflections on the "Postsocialist" Condition*, 11–40. New York: Routledge.

——. 1997b. "Heterosexism, Misrecognition, and Capitalism: A Response to Judith Butler." *Social Text* 52/53: 279–89.

——. 2003. "From Discipline to Flexibilization? Rereading Foucault in the Shadow of Globalization." *Constellations* 10 (2): 160–71.

Freedenberg, Molly. 2008. "Kink Dreams." *San Francisco Bay Guardian*, September 24.

Freud, Sigmund. (1905) 2000. *Three Essays on the Theory of Sexuality*. Rev. ed. Translated by James Strachey. New York: Basic.

——. (1919) 1955. "The Uncanny." In *The Standard Edition of the Complete Psychological Works of Sigmund Freud*. Volume XVII (1917–1919), *An Infantile Neurosis and Other Works*, translated under the general editorship of James Strachey, 217–56. London: Hogarth.

——. (1924) 1961. "The Economic Problem of Masochism." In *The Standard Edition of the Complete Psychological Works of Sigmund Freud*. Volume XIX (1923–1925), *The Ego and the Id and Other Works*, translated under the general editorship of James Strachey, 155–70. London: Hogarth.

——. (1927). 1961. "Fetishism." In *The Standard Edition of the Complete Psychological Works of Sigmund Freud*. Volume XXI (1927–1931), *The Future of an Illusion, Civilization and Its Discontents, and Other Works*, translated under the general editorship of James Strachey, 147–58. London: Hogarth.

Fritsch, Jane, and Katherine E. Finkelstein. 2001. "Charges Dismissed in Columbia Sexual Torture Case." *New York Times*, November 2.

Garreau, Joel. 1992. *Edge City: Life on the New Frontier*. New York: Anchor.

Gebhardt, Paul. (1969) 1995. "Sadomasochism." In *S&M: Studies in Dominance and*

Submission, rev. ed., edited by Thomas S. Weinberg, 41–45. Amherst, N.Y.: Prometheus.

Geertz, Clifford. 1973. "Deep Play: Notes on the Balinese Cockfight." In Clifford Geertz, *The Interpretation of Cultures: Selected Essays*, 412–53. New York: Basic.

Giroux, Henry A. 2004. "What Might Education Mean after Abu Ghraib: Revisiting Adorno's Politics of Education." *Comparative Studies of South Asia, Africa and the Middle East* 24 (1): 3–22.

Glick, Elisa. 2000. "Sex Positive: Feminism, Queer Theory, and the Politics of Transgression." *Feminist Review* 64 (Spring): 19–45.

Goldstein, Alyosha. 2008. "Where the Nation Takes Place: Proprietary Regimes, Antistatism, and U.S. Settler Colonialism." *South Atlantic Quarterly* 107 (4): 833–61.

Goldstein, Richard. 2004. "Bitch Bites Man! Why Lynndie England Is the Public Face of Torturegate." *Village Voice*, May 4.

Gordon, Avery, and Christopher Newfield. 1994. "White Philosophy." *Critical Inquiry* 20 (4): 737–57.

Graham, Bradley, and Josh White. 2004. "Top Pentagon Leaders Faulted in Prison Abuse." *Washington Post*, August 25.

Gray, Mary L. 2009. *Out in the Country: Youth, Media, and Queer Visibility in Rural America*. New York: New York University Press.

Grewal, Inderpal. 2006. "'Security Moms' in the Early Twenty-First-Century United States: The Gender of Security in Neoliberalism." *Women's Studies Quarterly* 34 (1–2): 25–39.

Gross, Jane. 1993. "Combating Rape on Campus in a Class on Sexual Consent." *New York Times*, September 25.

Grossman, William I. 1986. "Notes on Masochism: A Discussion of the History and Development of a Psychoanalytic Concept." *Psychoanalytic Quarterly* 55 (3): 379–413.

Grosz, Elizabeth. 1990. *Jacques Lacan: A Feminist Introduction*. New York: Routledge.

———. 1994. *Volatile Bodies: Toward a Corporeal Feminism*. Bloomington: Indiana University Press.

Halberstam, Judith. 1998. *Female Masculinity*. Durham: Duke University Press.

———. 2008. "The Anti-Social Turn in Queer Theory." *Graduate Journal of Social Science* 5 (2): 140–56.

Hale, C. Jacob. 1996. "Blurring Boundaries, Marking Boundaries: Who Is Lesbian?" *Journal of Homosexuality* 32 (1): 21–42.

———. 1997. "Leatherdyke Boys and Their Daddies: How to Have Sex without Women or Men." *Social Text*, no. 52/53: 225–38.

Han, Chong-suk. 2007. "They Don't Want To Cruise Your Type: Gay Men of Color and the Racial Politics of Exclusion." *Social Identities* 13 (1): 51–67.

Hanly, Margaret Ann Fitzpatrick, ed. 1995. *Essential Papers on Masochism*. New York: New York University Press.

Hanna, Cheryl. 2001. "Sex Is Not a Sport: Consent and Violence in Criminal Law." *Boston College Law Review* 42 (2): 239–90.

Hannigan, John. 1998. *Fantasy City: Pleasure and Profit in the Postmodern Metropolis*. New York: Routledge.

Haraway, Donna J. 1991. *Simians, Cyborgs, and Women: The Reinvention of Nature*. New York: Routledge.

Hardt, Michael, and Antonio Negri. 2001. *Empire*. Cambridge: Harvard University Press.

Hart, Lynda. 1998. *Between the Body and the Flesh: Performing Sadomasochism*. New York: Columbia University Press.

Hartigan, John. 1997. "Establishing the Fact of Whiteness." *American Anthropologist* 99 (3): 495–505.

Hartman, Chester W., with Sarah Carnochan. 2002. *City for Sale: The Transformation of San Francisco*. Rev. and updated ed. Berkeley: University of California Press.

Harvey, David. 1997. *The Condition of Postmodernity: An Enquiry into the Origins of Cultural Change*. Malden, Mass.: Blackwell.

——. 2005. *A Brief History of Neoliberalism*. New York: Oxford University Press.

Hein, Hilde. 1982. "Sadomasochism and the Liberal Tradition." In *Against Sadomasochism: A Radical Feminist Analysis*, edited by Robin R. Linden et al., 83–89. East Palo Alto, Calif.: Frog in the Well.

Hendrix, Anastasia. 2003. "Census: Bay Area Counties Shrink; Santa Clara, S.F. Lead U.S. in Drop in Population." *San Francisco Chronicle*, April 17.

Henkin, William A., and Sybil Holiday. 1996. *Consensual Sadomasochism: How to Talk about It and How to Do It Safely*. San Francisco: Daedalus.

Hennessy, Rosemary. 2000. *Profit and Pleasure: Sexual Identities in Late Capitalism*. New York: Routledge.

Herdt, Gilbert, ed. 1984. *Ritualized Homosexuality in Melanesia*. Berkeley: University of California Press.

——, ed. 1992. *Gay Culture in America: Essays from the Field*. Boston: Beacon.

Hersh, Seymour M. 2004. "Torture at Abu Ghraib." *New Yorker*, May 10, 42–47.

Higham, Scott, and Joe Stephens. 2004. "Punishment and Amusement." *Washington Post*, May 22.

Hollibaugh, Amber, and Cherríe Moraga. 1992. "What We're Rollin' Around in Bed With: Sexual Silences in Feminism: A Conversation toward Ending Them." In *The Persistent Desire: A Butch-Femme Reader*, edited by Joan Nestle, 243–53. Boston: Alyson.

hooks, bell. 1992. *Black Looks: Race and Representation*. Boston: South End.

Hopkins, Patrick D. 1994. "Rethinking Sadomasochism: Feminism, Interpretation, and Simulation." *Hypatia* 9 (1): 116–41.

——. 1995. "Simulation and the Reproduction of Injustice: A Reply." *Hypatia* 10 (2): 162–70.

Howe, Alyssa Cymene. 2001. "Queer Pilgrimage: The San Francisco Homeland and Identity Tourism." *Cultural Anthropology* 16 (1): 35–61.

Ingram, Gordon Brent, Anne-Marie Bouthillette, and Yolanda Retter, eds. 1997. *Queers in Space: Communities, Public Places, Sites of Resistance*. Seattle: Bay.

Jackson, John L. 2001. *Harlemworld: Doing Race and Class in Contemporary Black America*. Chicago: University of Chicago Press.

———. 2005. *Real Black: Adventures in Racial Sincerity*. Chicago: University of Chicago Press.

Jakobsen, Janet R. 2005. "Sex + Freedom = Regulation: Why?" *Social Text*, no. 84/85: 285–308.

Jameson, Fredric. 1992. *Postmodernism, or, the Cultural Logic of Late Capitalism*. Durham: Duke University Press.

Johnson, E. Patrick. 2003. *Appropriating Blackness: Performance and the Politics of Authenticity*. Durham: Duke University Press.

Johnson, V. M. 1999. *To Love, To Obey, To Serve: Diary of an Old Guard Slave*. Fairfield, Conn.: Mystic Rose.

Jonel, Marissa. 1982. "Letter from a Former Masochist." In *Against Sadomasochism: A Radical Feminist Analysis,* edited by Robin R. Linden et al., 16–22. East Palo Alto, Calif.: Frog in the Well.

Joseph, Miranda. 2002. *Against the Romance of Community*. Minneapolis: University of Minnesota Press.

Judd, Dennis, and Susan Fainstein, eds. 1999. *The Tourist City*. New Haven: Yale University Press.

Kamel, G. W. Levi. 1995. "Leathersex: Meaningful Aspects of Gay Sadomasochism." In *S&M: Studies in Dominance and Submission*, rev. ed., edited by Thomas S. Weinberg, 231–47. Amherst, N.Y.: Prometheus.

Kantrowitz, Arnie. 1991. "Swastika Toys." In *Leatherfolk: Radical Sex, People, Politics, and Practice*, edited by Mark Thompson, 193–209. Boston: Alyson.

Kingfisher, Catherine, and Jeff Maskovsky. 2008. "Introduction: The Limits of Neoliberalism." *Critique of Anthropology* 28 (2): 115–26.

Kipnis, Laura. 2000. "Adultery." In *Intimacy*, edited by Lauren Berlant, 9–47. Chicago: University of Chicago Press.

Klesse, Christian. 2007. "Racialising the Politics of Transgression: Body Modification in Queer Culture." *Social Semiotics* 17 (3): 275–92.

Krafft-Ebing, Richard von. (1886) 1999. *Psychopathia Sexualis: With Especial Reference to the Antipathic Sexual Instinct; A Medico-Forensic Study*. Edited by Brian King and translated from the twelfth and final edition. Burbank, Calif.: Bloat.

Krueger, Richard B. 2010a. "The *DSM* Diagnostic Criteria for Sexual Masochism." *Archives of Sexual Behavior* 39 (2): 346–56.

———. 2010b. "The *DSM* Diagnostic Criteria for Sexual Sadism." *Archives of Sexual Behavior* 39 (2): 325–345.

Kulick, Don. 1998. *Travesti: Sex, Gender, and Culture among Brazilian Transgendered Prostitutes*. Chicago: University of Chicago Press.

———. 2006. "Theory in Furs: Masochist Anthropology." *Current Anthropology* 47 (6): 933–52.

Kulick, Don, and Margaret Willson. eds. 1995. *Taboo: Sex, Identity, and Erotic Subjectivity in Anthropological Fieldwork*. New York: Routledge.

Kumar, Deepa. 2004. "War Propaganda and the (Ab)uses of Women: Media Constructions of the Jessica Lynch Story." *Feminist Media Studies* 4 (3): 297–313.

Lacan, Jacques. 1977. *Écrits: A Selection*. Translated by Alan Sheridan. New York: Norton.

Lacan, Jacques, with Juliet Mitchell and Jacqueline Rose, eds. 1985. *Feminine Sexuality: Jacques Lacan and the École Freudienne*. Translated by Jacqueline Rose. New York: W. W. Norton.

Lady Green. 1996. *The Compleat Spanker*. Emeryville, Calif.: Greenery.

Lancaster, Roger N. 1992. *Life Is Hard: Machismo, Danger, and the Intimacy of Power in Nicaragua*. Berkeley: University of California Press.

Langdridge, Darren, and Meg Barker, eds. 2007. *Safe, Sane and Consensual: Contemporary Perspectives on Sadomasochism*. New York: Palgrave Macmillan.

Langdridge, Darren, and Trevor Butt. 2005. "The Erotic Construction of Power Exchange." *Journal of Constructivist Psychology* 18 (1): 65–73.

Lapovsky-Kennedy, Elizabeth, and Madeline Davis. 1993. *Boots of Leather, Slippers of Gold: The History of a Lesbian Community*. New York: Penguin.

Lawrence, J. M. 2000. "Of Human Bondage: S&M Community Unites to Defend Paddleboro Martyrs." *Boston Herald*, October 27.

Leap, William L., ed. 1999. *Public Sex/Gay Space*. New York: Columbia University Press.

Lemke, Thomas. 2001. "'The Birth of Bio-Politics': Michel Foucault's Lectures at the Collège de France on Neo-Liberal Governmentality." *Economy and Society* 30 (2): 190–207.

Levitt, Eugene, Charles Moser, and Karen Jamison. 1994. "The Prevalence and Some Attributes of Females in the Sadomasochistic Subculture: A Second Report." *Archives of Sexual Behavior* 23 (4): 465–73.

Lewin, Ellen. 1993. *Lesbian Mothers: Accounts of Gender in American Culture*. Ithaca: Cornell University Press.

Lewin, Ellen, and William L. Leap, eds. 1996. *Out in the Field: Reflections of Lesbian and Gay Anthropologists*. Urbana: University of Illinois Press.

——. 2002. Introduction to *Out in Theory: The Emergence of Lesbian and Gay Anthropology*, edited by Ellen Lewin and William L. Leap, 1–15. Urbana: University of Illinois Press.

Linden, Robin Ruth. 1982. "Introduction: Against Sadomasochism." In *Against Sadomasochism: A Radical Feminist Analysis*, edited by Robin R. Linden et al., 1–15. East Palo Alto, Calif.: Frog in the Well.

Linden, Robin Ruth, Darlene R. Pagano, Diana E. H. Russell, and Susan Leigh Starr, eds. 1982. *Against Sadomasochism: A Radical Feminist Analysis*. East Palo Alto, Calif.: Frog in the Well.

Lingis, Alphonso. 2006. "The Effects of the Pictures." *Journal of Visual Culture* 5 (1): 83–86.

Lipsitz, George. 2006. *The Possessive Investment in Whiteness: How White People Profit from Identity Politics*. Philadelphia: Temple University Press.
Lorde, Audre, and Susan Leigh Starr. 1982. "Interview with Audre Lorde." In *Against Sadomasochism: A Radical Feminist Analysis*, edited by Robin R. Linden et al., 66–71. East Palo Alto, Calif.: Frog in the Well.
Lott, Eric. 1993. *Love and Theft: Blackface Minstrelsy and the American Working Class*. New York: Oxford University Press.
Love, Heather, ed. 2011. "Diary of a Conference on Sexuality, 1982." *GLQ* 17 (1): 49–78.
Low, Setha. 2003. *Behind the Gates: Life, Security, and the Pursuit of Happiness in Fortress America*. New York: Routledge.
Lowe, Donald M. 1995. *The Body in Late-Capitalist USA*. Durham: Duke University Press.
MacKendrick, Karmen. 1999. *Counterpleasures*. Albany: State University of New York Press.
Magister, Thom. 1991. "One among Many: The Seduction and Training of a Leatherman." In *Leatherfolk: Radical Sex, People, Politics, and Practice*, edited by Mark Thompson, 91–105. Boston: Alyson.
Mahmood, Saba. 2001. "Rehearsed Spontaneity and the Conventionality of Ritual: Disciplines of Salat." *American Ethnologist* 28 (4): 827–53.
———. 2004. *Politics of Piety: The Islamic Revival and the Feminist Subject*. Princeton: Princeton University Press.
Mains, Geoff. 1991. *Urban Aboriginals: A Celebration of Leathersexuality*. San Francisco: Gay Sunshine.
Manalansan, Martin F. 2003. *Global Divas: Filipino Gay Men in the Diaspora*. Durham: Duke University Press.
———. 2005. "Race, Violence, and Neoliberal Spatial Politics in the Global City." *Social Text*, no. 84/85: 141–55.
Marcucci, Michele R. 2005. "Bay Area Population Growth Seems Stunted." *Oakland Tribune*, April 15.
Martin, Biddy. 1994a. "Extraordinary Homosexuals and the Fear of Being Ordinary." *differences: A Journal of Feminist Cultural Studies* 6 (2–3): 100–126.
———. 1994b. "Sexualities without Genders and Other Queer Utopias," *Diacritics* 24 (2/3): 104–21.
Martin, Emily. 1992. "The End of the Body?" *American Ethnologist* 19 (1): 121–40.
———. 1994. *Flexible Bodies: Tracking Immunity in American Culture from the Days of Polio to the Age of AIDS*. Boston: Beacon.
Marx, Karl. (1867) 1990. *Capital: A Critique of Political Economy*. Vol. 1. Translated by Ben Fowkes. London: Penguin.
Maskovsky, Jeff. 2002. "Do We All 'Reek of the Commodity'? Consumption and the Erasure of Poverty in Lesbian and Gay Studies." In *Out in Theory: The Emergence of Lesbian and Gay Anthropology*, edited by Ellen Lewin and William L. Leap, 264–86. Urbana: University of Illinois Press.

McClintock, Anne. 1992. "Screwing the System: Sexwork, Race and the Law." *boundary 2* 19 (2): 70–95.
———. 1993. "Maid to Order: Commercial Fetishism and Gender Power." *Social Text*, no. 37: 87–116.
———. 1995. *Imperial Leather: Race, Gender, and Sexuality in the Colonial Conquest*. New York: Routledge.
McDougall, Marina, and Hope Mitnick. 1998. "Location: San Francisco." In *Reclaiming San Francisco: History, Politics, Culture*, edited by James Brook, Chris Carlsson, and Nancy J. Peters, 151–61. San Francisco: City Lights.
McKenzie, Jon. 2001. *Perform or Else: From Discipline to Performance*. New York: Routledge.
McRuer, Robert. 2006. *Crip Theory: Cultural Signs of Queerness and Disability*. New York: New York University Press.
Miller, Daniel. 1995. "Consumption as the Vanguard of History." In *Acknowledging Consumption: A Review of New Studies*, edited by Daniel Miller, 1–52. New York: Routledge.
Mirzoeff, Nicholas. 2006. "Invisible Empire: Visual Culture, Embodied Spectacle, and Abu Ghraib." *Radical History Review* 95 (Spring): 21–44.
Morris, Rosalind C. 1995. "All Made Up: Performance Theory and the New Anthropology of Sex and Gender." *Annual Review of Anthropology* 24:567–92.
———. 2007. "The War Drive: Image File Corrupted." *Social Text*, no. 91: 103–42.
Moser, Charles, and Peggy J. Kleinplatz. 2005. "*DSM-IV-TR* and the Paraphilias: An Argument for Removal." *Journal of Psychology and Human Sexuality* 17 (3–4): 91–109.
———, eds. 2006. *Sadomasochism: Powerful Pleasures*. Binghamton, N.Y.: Haworth.
Moser, Charles, and Eugene Levitt. 1987. "An Exploratory-Descriptive Study of a Sadomasochistically Oriented Sample." *Journal of Sex Research* 23 (3): 322–37.
Moser, Charles, and J. J. Madeson. 1996. *Bound to Be Free: The SM Experience*. New York: Continuum.
Muñoz, José Esteban. 1999. *Disidentifications: Queers of Color and the Performance of Politics*. Minneapolis: University of Minnesota Press.
———. 2007. "Cruising the Toilet: LeRoi Jones/Amiri Baraka, Radical Black Traditions, and Queer Futurity." *GLQ* 13 (2–3): 353–67.
———. 2009. *Cruising Utopia: The Then and There of Queer Futurity*. New York: New York University Press.
Mythen, Gabe. 2007. "Reappraising the Risk Society Thesis: Telescopic Sight or Myopic Vision?" *Current Sociology* 55 (6): 793–813.
Namaste, Ki. 1996. "Tragic Misreadings: Queer Theory's Erasure of Transgender Subjectivity." In *Queer Studies: A Lesbian, Gay, Bisexual, and Transgender Anthology*, edited by Brett Beemyn and Mickey Eliason, 183–203. New York: New York University Press.
Nelson, Diane M. 2001. "Phantom Limbs and Invisible Hands: Bodies, Prosthetics, and Late Capitalist Identifications." *Cultural Anthropology* 16 (3): 303–13.

Nestle, Joan, ed. 1992. *The Persistent Desire: A Butch-Femme Reader*. Boston: Alyson.

Newmahr, Staci. 2008. "Becoming a Sadomasochist: Integrating Self and Other in Ethnographic Analysis." *Journal of Contemporary Ethnography* 37 (5): 619–43.

——. 2011. *Playing on the Edge: Sadomasochism, Risk, and Intimacy*. Bloomington: Indiana University Press.

Newton, Esther. 1979. *Mother Camp: Female Impersonators in America*. Chicago: University of Chicago Press.

——. 1993. *Cherry Grove, Fire Island: Sixty Years in America's First Gay and Lesbian Town*. Boston: Beacon.

Nichols, Jeanette, Darlene Pagano, and Margaret Rossoff. 1982. "Is Sadomasochism Feminist? A Critique of the Samois Position." In *Against Sadomasochism: A Radical Feminist Analysis*, edited by Robin R. Linden et al., 137–46. East Palo Alto, Calif.: Frog in the Well.

Omi, Michael, and Howard Winant. 1994. *Racial Formation in the United States: From the 1960s to the 1990s*. New York: Routledge.

Ong, Aihwa. 2006. *Neoliberalism as Exception: Mutations in Citizenship and Sovereignty*. Durham: Duke University Press.

Ortner, Sherry B. 1996. *Making Gender: The Politics and Erotics of Culture*. Boston: Beacon.

Padilla, Mark. 2007a. *Caribbean Pleasure Industry: Tourism, Sexuality, and AIDS in the Dominican Republic*. Chicago: University of Chicago Press.

——, ed. 2007b. *Love and Globalization: Transformations of Intimacy in the Contemporary World*. Nashville, Tenn.: Vanderbilt University Press.

Parker, Paul. 2001. "Most Charges Dropped in S&M Party Hearing." *Providence Journal*, June 28.

Patton, Cindy, and Benigno Sánchez-Eppler, eds. 2000. *Queer Diasporas*. Durham: Duke University Press.

Pellegrini, Ann. 2002. "Consuming Lifestyle: Commodity Capitalism and Transformations in Gay Identity." In *Queer Globalizations: Citizenship and the Afterlife of Colonialism*, edited by Arnaldo Cruz and Martin F. Manalansan, 134–45. New York: New York University Press.

Person, Ethel Spector, ed. 1997. *On Freud's "A Child Is Being Beaten."* New Haven: Yale University Press.

Peters, Nancy J. 1998. "The Beat Generation and San Francisco's Culture of Dissent." In *Reclaiming San Francisco: History, Politics, Culture*, edited by James Brook, Chris Carlsson, and Nancy J. Peters, 199–215. San Francisco: City Lights.

Pincus, Walter. 2004. "Iraq Tactics Have Long History with U.S. Interrogators." *Washington Post*, June 13.

Plant, Bob. 2007. "Playing Games/Playing Us: Foucault on Sadomasochism." *Philosophy and Social Criticism* 33 (5): 531–61.

Portillo, Tina. 1991. "I Get Real: Celebrating My Sadomasochistic Soul." In *Leatherfolk: Radical Sex, People, Politics, and Practice*, edited by Mark Thompson, 49–55. Boston: Alyson.

Povinelli, Elizabeth A. 2006. *The Empire of Love: Toward a Theory of Intimacy, Genealogy, and Carnality*. Durham: Duke University Press.

Preston, John. 1991. "What Happened?" In *Leatherfolk: Radical Sex, People, Politics, and Practice*, edited by Mark Thompson, 210–20. Boston: Alyson.

Puar, Jasbir K. 2005. "On Torture: Abu Ghraib." *Radical History Review* 93 (Fall): 13–38.

Puar, Jasbir K., and Amit S. Rai. 2002. "Monster, Terrorist, Fag: The War on Terrorism and the Production of Docile Subjects." *Social Text*, no. 72: 117–48.

Putnam, Robert D. 2000. *Bowling Alone: The Collapse and Revival of American Community*. New York: Simon and Schuster.

Rabinow, Paul, and Nikolas Rose. 2006. "Biopower Today." *Biosocieties* 1 (2): 195–217.

Raine, George. 1999. "Making Sense of Multimedia Gulch: Digital Mecca Is Changing the City in Just about Every Way Imaginable." *San Francisco Examiner*, October 31.

Ramírez, Horacio N. Roque. 2003. "'That's My Place!': Negotiating Racial, Sexual, and Gender Politics in San Francisco's Gay Latino Alliance, 1975–1983." *Journal of the History of Sexuality* 12 (2): 224–58.

Rapoport, Lynn. 2005. "Is San Francisco Still a Gay Mecca?" *San Francisco Bay Guardian*, June 22.

Reid-Pharr, Robert. 2001. *Black Gay Man: Essays*. New York: New York University Press.

Reinisch, June M., with Ruth Beasley. 1990. *The Kinsey Institute New Report on Sex: What You Must Know to Be Sexually Literate*. Edited and compiled by Debra Kent. New York: St. Martin's.

Reti, Irene. 1993a. Introduction to *Unleashing Feminism: Critiquing Lesbian Sadomasochism in the Gay Nineties*, edited by Irene Reti, 1–3. Santa Cruz, Calif.: Herbooks.

——, ed. 1993b. *Unleashing Feminism: Critiquing Lesbian Sadomasochism in the Gay Nineties*. Santa Cruz, Calif.: Herbooks.

Reynolds, Dawn. 2007. "Disability and BDSM: Bob Flanagan and the Case for Sexual Rights." *Sexuality Research and Social Policy* 4 (1): 40–52.

Richter, Judy. 2009. "Infinity's Breathtaking Views Just the Start." *San Francisco Chronicle*, May 17.

Richters, Juliet, Richard O. De Visser, Chris E. Rissel, Andrew E. Grulich, and Anthony M. A. Smith. 2008. "Demographic and Psychosocial Features of Participants in Bondage and Discipline, 'Sadomasochism' or Dominance and Submission (BDSM): Data from a National Survey." *Journal of Sexual Medicine* 5 (7): 1660–68.

Ridinger, Robert. 2006. "Negotiating Limits: The Legal Status of SM in the United States." *Journal of Homosexuality* 50 (1–2): 189–216.

Rofel, Lisa. 2007. *Desiring China: Experiments in Neoliberalism, Sexuality, and Public Culture*. Durham: Duke University Press.

Rose, Nikolas. (1999) 2007. *Powers of Freedom: Reframing Political Thought*. Cambridge: Cambridge University Press.
——. 2007. *The Politics of Life Itself: Biomedicine, Power, and Subjectivity in the Twenty-First Century*. Princeton: Princeton University Press.
Rubenstein, Steve. 2007. "Ex-Armory Turns into Porn Site." *San Francisco Chronicle*, January 13.
Rubin, Gayle. 1984. "Thinking Sex: Notes for a Radical Theory of the Politics of Sexuality." In *Pleasure and Danger: Exploring Female Sexuality*, edited by Carole S. Vance, 267–319. Boston: Routledge and K. Paul.
——. 1987. "The Leather Menace: Comments on Politics and S/M." In *Coming to Power: Writings and Graphics on Lesbian S/M*, 3rd ed., edited by Samois, 194–229. Boston: Alyson.
——. 1991. "The Catacombs: A Temple of the Butthole." In *Leatherfolk: Radical Sex, People, Politics, and Practice*, edited by Mark Thompson, 119–41. Boston: Alyson.
——. 1994. "Milestones of Modern Whipmaking." *DungeonMaster* 48 (March): 22–23.
——. 1995. "Visions of Paradise: SM Communities (and Their Limitations)." *Cuir Underground*, 1 (8): 1–2.
——. 1996. "The Outcasts: A Social History." In *The Second Coming—A Leatherdyke Reader*, edited by Pat Califia and Robin Sweeney, 339–46. Los Angeles: Alyson.
——. 1997. "Elegy for the Valley of the Kings: AIDS and the Leather Community in San Francisco, 1981–1996." In *In Changing Times: Gay Men and Lesbians Encounter HIV/AIDS*, edited by John H. Gagnon, Martin P. Levine, and Peter M. Nardi, 101–44. Chicago: University of Chicago Press.
——. 1998. "The Miracle Mile: South of Market and Gay Male Leather 1962–1997." In *Reclaiming San Francisco: History, Politics, Culture*, edited by James Brook, Chris Carlsson, and Nancy J. Peters, 247–72. San Francisco: City Lights.
——. 2004. "Samois." *Leather Times: News from the Leather Archives and Museum* (Spring): 3–7.
——. 2011. "Blood Under the Bridge: Reflections on 'Thinking Sex.'" *GLQ* 17 (1): 15–48.
Rudy, M. Kathy. 1998. "Sex Radical Communities and the Future of Sexual Ethics." In *Lesbian Sex Scandals: Sexual Practices, Identities, and Politics*, edited by Dawn Atkins, 133–42. New York: Harrington Park.
"Rumsfeld Testifies Before Senate Armed Services Committee." 2004. *Washington Post*, May 7.
Samois, ed. (1981) 1987. *Coming to Power: Writings and Graphics on Lesbian S/M*, 3rd ed. Boston: Alyson. Third Edition.
Samuels, Ellen Jean. 2003. "My Body, My Closet: Invisible Disability and the Limits of Coming-Out Discourse." *GLQ* 9 (1–2): 233–55.
Savran, David. 1998. *Taking It Like a Man: White Masculinity, Masochism, and Contemporary American Culture*. Princeton: Princeton University Press.
Sawhney, Deepak Narang, ed. 1999. *Must We Burn Sade?* Amherst, N.Y.: Humanity.

Scarry, Elaine. 1985. *The Body in Pain: The Making and Unmaking of the World*. New York: Oxford University Press.

Scelfo, Julie, and Rod Nordland. 2004. "Beneath the Hoods: Many of the Tortured at Abu Ghraib Were Common Criminals, Not Terrorists." *Newsweek*, July 19, 41–42.

Schechner, Richard. 1985. *Between Theater and Anthropology*. Philadelphia: University of Pennsylvania Press.

——. 2001. "Performance Studies in/for the 21st Century." *Anthropology and Humanism* 26 (2): 158–66.

Scheper-Hughes, Nancy. 2002a. "Bodies for Sale—Whole or in Parts." In *Commodifying Bodies*, edited by Nancy Scheper-Hughes and Loïc Wacquant, 1–8. London: Sage.

——. 2002b. "The Ends of the Body: Commodity Fetishism and the Global Traffic in Organs." *SAIS Review* 22 (1): 61–80.

Schlesinger, James R., et al. 2004. *Final Report of the Independent Panel to Review Department of Defense Detention Operations*. Arlington, Va.: Independent Panel to Review DoD Detention Operations. http://www.defense.gov/news/Aug2004/d20040824finalreport.pdf.

Schlichter, Annette. 2004. "Queer at Last? Straight Intellectuals and the Desire for Transgression." *GLQ* 10 (4): 543–64.

Scott, Gini Graham. 1993. *Erotic Power: An Exploration of Dominance and Submission*. New York: Citadel.

Sedgwick, Eve Kosofsky. 1990. *Epistemology of the Closet*. Berkeley: University of California Press.

——. 1993a. "Queer Performativity: Henry James's *The Art of the Novel*." *GLQ* 1 (1): 1–16.

——. 1993b. *Tendencies*. Durham: Duke University Press.

Serrano, Richard A., and Patrick J. McDonnell. 2004. "Witness Faults Actions of Prison Interrogators." *Los Angeles Times*, May 13.

"Sex, Sexism Drive Prison Coverage." 2004. *Toronto Star*, May 9.

Shah, Nayan. 2001. *Contagious Divides: Epidemics and Race in San Francisco's Chinatown*. Berkeley: University of California Press.

Sharp, Lesley A. 2000. "The Commodification of the Body and Its Parts." *Annual Review of Anthropology* 29: 287–328.

Simon, Jonathan. 2002. "Taking Risks: Extreme Sports and the Embrace of Risk in Advanced Liberal Societies." In *Embracing Risk: The Changing Culture of Insurance and Responsibility*, edited by Tom Baker and Jonathan Simon, 177–208. Chicago: University of Chicago Press.

Sims, Karen, and Rose Mason, with Darlene Pagano. 1982. "Racism and Sadomasochism: A Conversation with Two Black Lesbians." In *Against Sadomasochism: A Radical Feminist Analysis*, edited by Robin R. Linden et al., 99–105. East Palo Alto, Calif.: Frog in the Well.

Singer, Linda. 1993. *Erotic Welfare: Sexual Theory and Politics in the Age of Epidemic*. Edited by Judith Butler and Maureen MacGrogan. New York: Routledge.

Sjoberg, Laura. 2007. "Agency, Militarized Femininity and Enemy Others: Observations from the War in Iraq." *International Feminist Journal of Politics* 9 (1): 82–101.

Soble, Alan. 1997. "Antioch's 'Sexual Offense Policy': A Philosophical Exploration." *Journal of Social Philosophy* 28 (1): 22–36.

Solnit, Rebecca, and Susan Schwartzenberg. 2000. *Hollow City: The Siege of San Francisco and the Crisis of American Urbanism*. London: Verso.

Sontag, Susan. 2004. "Regarding the Torture of Others." *New York Times Magazine*, May 23, 25–29, 42.

Sorkin, Michael, ed. 1992. *Variations on a Theme Park: The New American City and the End of Public Space*. New York: Hill and Wang.

Stear, Nils-Hennes. 2009. "Sadomasochism as Make-Believe." *Hypatia* 24 (2): 21–38.

Steinberg, David. 2003. "No Apologies: The Story of Jack McGeorge." *Spectator*, January 10.

Steyn, Mark. 2002. "The UN's Foray into Saddamasochism." *National Post*, December 2.

Stoler, Ann Laura. 1995. *Race and the Education of Desire: Foucault's* History of Sexuality *and the Colonial Order of Things*. Durham: Duke University Press.

———. 2002. *Carnal Knowledge and Imperial Power: Race and the Intimate in Colonial Rule*. Berkeley: University of California Press.

Stoller, Robert J. 1991. *Pain and Passion: A Psychoanalyst Explores the World of S & M*. New York: Plenum.

Stryker, Susan. 2008. "Dungeon Intimacies: The Poetics of Transsexual Sadomasochism." *Parallax* 14 (1): 36–47.

Stryker, Susan, and Jim Van Buskirk. 1996. *Gay by the Bay: A History of Queer Culture in the San Francisco Bay Area*. San Francisco: Chronicle.

Taussig, Michael T. 1993. *Mimesis and Alterity: A Particular History of the Senses*. New York: Routledge.

Taylor, Gary W., and Jane M. Ussher. 2001. "Making Sense of S&M: A Discourse Analytic Account." *Sexualities* 4 (3): 293–314.

Thomas, Calvin, Joseph O. Aimone, and Catherine A. F. MacGillivray, eds. 2000. *Straight with a Twist: Queer Theory and the Subject of Heterosexuality*. Urbana: University of Illinois Press.

Thompson, Mark, ed. 1991. *Leatherfolk: Radical Sex, People, Politics, and Practice*. Boston: Alyson.

Townsend, Anthony. 2001. "The Internet and the Rise of the New Network Cities, 1969–1999." *Environment and Planning B: Planning and Design* 28 (1): 39–58.

Truscott, Carol. 1990. "San Francisco: A Reverent, Non-Linear, Necessarily Incomplete History of Its SM Community." *Sandmutopia Guardian*, no. 8, 6–12.

Turner, Victor. 1980. "Social Dramas and Stories about Them." *Critical Inquiry* 7 (1): 141–68.

———. 1986. *The Anthropology of Performance*. New York: PAJ.

US Department of Labor. 2008. *Occupational Outlook Handbook, 2008–2009*. New York: McGraw-Hill.

Vadas, Melinda. 1995. "Reply to Patrick Hopkins." *Hypatia* 10 (2): 159–61.

Valentine, David. 2003. " 'I Went to Bed with My Own Kind Once': The Erasure of Desire in the Name of Identity." *Language and Communication* 23 (2): 123–38.

——. 2007. *Imagining Transgender: An Ethnography of a Category*. Durham: Duke University Press.

Vance, Carole S., ed. 1984. *Pleasure and Danger: Exploring Female Sexuality*. Boston: Routledge and K. Paul.

Wagner, Sally Roesch. 1982. "Pornography and the Sexual Revolution: The Backlash of Sadomasochism." In *Against Sadomasochism: A Radical Feminist Analysis*, edited by Robin R. Linden et al., 23–40. East Palo Alto, Calif.: Frog in the Well.

Walker, Alice. 1982. "A Letter of the Times, or Should This Sado-Masochism Be Saved?" In *Against Sadomasochism: A Radical Feminist Analysis*, edited by Robin R. Linden et al., 205–9. East Palo Alto, Calif.: Frog in the Well.

Walker, Richard. 1996. "Another Round of Globalization in San Francisco." *Urban Geography* 17 (1): 60–94.

Walters, Suzanna Danuta. 1996. "From Here to Queer: Radical Feminism, Postmodernism, and the Lesbian Menace (Or, Why Can't a Woman Be More like a Fag?)." *Signs* 21 (4): 830–69.

Warner, Michael, ed. 1993. *Fear of a Queer Planet: Queer Politics and Social Theory*. Minneapolis: University of Minnesota Press.

——. 1999. *The Trouble with Normal: Sex, Politics and the Ethics of Queer Life*. New York: Free Press.

——. 2002. *Publics and Counterpublics*. New York: Zone.

Weeks, Jeffrey. 1977. *Coming Out: Homosexual Politics in Britain, from the Nineteenth Century to the Present*. New York: Quartet.

——. 1995. "History, Desire, and Identities." In *Conceiving Sexuality: Approaches to Sex Research in a Postmodern World*, edited by Richard Parker and John H. Gagnon, 33–50. New York: Routledge.

Weinberg, Martin, Colin Williams, and Charles Moser. 1984. "The Social Constituents of Sadomasochism." *Social Problems* 31 (4): 379–89.

Weinberg, Thomas S. 1987. "Sadomasochism in the United States: A Review of Recent Sociological Literature." *Journal of Sex Research* 23 (1): 50–69.

——. 1995. "Sociological and Social-Psychological Issues in the Study of Sadomasochism." In *S&M: Studies in Dominance and Submission*, rev. ed., edited by Thomas S. Weinberg, 289–303. Amherst, N.Y.: Prometheus.

Weinberg, Thomas S., and G. W. Levi Kamel. 1995. "S&M: An Introduction to the Study of Sadomasochism." In *S&M: Studies in Dominance and Submission*, rev. ed., edited by Thomas S. Weinberg, 15–24. Amherst, N.Y.: Prometheus.

Weiss, Margot. 2006a. "Mainstreaming Kink: The Politics of BDSM Representation in US Popular Media." *Journal of Homosexuality* 50 (2–3): 103–32.

——. 2006b. "Working at Play: BDSM Sexuality in the San Francisco Bay Area." *Anthropologica* 48 (2): 229–45.

——. 2008. "Gay Shame and BDSM Pride: Neoliberalism, Privacy and Sexual Politics." *Radical History Review* 100 (Winter): 87–101.

——. 2009. "Rumsfeld! Consensual BDSM and 'Sadomasochistic' Torture at Abu Ghraib." In *Out in Public: Reinventing Lesbian/Gay Anthropology in a Globalizing World*, edited by Ellen Lewin and William L. Leap, 180–201. Chichester, England: Wiley-Blackwell.

Wekker, Gloria. 2006. *The Politics of Passion: Women's Sexual Culture in the Afro-Surinamese Diaspora*. New York: Columbia University Press.

Weston, Kath. 1991. *Families We Choose: Lesbians, Gays, Kinship*. New York: Columbia University Press.

——. 1995a. "Get Thee to a Big City: Sexual Imaginary and the Great Gay Migration." *GLQ* 2 (3): 253–77.

——. 1995b. "Theory, Theory, Who's Got the Theory? Or, Why I'm Tired of That Tired Debate." *GLQ* 2 (4): 347–49.

——. 1998. *Long Slow Burn: Sexuality and Social Science*. New York: Routledge.

Weymouth, T., and Society of Janus. 1999. *Society of Janus: 25 Years*. Rev. ed. Prepared for SOJ 25, September 24–25. San Francisco: Society of Janus. http://soj.org/blogs/history/.

White, Josh. 2008. "Army Officer Is Cleared in Abu Ghraib Scandal." *Washington Post*, January 10.

Wiegman, Robyn. 1999. "Whiteness Studies and the Paradox of Particularity." *boundary 2* 26 (3): 115–50.

——. 2002. "The Progress of Gender: Whither 'Women'?" In *Women's Studies on Its Own*, edited by Robyn Wiegman, 106–40. Durham: Duke University Press.

Williams, Linda. 1989. *Hard Core: Power, Pleasure, and the "Frenzy of the Visible."* Berkeley: University of California Press.

Williamson, Dianne. 2004. "Horrors of War Tar Women, Too; Soldiers' Abuses in Iraq Appalling, Un-American." *Worcester (Mass.) Telegram and Gazette*, May 9.

Winant, Howard. 1997. "Behind Blue Eyes: Whiteness and Contemporary U.S. Racial Politics." In *Off White: Readings on Race, Power, and Society*, edited by Michelle Fine et al., 40–53. New York: Routledge.

Wiseman, Jay. 1998. *SM 101: A Realistic Introduction*. San Francisco: Greenery.

Wolfe, Mark. 1999. "The Wired Loft: Lifestyle Innovation Diffusion and Industrial Networking in the Rise of San Francisco's Multimedia Gulch." *Urban Affairs Review* 34 (5): 707–28.

Wolf-Powers, Laura. 2001. "Information Technology and Urban Labor Markets in the United States." *International Journal of Urban and Regional Research* 25 (2): 427–37.

Wollenberg, Charles. 1985. *Golden Gate Metropolis: Perspectives on Bay Area History*. Berkeley: University of California Press.

Woltersdorff, Volker. 2011. "Paradoxes of Precarious Sexualities: Sexual Subcultures under Neo-liberalism." *Cultural Studies* 25 (2): 164–82.

Zaloom, Caitlin. 2004. "The Productive Life of Risk." *Cultural Anthropology* 19 (3): 365–91.

Zussman, Mira. 1998. "Shifts of Consciousness in Consensual S/M, Bondage, and Fetish Play." *Anthropology of Consciousness* 9 (4): 15–38.

INDEX

Italicized page numbers indicate illustrations.

MARGOT WEISS is assistant professor of American studies and anthropology at Wesleyan University.

Library of Congress Cataloging-in-Publication Data
Weiss, Margot Danielle
Techniques of pleasure : BDSM and the circuits of sexuality / Margot Weiss.
p. cm.
Includes bibliographical references and index.
ISBN 978-0-8223-5145-0 (cloth : alk. paper)
ISBN 978-0-8223-5159-7 (pbk. : alk. paper)
1. Sadomasochism—California—San Francisco Bay Area.
2. Bondage (Sexual behavior)—California—San Francisco Bay Area.
3. Sex—Social aspects.
4. Sex—Political aspects.
I. Title.
HQ79.W45 2012
306.77′5097946—dc23
2011027662